Complete Home Guide to All the Vitamins

by Ruth Adams

Larchmont Books
New York

Eighth Printing: August 1979
Seventh Printing: March 1979
Sixth Printing: January 1978
Fifth Printing: October 1977
Fourth Printing: November 1976
Third Printing: June 1975
Second Printing: March 1973
First Printing: November 1972

ISBN 0-915962-05-5

**THE COMPLETE HOME GUIDE
TO ALL THE VITAMINS**

Copyright © Larchmont Books, 1972, 1976

Printed in the United States of America

LARCHMONT BOOKS
*6 East 43rd Street
New York, N.Y. 10017*

Contents

3

VITAMIN C

VITAMIN D

VITAMIN E

VITAMIN K

Foreword

SOME MONTHS AGO I received a long-distance telephone call from a man who wished to have me resolve a question. This type of request is not uncommon in our office. What made this particular incident unique was the fact that the caller is a very prominent man, famous enough to appear in the newspapers across the nation almost daily.

Clearly, as one might expect, anyone of such stature can certainly afford the best medical counsel. Anyhow, the question he wished resolved was "Should I take vitamins?"

The real reason for the call was that he had already queried his three attending physicians. His internist said, "Absolutely no, if you do, you will get kidney stones!" His urologist responded with, "It really doesn't matter, you will simply excrete what you don't need." Finally, his ear-nose-throat specialist said, "I insist that you take vitamins daily." Which makes for a convenient array of answers, the only spectrum of answers, absolutely yes, absolutely no, and it really doesn't matter.

Had the famous patient-caller or any of his physicians read this book, there would have been no need for the question and, hence, no justification for the confusing answers.

E. Cheraskin, M.D., D.M.D.
Department of Oral Medicine
Medical Center, School of Dentistry
University of Alabama
Birmingham, Alabama
July 31, 1972

CHAPTER 1

What Are Vitamins?

I CAN'T take vitamins. They give me heartburn."

"I never take vitamins. I've heard they make you fat."

"What vitamins will cure the disease I've got?"

"I'm allergic to vitamins, so I can't eat anything that contains Vitamin C."

"I eat a good, well-balanced diet. Why should I take vitamins?"

"I have no faith in vitamins. Something that comes in a tiny pill couldn't possibly do anything important for your health."

"Don't vitamins have calories? Won't they make me fat?"

Statements like these illustrate the confusion many of us are in when it comes to vitamins. We think of them as something like starches, fats, or proteins, and we imagine that we may need some of them, but not all of them. And, unfortunately, we tend to think of each vitamin as related to the prevention or cure of some specific disease.

Vitamins are not the same thing as starches, fats and proteins. We do not eat them in quantity and take them or not take them according to whether we feel hungry for that particular one on a certain day.

Vitamins are chemical substances which are necessary in extremely small amounts to bring about certain chemical changes or reactions in our bodies. They combine with other substances—minerals, proteins, enzymes, or, perhaps, all three—to change something chemically. Generally speaking, vitamins cannot be made by the body but must be obtained from food.

Carbohydrates (starches and sugars) and fats are energy-providing foods. Proteins are building, repairing and protective foods. Vitamins help to process carbohydrates, fats and proteins so that they can perform their functions. In *Bridges Dietetics for the Clinician*, vitamins are defined as "substances which differ widely in chemical nature and physiologic function. They have the one common characteristic of being non-mineral substances required in relatively small amounts for the maintenance of normal structure and function of body tissues." Note that important word "required". It is impossible to sustain life without vitamins—without *all* the essential vitamins.

To put it more simply, carbohydrates, proteins and fats could not be used, broken down in digestion and later built into cells, turned into energy or stored in the body without a long chain of chemical reactions which must take place to transform cells of plants or food animals into human cells. Vitamins play an important part in this process, along with minerals, which are present in food and water, and hormones, which are manufactured by body glands. Vitamins occur naturally in food, and the charts throughout this book show the amounts of the vitamins in various types of foods.

A food rich in carbohydrate contains plenty of the vitamins and minerals necessary for processing that carbohydrate. If it did not, our ancestors would never have grown to maturity and had children. Protein food is accompanied naturally by the vitamins and minerals our bodies must have to deal healthfully with protein. In fatty foods, we find the vitamins, minerals and other substances we must have to deal with fats in food.

Most vitamins are manufactured by plants. We do not know exactly what functions they perform for plants. One vitamin which is almost non-existent in plants, however, is vitamin D. It is produced in human tissues by the action of sunlight on the skin. Recently some nutrition researchers have asked that vitamin D be classified as a hormone rather than a vitamin, since it is manufactured in the bodies of animals, rather than in plants.

This illustrates the great difference between a vitamin and a protein or a starch. Obviously, you could not obtain either of these from sunlight. They have bulk. You must obtain quite a large quantity of them, right there before you on a plate, in order to be well nourished. All vitamins exist and are needed only in extremely small amounts, generally speaking.

For instance, the recommended amount of protein needed by an adult male is 56 grams; for an adult woman, 46 grams. A serving of lean beef contains about 25 grams of protein. The recommended amount of B1 (thiamine) required in a day is one to one and a half milligrams. A milligram is one-thousandths of a gram. Some vitamins are needed in such small amounts that we measure them in micrograms. This is one-millionth of a gram. Vitamin B12 is one of these. If you have taken vitamin B12 in a pill, you have noticed that the pill is quite small but not microscopic. It contains a filler, in addition to the vitamin, to give it enough bulk so that it can be handled easily.

It is, for the most part, impossible to relate any one vitamin to any one disease, except for those disorders which we know are directly caused by a shortage of some vitamin. Scurvy is the disease that results when one lacks vitamin C. Beriberi is the disease that results when one lacks one of the B vitamins. Pellagra indicates lack of another B vitamin. Rickets is a crippling disease involving lack of vitamin D and/or calcium. In this case, both the vitamin and the mineral are important.

Today, we are apt to suffer most from what we call *sub-clinical deficiencies*, which means that we may be deficient in several vitamins or minerals—not enough to develop one of the classic deficiency diseases—but enough to result in chronic ill health, plus susceptibility to more serious conditions.

WHAT ARE VITAMINS?

Said the authors of *Clinical Nutrition*: "Most physicians are familiar with the signs of advanced ... deficiency disease as they occur in classical starvation, protein deficiency, osteomalacia, rickets, scurvy, pellagra and beriberi. Most malnutrition, however, is not of this advanced, easily recognized variety, but is manifested by signs less fully developed, less severe, or less acute than the classical textbook descriptions imply. Those lesser signs are frequently overlooked."

If you lack one vitamin, you are probably deficient in a number of others as well. And you may not be getting enough protein or minerals either. So taking a pill that adds just one vitamin to your diet will probably not accomplish very much.

Do vitamins make you fat? Considering the complexity of the activity vitamins create and the small amounts of them in food, how could they possibly make you fat? Anyone who gets fat from eating too much starch or fat is involved with whole platefuls of such foods, meal after meal. A milligram or so of a vitamin weighs almost nothing. In addition, its function is not to provide energy or to store fat, so no vitamin could possibly cause anyone to gain weight.

It *is* true that people who are very thin and rundown, those who have not eaten enough for years, may gain weight when they are given enough nourishing food plus vitamins. The vitamins go to work immediately to process the food so that it is available to create energy or to build and replace cells.

On the contrary, there is considerable evidence that one reason for our nationwide problem of overweight is simply that we are not getting enough vitamins, minerals and other nutrients from our daily meals. So we suffer from pathological hunger. This means that we continue to crave and to gorge on empty-calorie foods, because we are actually hungry for the good, solid nutrients we need. Adding vitamins and minerals in good quantity may help to relieve this unnatural hunger and help us to reduce.

11

Can you be allergic to vitamins? Hardly. If you can't eat oranges, is there any reason to believe that it's the vitamin C in the orange that causes your difficulty? If you were really allergic to vitamin C and could not eat a mouthful of food that contains it, you would have died long ago of scurvy. You cannot live any length of time without vitamin C, and it is not stored to any extent in your body.

Of course, you might be allergic to the filler or binder in a vitamin tablet or capsule. If your doctor thinks this may be the case, try to ascertain from the manufacturer what kind of filler they use, or try another brand of vitamin.

Is it true that, if you get a well-rounded diet, you don't need vitamins? Possibly, depending on the person. Many of us, down through the millions of years while the human race has developed, have inherited a need for much larger amounts of vitamins than other people need, even among our own families. And what happens when the vitamins and minerals are removed from food by processing and we eat the depleted food? What happens when you eat food rich in starch from which most or all of the B vitamins have been taken? B vitamins are essential for processing the starch in foods.

White sugar is such a food. It contains no vitamins and almost no minerals. So, whenever you eat sugar, you may be creating a slight vitamin B deficiency in your body. The more sugar you eat, the more B vitamins you need. Almost all the B vitamins are removed from most cereals and grains used in baking. Only a few of the vitamins are restored synthetically by "enriching" the cereal or flour. And we do not as yet know much about the importance of those vitamins which are removed in the milling and are not put back in the finished product.

Surveys have shown that more than half the calories of the average American diet are made up of foods whose base is white sugar or refined cereals and flours. Isn't it possible, from this fact alone, that many of us desperately need to supplement our diets with the B vitamins?

The best source of vitamin E is also wholegrain cereals

and breads. Most vitamin E is removed when the grain is refined, and nothing is done about restoring that which is lost. Can anyone say with justice that we should not take vitamin E or wheat germ products to help restore to our bodies this naturally occurring vitamin which is lost in processing? Dr. Evan Shute, founder of the Shute Clinic in London, Ontario, Canada, and one of the world's leading authorities on the vitamin, regularly treats heart patients with massive doses of vitamin E. He states:

"One uses vitamin B1 to prevent neuritis because it has been found to cure neuritis.

"One uses vitamin B2 to prevent certain symptoms of riboflavin (vitamin B2) deficiency, because it has been shown to cure them.

"One uses niacin (vitamin B3) to prevent pellagra because it has been found so valuable in treating pellagra. . . .

"One uses vitamin K to prevent hemorrhagic disease of the newborn because it cures hemorrhagic disease of the newborn.

"Could vitamin E be the sole exception to the rule that vitamins tend to prevent what they relieve? . . . Why wait for your coronary (heart attack)? Why not prevent it?"

It seems more than just coincidental that heart attacks became the leading cause of death in the Western world about 30 to 40 years after refined cereals, sugar and flour became staples, making up about half of the average diet.

What about "having faith in vitamins?" Faith has to do with religion, not science. The necessity for vitamins is not a matter of faith. It's a matter of scientific fact that living things must have certain vitamins to survive. Don't think of vitamins as something magic in which you should or should not "have faith". Think of them as essential substances which exist in all natural foods and which perform certain functions in your body which cannot be performed by anything else.

How large a package they come in (like brewers yeast or wholegrain flour) or how small (like a 5-microgram tablet of vitamin B12) is not of the slightest importance. What is important is that you must have them. If you read labels carefully and take the suggested amounts, you cannot possibly get too much of any of them.

Vitamins are divided into two groups on the basis of their solubility. The fat-soluble vitamins are A, D, E and K. The water-soluble vitamins are C and the B complex.

In the United States, the following vitamins are listed officially as vitamins, and recommendations for daily amounts are provided officially for most of them:

Vitamin A

The B complex of vitamins:

    B1 (Thiamine)

    B2 (Riboflavin)

    B3 (Niacin)

    B6 (Pyridoxine)

    Pantothenic acid

    Biotin

    Folic Acid or Folacin

    B12 Cobalamine

    Choline

(Two other vitamin-like substances associated with the B complex are: Inositol and Para-Amino-Benzoic Acid.)

Vitamin C (Ascorbic Acid)

Vitamin D (Calciferol)

Vitamin E (Alpha Tocopherol)

Vitamin K (Menadione)

Vitamin research is proceeding in many laboratories in many parts of the world. Perhaps more vitamins will eventually be discovered. The Russians, for instance, already recognize a substance in the B complex which they call vitamin B15 and they are using it in many interesting ways. But from the layman's point of view, the vitamins listed above are the only ones that need to concern you.

For the record, here are the minerals currently considered essential for human nutrition: calcium, zinc, phosphorus, iron potassium, sodium, iodine and magnesium. In addition, certain trace minerals (that is, they occur in only traces in foods and soil) are vital to human needs, although the amounts have not yet been determined. These include copper, cobalt, manganese and others.

CHAPTER 2

Officially, How Much of Each Vitamin Do You Need?

THE OFFICIAL BUREAU which decides these things publishes a booklet on the recommended dietary allowances, by which is meant how much you and I need of the various vitamins and minerals. This book, titled, *Recommended Dietary Allowances*, is written by experts in the field of nutrition—university scientists and professors who have studied the subject for many years. The book is published by the National Academy of Sciences—National Research Council. It lists many scientific papers and books which were consulted by the committee in order to reach their conclusions.

The chart on pages 18, 19 (shortened a bit for simplicity) shows their recommendations. Most of us non-scientists need considerable explanation in order to know what such a chart is all about. First, why aren't all the vitamins and minerals listed? What about the rest of the B vitamins, potassium, vitamin K? What does the chart mean when it says "designed for the maintenance of good nutrition of practically all healthy people in the U.S.A.?" Does the chart mean that, if you get the recommended amount of every vitamin and mineral listed, you will be healthy no matter what else you do or do not eat?

Let's try to answer some of these questions, for if you plan to use the information about individual vitamins which we give you later in this book, you will want to know how to use this chart.

Officially recommended allowances are made for only the nutrients listed in the chart. The experts agree that things like potassium, the other B vitamins and vitamin K are essential to life and health. We must get them in our food or we cannot survive. But even after years of research, scientists simply do not know how much the average healthy person needs of each of these nutrients and others like the trace minerals—which is a story all by itself.

Until 1968 the NAS-NRC experts did not consider vitamin E essential to good health and did not list a recommended allowance for it. Although they knew that we must get iodine in our food they had no suggested allowance for this element. Magnesium, too, was ignored in their recommendations, although they were aware that this mineral is essential.

In the case of vitamin E, any official recommendations must be made with one thing in mind: some people are at present taking, under doctor's orders, quite large amounts of the unsaturated fats, in an effort to keep their blood cholesterol levels low. The more unsaturated fats anyone is taking, the more vitamin E he needs. The processing and refining of modern cereals and flours removes most of the vitamin E. So people who make sure they eat cereals and bread which are completely wholegrain and folks who eat lots of seeds, nuts, wheat germ and salad oils may be getting enough of this vitamin, while others who eat white bread and refined cereals and avoid other good sources of vitamin E may not be getting enough.

Vitamin K is another nutrient for which human requirements can not be arrived at because some vitamin K may be manufactured by beneficial bacteria in the digestive tract. The authors say that different people have different kinds of bacterial activity in their digestive tracts, so there is no way of knowing how much vitamin K each individual is

FOOD AND NUTRITION BOARD, NATIONAL ACADEMY OF SCIENCES—NATIONAL RESEARCH COUNCIL RECOMMENDED DAILY DIETARY ALLOWANCES. Revised 1974

							FAT-SOLUBLE VITAMINS		
AGE (years)	WEIGHT (kg)	(lbs)	HEIGHT (cm)	(in)	ENERGY (kcal)	PROTEIN (g)	VITAMIN A ACTIVITY (IU) (IU)	VITAMIN D (IU)	VITAMIN E ACTIVITY (IU)
Infants									
0.0-0.5	6	14	60	24	kg x 117	kg x 2.2	420 1.400	400	4
0.5-1.0	9	20	71	28	kg x 108	kg x 2.0	400 2.000	400	5
Children									
1-3	13	28	86	34	1,300	23	400 2.000	400	7
4-6	20	44	110	44	1,800	30	500 2.500	400	9
7-10	30	66	135	54	2.400	36	700 3.300	400	10
Males									
11-14	44	97	158	63	2,800	44	1.000 5.000	400	12
15-18	61	134	172	69	3,000	54	1.000 5.000	400	15
19-22	67	147	172	69	3,000	54	1.000 5.000	400	15
23-50	70	154	172	69	2,700	56	1.000 5.000		15
51+	70	154	172	69	2,400	56	1.000 5.000		15
Females									
11-14	44	97	155	62	2,400	44	800 4.000	400	12
15-18	54	119	162	65	2,100	46	800 4.000	400	12
19-22	58	128	162	65	2,100	46	800 4.000	400	12
23-50	58	128	162	65	2.000	46	800 4.000		12
51+	58	128	162	65	1.800	46	800 4.000		12
Pregnant					+300	+30	1.000 5.000	400	15
Lactating					+500	+20	1.200 6.000	400	15

a The allowances are intended to provide for individual variations among most normal persons as they live in the United States under usual environmental stresses. Diets should be based on a variety of common foods in order to provide other nutrients for which human requirements have been less well defined. See text for more detailed discussion of allowances and of nutrients not tabulated. See Table I (p. 6) for weights and heights by individual year of age.

b Kilojoules (kJ) = 4.2 × kcal.

c Retinol equivalents.

d Assumed to be all as retinol in milk during the first six months of life. All subsequent intakes are assumed to be half as retinol and half as B-carotene when calculated from

HOW MUCH DO YOU NEED?

Designed for the maintenance of good nutrition of practically all healthy people in the U.S.A.

WATER-SOLUBLE VITAMINS							MINERALS					
ASCORBIC ACID (mg)	FOLACIN (ug)	NIACIN (mg)	RIBOFLAVIN (mg)	THIAMIN (mg)	VITAMIN B6 (mg)	VITAMIN B12 (ug)	CALCIUM (mg)	PHOSPHORUS (mg)	IODINE (ug)	IRON (mg)	MAGNESIUM (mg)	ZINC (mg)
35	50	5	0.4	0.3	0.3	0.3	360	240	35	10	60	3
35	50	8	0.6	0.5	0.4	0.3	540	400	45	15	70	5
40	100	9	0.8	0.7	0.6	1.0	800	800	60	15	150	10
40	200	12	1.1	0.9	0.9	1.5	800	800	80	10	200	10
40	300	16	1.2	1.2	1.2	2.0	800	800	110	10	250	10
45	400	18	1.5	1.4	1.6	3.0	1,200	1,200	130	18	350	15
45	400	20	1.8	1.5	2.0	3.0	1,200	1,200	150	18	400	15
45	400	20	1.8	1.5	2.0	3.0	800	800	140	10	350	15
45	400	18	1.6	1.4	2.0	3.0	800	800	130	10	350	15
45	400	16	1.5	1.2	2.0	3.0	800	800	110	10	350	15
45	400	16	1.3	1.2	1.6	3.0	1,200	1,200	115	18	300	15
45	400	14	1.4	1.1	2.0	3.0	1,200	1,200	115	18	300	15
45	400	14	1.4	1.1	2.0	3.0	800	800	100	18	300	15
45	400	13	1.2	1.0	2.0	3.0	800	800	100	18	300	15
45	400	12	1.1	1.0	2.0	3.0	800	800	80	10	300	15
60	800	+2	+0.3	+0.3	2.5	4.0	1,200	1,200	125	18+	450	20
80	600	+4	+0.5	+0.3	2.5	4.0	1,200	1,200	150	18	450	25

international units. As retinol equivalents, three fourths are as retinol and one fourth as B-carotene.

c Total vitamin E activity, estimated to be 80 percent as a-tocopherol and 20 percent other tocopherols. See text for variation in allowances.

f The folacin allowances refer to dietary sources as determined by *Lactobacillus casei* assay. Pure forms of folacin may be effective in doses less than one fourth of the recommended dietary allowance.

g Although allowances are expressed as niacin, it is recognized that on the average 1 mg of niacin is derived from each 60 mg of dietary tryptophan.

h This increased requirement cannot be met by ordinary diets; therefore, the use of supplemental iron is recommended.

manufacturing for himself, inside, and how much, therefore, should be included in his food.

Then, too, each person has a different pattern of absorbing this important vitamin, which is essential for the proper clotting of the blood. Some people may eat food rich in vitamin K, but absorb little of it, while others may require very little, but may just happen to like foods in which there is lots of vitamin K and may be able to absorb it very well.

Iodine is a mineral essential for the proper functioning of the thyroid gland, whose hormones perform life-saving and life-preserving work in the body of each of us. Supposedly, people who use iodized salt and/or eat plenty of fish and seafood get enough iodine. But folks who live far inland and eat food grown locally do not get much iodine in their meals, unless they eat plenty of fish, for iodine is absent from inland soils. We are told that the average adult needs about 50 to 75 micrograms of iodine to scrape through. To insure a margin of safety, daily intake of 100-150 micrograms is suggested. What about people who don't use much salt of any kind, let alone iodized salt? Are they likely to be short on iodine?

Lack of vitamin C is known to cause the disease called scurvy. We have known this for many years. So much research has been done on vitamin C that experts feel pretty certain the amounts of vitamin C recommended in the official chart will prevent scurvy. However, there is a great deal of evidence that much larger amounts of this essential vitamin may be necessary for abundant good health. Recently the world-famous biologist, Linus Pauling, suggested in his book, *Vitamin C and the Common Cold*, that most of us need vitamin C in massive doses to prevent colds the year round. He justified this theory by reminding us that human beings are almost the only animal which does not manufacture its own vitamin C. In the early days of man's history on earth he must have gotten immense amounts of this vitamin from the fresh, green fruits, berries and leaves which made up a large part of his diet then.

HOW MUCH DO YOU NEED?

Following the publication of Dr. Pauling's book, other scientists confirmed his theory, many physicians and lay people wrote in medical and lay journals of their own experiences taking massive doses of vitamin C with nothing but excellent results so far as good health is concerned.

So the generally accepted precept "Get a little orange juice (or fake orange juice) at breakfast every morning and that will take care of your vitamin C needs" falls quite a bit short of what is currently being discussed in regard to optimum amounts of vitamin C.

Officially, we know that needs for vitamin C rise as stresses mount. What do we mean by stress? Illness, colds, chronic conditions of ill health, the effects of many drugs. Almost everything in our modern environment would classify as "stress" these days: noise, air pollution, water pollution, smoking, chemicals in food, worry over family affairs or even the perennial bad news on the evening news report.

Tests have shown that merely driving through heavy traffic on a busy throughway going to work is a form of stress which influences blood pressure, blood sugar, nerves, heart action and, possibly, the fate of vitamin C stores in the body. As a matter of fact, can you think of anybody you know who is not under some kind of "stress"? Hence should not everybody perhaps be getting lots more vitamin C than the recommended amount?

Iron is another nutrient essential for good health. It is not a vitamin, but a mineral. We bring it up here because it is on the chart of *Recommended Dietary Allowances*. Can we all feel comfortable about the amount of iron we get? Not at all. Officially, we are told there are no definite studies to determine to what extent iron deficiency anemia exists in the U.S. population. So no one knows whether there are large or small numbers of people who are not getting, in their food, the recommended amount of iron.

Many surveys have shown that there are serious iron shortages, probably in several age groups, especially teenagers, women and older folks. Recently so much concern has arisen over the fact that everyday food may not give enough iron for protection, that nutrition specialists are debating the addition of large amounts of iron to white bread. As this book is written the final decision has not been made.

Official recommendations in the chart on pages 18, 19, *Recommended Dietary Allowances*, are planned for a healthy man 22 years old, who weighs about 140 pounds and a healthy woman about 22 years old who weighs about 116 pounds. These imaginary "average" people lead fairly active lives, they live in moderate climates. Of course for everyone in the country who does not fall into one of these categories, "adjustments must be made", say the experts who decided on these allowances.

Literally nobody knows what that means. For nobody knows but you how active you are, what and how much you eat, how healthy you are, what stresses you are under, and what you may have inherited in the way of special needs for one nutrient or another.

Does this mean you may need twice or three times more of some nutrient than someone else in your family needs? Of course. Or you may need less, or you may need twenty or thirty times more! This happens regularly with laboratory animals which have been bred to be as much alike as possible. Human beings vary much more than these animals in their individual biological needs.

So your husband or wife, sister or brother, mother or father may get along perfectly well with no more vitamins or minerals than they get at mealtime, but *you* may need far, far more of this or that vitamin or any other nutrient. What makes the difference? Your hereditary background which may make your natural need for one or more nutrients much higher than average. Or the circumstances of your past or present life which may dictate the necessity for larger amounts of some nutrients. Perhaps you do not assimilate or absorb your food well. Perhaps you are exposed to greater than average amounts of stress. Perhaps you have had accidents, burns or operations which have greatly increased your need for some nutrients.

Dr. Roger J. Williams, eminent biologist and vitamin researcher of Clayton Biological Foundation, at the University of Texas, recently published a book on something which he calls "super-nutrition". Dr. Williams says that no living things have ever been studied who were living under absolutely optimal conditions of nutrition because we are not even sure what such conditions might be. If or when we finally have the knowledge to determine just which nutrients are needed and in what amounts, when we finally know just what the perfect diet is, we may be able to produce in everyone a state of "supernutrition" which might bring about such excellent health that we would live longer, happier, much more abundant and productive lives just because we were so perfectly nourished! It is indeed a perfection for which we should strive.

Is there any way for you to find out, at this moment, just what your own nutritional state is? Can you take some kind of test, or ask your doctor? In general, some physicians may recognize some of the gross symptoms of malnutrition: the bleeding gums and aching bones of scurvy, the skin disorders and mental depression of pellagra, a vitamin B deficiency disease, and so on. But, in general, most physicians are unfamiliar with these symptoms and seldom think of diagnosing any condition as a nutritional deficiency.

There are some very complicated and expensive tests used in official surveys to determine just what the state of one's nutrition is, in regard to B vitamins, vitamin A and so on. But these are not available, generally, in physicians' offices. So there is no way for you to know absolutely whether you are short on this or that vitamin or mineral. And, in fact, it is almost axiomatic to say that no one is ever short on just one vitamin or mineral. The kind of diet that would produce such a deficiency state would almost certainly be short on lots of other nutrients as well.

What does the official chart mean when it says it is designed for "practically all healthy people"? If you are perfectly healthy, then you may be able to get along on these recommended amounts of protein, vitamins and minerals. This means that you do not suffer from headaches, tooth decay, indigestion, constipation, falling hair, baldness, overweight or underweight, to say nothing of the far more serious disorders like diabetes, high blood pressure, heart trouble, colitis, cancer, mental illness, cataract, and so on. On this basis do you know anyone who is perfectly healthy?

National health statistics show that more than 50 million Americans suffer from some form of serious chronic illness: diabetes, epilepsy, multiple sclerosis, mental illness, circulatory and heart ailments and so on. Fifty percent of them are under the age of 45. So just who *is* this completely healthy individual for whom the recommended dietary allowances are designed?

If you are one of the many who cannot qualify as being completely healthy, would it not be wise to provide yourself with a form of health insurance, much as you might buy fire insurance, in the form of added nutrients? Isn't it possible that you may need considerably more of some or all of the nutrients listed?

Perhaps someone among your friends or family has derided you for taking food supplements. Chances are they quote some newspaper columnist who says, "The person who eats a good diet gets plenty of vitamins and minerals." The next time you get into such a discussion quote the official booklet on vitamin and mineral needs which states on almost every page that *individual* needs for things like vitamins and minerals cannot be estimated. The official estimates are very general. Deviations from the recommended nutrient allowances are significant only in terms of the *individual's* total health status.

Sure, eat the best possible diet you can afford. Be sure to include in this diet ample amounts of the four basic groups of foods which should be eaten every day: meats, fish, poultry, eggs, milk, cheese, yogurt and other dairy products; the seed foods like whole grain cereals, nuts, seeds, beans and legumes; fresh fruits and vegetables, especially those which are bright yellow or bright green. Eat as many foods as possible that have been organically grown, for in this way you can avoid ingesting many pesticide residues and some of the 10,000 or so chemicals which pollute our food supply, which are added either intentionally or somehow get into the food as remnants of pollution.

In addition to this good diet, just in case you're one of those people who have much greater than average nutritional needs or just in case you want to prevent some chronic illness or condition that has victimized other members of your family or circle of friends, why not use vitamin and mineral supplements as health insurance? What's to be lost?

The 128-page NAS booklet, *Recommended Dietary Allowances*, is available from the Printing and Publishing Office, National Academy of Sciences, 2101 Constitution Avenue, Washington, D.C. 20418. Price $2.50. If you order it, keep in mind when you read it that the RDA's it discusses are very general estimates for "practically all healthy people." (How many really healthy people do you know?) They are not meant to be optimal or ideal intakes, nor recommendations for an ideal diet.

Even the authors of the NAS booklet recognize that each individual is different and that nutritional requirements may vary by wide margins, depending on the state of past and present health, inherited need for larger amounts of one nutrient or many, and the everyday stresses which may take much greater toll of one or another individual.

CHAPTER 3

Are You Deficient
in Vitamins
and Minerals?

How CAN YOU tell if you need to supplement your diet with vitamins and minerals? As you will discover in other places in this book, many circumstances of life, health, disease, working conditions, inheritance, stress, exposure to drugs or chemicals, unwise reducing diets, unwise choice of foods and many other things help to determine whether or not you need vitamin and mineral supplements.

Perhaps most important of all is your inherited make-up. You may inherit, or for some other reason have, a far greater need for one or many vitamins than those around you—even members of your own family. No physical examination will reveal this to you. You must discover it for yourself. If you find that you have chronically some or many of the symptoms of a deficiency in this or that vitamin, it's up to you to try supplementing your diet with that vitamin or those vitamins and see if better health results. It won't come about overnight. Vitamins are not drugs. It takes quite a while to repair damage that you may have been doing to yourself for many years. Don't expect overnight relief from symptoms.

In the May, 1974 issue of *Geriatrics* Samuel Dreizen, DDS, MD, of the University of Texas, lists what he believes are the most easily recognizable symptoms of vitamin deficiency in older folks. What he says is just as likely to be true of younger folks if they have been eating unwisely for most of their lives.

"The earliest evidence of malnutrition in the elderly," says Dr. Dreizen, "is a conglomerate of nonspecific complaints that coincide in time with the subclinical phase of nutritive failure." They include such things as: lack of appetite, abdominal discomfort, anxiety, backache, confusion, decreased work output, depression, indigestion, fatigue, headache, insomnia, irritability, lassitude, muscle pain, muscle weakness, nervousness, palpitations (fluttering or noticeable throbbing of the heart), "pins and needles" in arms and legs, lack of ability to concentrate. These symptoms differ from person to person and we must not make the mistake of thinking that all fatigue or all headaches and so on are due to vitamin deficiency.

In terms of individual vitamins, we remind you that a deficiency in one vitamin is almost impossible, unless you have been eating a most peculiar diet. Eating day after day a diet which produces deficiency in one vitamin will almost certainly produce deficiency in many, for the obvious reason that foods which are good sources of one vitamin are good sources of other vitamins as well. And foods which lack one B vitamin, pyridoxine, let's say, are bound to be short on all those other B vitamins which occur along with it in the B vitamin complex. Such foods also lack iron, potassium and magnesium.

Chances are you will not be aware of a vitamin deficiency until it is quite far advanced. Eyes and skin show symptoms of deficiency first. If you have trouble seeing in dim light this is night blindness which is a symptom of vitamin A deficiency. If the surface of the eye is dry, and bright lights are almost unbearable, this is a disorder called xerophthalmia caused by lack of vitamin A.

The skin gets horny in someone deficient in vitamin A— rough, dry and toad-like. Where each little hair grows on the skin there is likely to be a horny nodule—perhaps on shoulders, arms, chest, back and buttocks.

If you lack the B vitamin thiamine you may have neuritis which is inflammation of a nerve close to the surface, usually beginning in feet or legs. You may have leg cramps, weakness, "pins and needles", tenderness of the calf, atrophy of muscles. The same kind of pain may be present in hands as well. Edema, or swelling, is also a symptom of thiamine deficiency. It begins in the legs and moves up. The heart may also be involved, with pain, shortness of breath, rapid heart beat. Once again—these are symptoms which may occur due to other reasons as well. But they will almost certainly occur in someone not getting enough thiamine.

Riboflavin is another B vitamin which is rather scarce in the diets of people who don't use dairy products or liver. Most common symptoms of deficiency appear in lips, tongue, eyes, and skin. A white substance appears at the corners of the mouth, lips may be reddened and may show many little vertical lines. In a woman, lipstick tends to melt and run in these little grooves.

The tongue may be swollen or purplish red or magenta. Eyes may suffer from conjunctivitis, inflamed eyelids, tearing, discomfort in bright light, burning and itching, changes in the color of the iris. The skin may become scaly and greasy at the corners of the nostrils, the eyelids, the bridge of the nose, chin or forehead. Or the deficiency may produce eczema in the scrotum or vulva.

If you lack vitamin B3 (niacin) you will have the same troubles that accompany pellagra: skin, digestive tract and nervous troubles. Skin troubles start out a little like sunburn, red and itchy. They may blister, then flake. Digestive troubles may occur anywhere from the mouth to the anus. The tongue may be swollen and red, the mouth tissues ulcerated. The lining of the stomach or any part of the intestinal tract may be inflamed. In advanced cases severe diarrhea occurs. Nervous troubles may include painful neuritis or many mental symptoms which, in advanced cases, may involve confusion, memory loss, disorientation and confabulation which means the confused recital of things that never happened.

You may recognize some symptoms you have seen in older folks around you. Is it possible they have occurred because of niacin deficiency? Of course it is, even though these older people have plenty to eat. They may lack appetite or they may choose foods which are drastically short on vitamins and minerals. There is a good chance the doctors will not recognize these symptoms as vitamin deficiency. But there is ample evidence that such symptoms can be prevented by nothing more difficult or expensive than massive doses of the missing vitamins.

Folic acid is another B vitamin, lack of which produces a kind of anemia which can be fatal. Symptoms appear in the mouth, with inflamed tongue and other mouth tissues. Any part of the digestive tract can be affected, with diarrhea and lack of absorption. Lack of vitamin B12 produces another kind of anemia which can also be fatal—pernicious anemia. The victim of this disease is pale, lacks appetite, has many digestive disorders and heart problems, neuritis, "pins and needles", a peculiar gait. The tongue and mouth may be very pale or fiery red. Tongue may be sore or ulcerated. The only possible remedy is plenty of vitamin B12. In older people it is often advisable to have injections of this vitamin because they may lack ability to absorb it from the intestine.

Lack of vitamin C produces symptoms that are almost universal among older people: lassitude, weakness, irritability and an almost unnoticeable loss of weight. Slight injuries produce big black and blue marks. Legs, arms, face and neck may show tiny hemorrhages under the skin. The gums and teeth are most frequently and most seriously affected. Gums swell, become congested, dark or purplish. They bleed, either spontaneously or with only a touch of a toothbrush or a fork. Teeth may loosen and have to be pulled. Is it possible that everybody suffering from "pyorrhea" is actually short on vitamin C? Quite possible. In many cases bleeding gums and loosening teeth can be corrected almost overnight by large doses of vitamin C.

Lack of iron in the diet produces anemia, with pallor and listlessness. Other specialists in nutrition have reported that there is widespread anemia among older people, due to lack of iron in their diets. Weakness, easy fatigability, irritability, sore mouth and sore tongue as well as longitudinal ridging of the fingernails are symptoms.

Deficiency in the mineral magnesium may occur in someone not getting enough of it in food or in someone who loses it or does not absorb it due to other disorders: chronic kidney disease, diuretics given by doctors for high blood pressure or other conditions, prolonged vomiting or diarrhea. Symptoms of lack of magnesium are muscle tremors, spasms of the wrists or ankles, involuntary movements, delirium or convulsions.

Lack of calcium results in bone softening or osteoporosis. This very common disorder of older folks may be accompanied by low back pain, muscle spasms, decrease in height, bone deformities, and a tendency of spontaneous fractures of bone.

Not getting enough protein can produce edema or swelling. It can also produce pellagra, nutritional liver disease and a fatal anemia. "All are invariably complicated by deficiencies of other essential nutrients," says Dr. Dreizen. Generally speaking, high protein foods also contain the most B vitamins and minerals. So if your diet is short on protein you will lack these other nutrients as well. Just making sure you get enough high protein foods (meat, fish, poultry, eggs, dairy products, wholegrain cereals and seeds) provides for mineral and B vitamin needs as well. Vitamin C and vitamin A, along with many minerals, occur mostly in fruits and vegetables, although liver is an excellent source of both.

If you have one or several of these symptoms, how can you correct it and how safe can you feel about taking large doses of vitamins? First of all, correct your diet. Eliminate every food that is worthless nutritionally. This means most desserts and everything that contains white sugar. Use only whole grain cereals, bread and flour. Eat plenty of high protein foods, plus fruits and vegetables. Vitamin C and the B vitamins are water-soluble. Any excess is harmlessly excreted. If you have symptoms like those listed above, chances are you need large doses of vitamins to correct them. Vitamin A has produced temporary unpleasant symptoms when extremely large doses are taken over long periods of time because it is fat soluble, hence stored in the body. No adult has ever had any trouble with 50,000 units daily, which is ten times the official recommended allowance.

But don't fool yourself into thinking you can cure symptoms like the ones outlined here by eating the same old deficient diet you have been eating and just adding some vitamins. The protein is just as essential as the vitamins and minerals. And you must get the protein from food—the same nutritious food which provides the most in the way of vitamins and minerals.

CHAPTER 4

Vitamin Thieves
Are at Work
All About Us

LET'S SAY YOUR diet contains plenty of all the known vitamins and you are quite sure you don't have any inherited special needs for larger than average amounts. Are you aware of the fact that many things you encounter in daily life may be inactivating or destroying those vitamins before they have a chance to do you any good?

Vitamins disappear rapidly from fresh foods that have been cut, chopped or otherwise exposed to air. Some vitamins are destroyed by heat, some by light, some by steam, some by soaking foods in water. Rancid fats destroy fat-soluble vitamins either in food or in the digestive tract. In addition to all this, many modern chemicals are extremely destructive of vitamins.

To take just one modern poison—a widely used, almost everpresent one in daily life, nicotine. No one knows for certain just how continuous, heavy exposure to cigarette smoke may operate to produce cancer, heart attacks, emphysema, Buerger's Disease and the many other conditions that appear to be closely related to heavy smoking. It seems quite possible that one reason for the damage may be that cigarette smoke destroys a very important vitamin.

As long ago as 1952 American researchers knew that nicotine added to a sample of whole blood in a test tube decreased the vitamin C content of that blood by 24 to 31 percent. As long ago as 1941 a German scientist demonstrated that vitamin C levels are much lower in the blood of heavy smokers than in the blood of those who do not smoke at all.

A Canadian physician, Dr. W.J. McCormick, wrote in the October 1954 issue of *Archives of Pediatrics* that he believes lack of vitamin C may be one factor that predisposes to cancer. Smoking may have three effects on health, says Dr. McCormick, all of them relating to susceptibility to cancer. Exposure to the tobacco tars accumulating in the lungs causes a vitamin C deficiency in the very area where the tissues have been broken down by this exposure. Vitamin C is essential for prompt and effective healing. But it is not available at the cell level in the lungs. Then, too, smoking may have destroyed the body's store of vitamin C, so not nearly enough of the vitamin to heal these tissues can be brought by the blood to the lungs.

Finally, people who smoke seem to need stimulating drinks like coffee, tea or soft drinks, rather than fruit juice which is rich in vitamin C. Dr. McCormick goes on to say that he has tested the vitamin C blood level of close to 6,000 patients and has never yet found a smoker with normal levels of vitamin C.

In the March 9, 1963 issue of *The Lancet*, a British medical publication, three scientists described their experiment with smokers and vitamin C. They say they have confirmed the fact that vitamin C is destroyed in a test tube when tobacco smoke comes into contact with it. Then they tested the blood levels of vitamin C in volunteers who smoked one cigarette every half hour and in volunteers who smoked 19 to 25 cigarettes within six hours. They could find no evidence of vitamin C being destroyed, they say. But when they tested the vitamin C level in the blood of long-term smokers and compared it to that of non-smokers, they found that the levels were considerably lower in the blood of those who had smoked for some time. They go on to say, "There was no evidence ... that the difference in blood-vitamin levels was due to a larger intake of vitamin C among the non-smokers."

In other words, non-smokers were not getting more vitamin C in their food than the smokers. They were simply getting the benefit of the vitamin C they did eat. But the smokers—eating the same amount of vitamin C—were losing so much of it, due to smoking, that they consistently showed lower blood levels of the vitamin than the non-smokers.

We do not know as yet all the functions of vitamin C in the body. We do know that they include the following. Vitamin C is essential for us to use properly two kinds of amino acids or forms of protein. It also helps the body to use a B vitamin, folic acid. It is believed that vitamin C carries hydrogen, an important substance, to every cell. It enhances the absorption of iron from the intestine.

In addition, vitamin C is necessary for the formation of the substance between cells—the biological glue that literally holds our bodies together. It is essential for the swift and successful knitting of broken bones and healing of wounds. It maintains the walls of the capillaries, the smallest of the blood vessels. It is essential for healing burns where new intercellular cement must be created to replace what has been destroyed.

These are only some of the functions of this extremely important vitamin. No other substance, vitamin or mineral, can be substituted for vitamin C. It seems abundantly clear that, in any individual whose blood levels of vitamin C are consistently too low, year after year, all these functions will be impaired to some extent. Do you see now why smokers are likely to suffer from many ailments, some of them quite well known to doctors, some more mysterious, because we just don't know enough as yet to relate them to a lack of vitamin C in the blood?

Nor do we know what other nutrients may be inactivated or destroyed by the nicotine in cigarettes. There

.is now evidence that one eye condition, caused by smoking and drinking, is nutritional in origin. Amblyopia is a condition where vision is dim, with no organic reason for it. According to a writer in *Archives of Ophthalmology* for September 1963, there is no convincing evidence that this condition is the direct result of poisoning by nicotine or alcohol. Rather "it is concluded that the primary cause is probably nutritional."

According to a South African physician, writing in *The Lancet* for October 19, 1963, tobacco amblyopia is cured (note that word—cured) by vitamin B12, even though the individual goes on smoking and even though his blood levels do not indicate that he has any deficiency in this vitamin.

For people who cannot or will not give up smoking, large amounts of vitamin C taken every day will perhaps mitigate some of the damage being done. And the most helpful thing we learn from the story of vitamin C and smoking is that exposure to every-day poisons destroys some vitamins. The best way to protect yourself is to guard against such exposure if you can. This means avoid, as much as you can, everything in modern life that you know is or could be toxic: drugs, insecticides, weed killers, chemicals in food, household products like strong cleansers and paint removers, industrial solvents, dusts and sprays of all kinds. If there is any question about the safety of any product and you can possibly avoid using it—do so.

Since it is quite impossible, however, to avoid all such poisons, the best protection is an abundance of vitamins and minerals. Make sure you are getting more than you may need as added insurance against vitamin thieves, which you cannot avoid. Here are some other destroyers of vitamins. How many of these play an important part in your life or that of your family?

Antibiotics destroy B vitamins in the digestive tract.

Mineral oil destroys fat-soluble vitamins A, D, E and K.

Drugs containing mercury, procaine, gold or lead destroy vitamin C.

Bicarbonate of soda in food destroys vitamin B in the stomach.

Aspirin and barbiturates destroy vitamins.

Benzene, a solvent, destroys vitamins.

Lindane, an insecticide, destroys vitamins.

Other pesticides destroy other vitamins.

Raw fish destroys the B vitamin thiamine.

Raw egg white in excess destroys the B vitamin biotin.

Chlorine and other bleaches destroy vitamin E.

Antihistamines and sulfa drugs destroy vitamin C.

The following are antagonists to vitamin D—that is, they tend to destroy it: toxisterol, phytin in many fibrous vegetables and grains, phlorizin (from the bark and fruit of certain trees), cortisone and cortisol (drugs), thyrocalcitonin (a drug).

These are antagonists to vitamin E: any oxidants, cod liver oil, thyroxine (a drug).

These are antagonists to vitamin K: the drugs dicoumarol, sulfonamides, antibiotics, a certain drug form of vitamin E, aspirin preparations, warfarin, a drug given to prevent the formation of clots.

No one has investigated how many other vitamin "enemies" are present in any of the chemical pollutants to which we are exposed these days. If we were living in Eden, a pure, pristine, unpolluted paradise, we would not have to worry about vitamin enemies. But we're not. They are all around us and we have yet to discover how much harm they have done or can do in the future.

CHAPTER 5

Getting the Most
Out of Your
Vitamins

You bring the bottles home from the health food store and put them away. The label indicates the amount to take each day relevant to the present official Dietary Allowances. But how do you know when to take them? Should you take them all at the same time, or spaced out through the day? Are some of them incompatible with others? Will one vitamin possibly cancel out the good effects of another? Is there danger of getting too much? If you take the amount indicated on the label can you be certain this is enough to answer your individual needs? What is the best way to store vitamins and for how long?

Studies seem to show that vitamin and mineral supplements are best absorbed and used if they are taken at breakfast. That means, with breakfast while you are eating, or shortly before or after breakfast. Apparently in the body's rested state in early morning, all body processes are purring along at their best and the vitamins and minerals get to the appointed spot and do their best work, most economically, when they are taken at breakfast.

If you don't eat breakfast, now is a good time to begin this very healthful habit. Your body has been on a 12- to 14-hour fast. Feed it! Feed it a good high protein breakfast that will stay with you until lunch time so you won't be tempted to sneak some sugary goody at coffee break. Vitamin and mineral supplements are food, not medicine. So they should be taken along with food, for every one of them has a number of important functions dealing directly with food. That is their purpose—to guide your food in the paths it should go, right through all the complicated body machinery into each cell and then into every activity that cell engages in. So always take your vitamins with food. Lunchtime is best, if you can't manage to take them at breakfast.

What about spacing them out during the day? In the case of the fat soluble vitamins—A, D and E—these are stored in your body, so there is no need to worry whether they will be present when they are needed most. If you are taking them regularly, they will be there, stored in fatty tissues or in your liver or wherever their storehouse is. With the water-soluble vitamins—C and all B vitamins—these are not stored to any great extent, so it is important that you get them every day. Body metabolism tends to excrete things on a four-hour basis. That is, it takes about four hours for any substance that has completed its tasks to be excreted in urine. So if you are taking large amounts of vitamin C or some of the B vitamins, it is best to divide the dosages to allow for this body activity. If you want to keep your cells flooded with vitamin C, it's best to space out the tablets every four hours or so.

Is there any chance that some vitamins and minerals are not compatible—that you should not take them together? No. Vitamins and minerals occur together in food where they certainly do not cancel one another out. Instead they work so closely together that scientists have discovered some of them can actually substitute for others, in emergencies. In cases of scurvy, for example. Laboratory animals which are getting enough of the B vitamins can somehow substitute them for vitamin C, so that they do not get scurvy as soon as those animals which are not getting so much vitamin B.

It is true, however, that certain forms of iron interfere with the body's store of vitamin E. This is medicinal iron—not the kind that is found in food supplements or in iron-rich foods like wheat germ. If you are taking iron pills prescribed by your doctor, chances are that this iron is in the form that interferes with vitamin E absorption. This does not mean that anything terrible will happen if you take the two pills at the same time, but you will probably be wasting some of the vitamin E. So, to be economical, take the iron pill in the morning and the vitamin E at night or vice versa, so that they will not be in your digestive tract at the same time.

Is there danger of getting too much of the vitamins? In the case of vitamin A and vitamin D, yes. A number of cases have been reported in medical literature, almost all of them involving mothers who have misinterpreted the label on a vitamin D bottle and given it as if it were cod liver oil. And there have been cases—mostly resulting from doctor's prescriptions—where people have taken too much vitamin A over long periods of time and have had quite serious side effects. These disappeared when the vitamin was discontinued, so there is no doubt that the vitamin caused the damage. But it was not permanent.

In any case, your vitamin intake should depend on your needs. If you are a devotee of vegetable juices and regularly quaff large glasses of carrot or spinach juice, you are getting enormous amounts of vitamin A in these juices. If you love liver, carrots, sweet potatoes, squash, watercress and other bright yellow or bright green foods, you are getting very large amounts of vitamin A in these foods. So you need less of this vitamin in supplements than does the person who avoids foods like these and lives mostly on meat, potatoes and desserts.

In general, 10,000 units of vitamin A taken in a supplement every day have never caused any trouble and many people feel their best while taking 20,000 units daily. Medical men have reported giving as much as 50,000 units daily to treat certain conditions harmlessly. On your own, it's best to stick with something around 10,000 units. If you need more vitamin A, get it in the highly nutritious foods mentioned above.

Vitamin C and the B vitamins are water soluble, hence any excess is excreted harmlessly. A number of physicians and psychiatrists are now recommending massive doses of vitamin C to prevent colds, counteract cholesterol, fight infections and perform many other beneficial acts for the health seeker. Dr. Fred Klenner, who has been giving massive doses of vitamin C for longer than any other physician, says, "I have taken 10 grams to 20 grams (10,000 to 20,000 milligrams) of vitamin C daily for the past 10 years with nothing but beneficial results. With these doses at least three glasses of milk—regular, skimmed or buttermilk—should be taken every day. I have several hundred patients who have taken 10 grams or more of vitamin C daily for three to 15 years. Ninety percent of these never have colds; the other need additional ascorbic acid (vitamin C)."

Dr. Klenner sometimes gives as much as 150 grams intravenously in 24 hours to counteract such things as carbon monoxide or barbiturate poisoning. He gives enormous doses of the vitamin to combat all virus infections. In his fine book, *The Healing Factor, Vitamin C Against Disease*, Dr. Irwin Stone presents evidence that seems to show the versatility of large doses of vitamin C in preventing many common disorders—allergies, asthma, cancer, arthritis, strokes, ulcers and so on.

During the past few years researchers and physicians who doubt the effectiveness of vitamin C and vitamin E in preventing and treating many conditions of ill health have prophesied grim results—everything from kidney stones to prolonged fatigue. But somehow none of these predictions have materialized. Today hundreds of thousands of people are taking vitamin C in large doses and vitamin E in large doses with no results but beneficial ones. In the case of vitamin E, some high blood pressure patients may experience a temporary but uncomfortable rise in pressure if they begin abruptly with a large dose, so they should start with small amounts and increase them gradually.

How should you store your vitamin and mineral supplements and how long can you keep them? Vitamin and mineral supplements, like any other food, deteriorate with time, of course. If one leaves his bottle of vitamin C in a hot sunlit room, with lid off, for months at a time, he should expect to find some deterioration in quality. Like other perishable foods, vitamins should be treated gently and carefully. Light destroys some vitamins. Heat is destructive of others. Sealing the bottles they are packed in guarantees the freshness of the products you buy.

Once you have broken the seal, it is best to store your supplements in a cool spot—the refrigerator if possible. This prevents light from getting to those which are light sensitive and guarantees that differences in daily temperature will not affect the quality of your products.

How long can you keep them? Use your good judgment. Just as you would not expect a loaf of bread or an apple to keep forever, so you cannot expect your vitamin supplements to keep forever even under the most favorable conditions. Generally speaking, food supplements made today have been manufactured with every precaution to guarantee their freshness and quality. The careful way you store them will do much to retain that quality.

CHAPTER 6

Reading Labels
on Vitamin and
Mineral Supplements

Do YOU GET confused trying to figure out what all those
tiny words and figures mean on the labels of food
supplements? Some vitamins and minerals are spoken of in
terms of milligrams or micrograms, some in terms of
International Units. What's the difference or is there any?

Why do scientists use such confusing words and how is
the average layman expected to find his way through this
clutter of unfamiliar terms and meaningless figures? Why
do some of the ingredients of a supplement have notes after
them stating "the need for this vitamin in human nutrition
has not been established"? Why are there combinations of
things—like an iron pill which is called "ferrous gluconate"
or a pantothenic acid pill called "calcium pantothenate"?
Why don't the labels tell you exactly how much to take,
instead of just saying "one tablet provides such and such a
percentage of the daily requirement"?

These are some of the questions that arise, especially
among people who are just beginning to supplement their
diets with vitamins and minerals. The answers are not
really as difficult to come by as you might think. Keep in
mind that some of the vitamins are fat-soluble—that is,
they dissolve in fats but not in water. And some of them are

water soluble—they dissolve in water but not in fats. The fat-soluble vitamins are A, D, E and K. The water soluble ones are all the B vitamins and vitamin C. These are always listed in terms of milligrams or, in the case of some B vitamins, micrograms. Proteins, carbohydrates and fats are needed in relatively large quantities, so they are spoken of in terms of grams.

A milligram in one-thousandth of a gram. A microgram is one millionth of a gram. A gram is 1/28th of an ounce. Chemists must work in terms of grams, milligrams and micrograms. That's the way the laboratory apparatus is made, so we must put up with it and learn to read labels in these terms.

One reason why the fat-soluble vitamins are expressed in terms of International Units is that each of them consists of several compounds. Thus one International Unit of vitamin A (fat soluble) includes some retinol, some retinyl acetate and some carotene. So experts from the World Health Organization and official bodies of various countries have decided to apply the term International Unit to a measured amount of each of these three.

Vitamin D (fat soluble) exists in two forms: vitamin D2 (ergocalciferol) and vitamin D3 (cholecalciferol). Vitamin D3 is the natural vitamin which is formed in the deep layers of the skin when exposed to sunlight. Vitamin D2 is made by exposing a plant compound to ultraviolet light. This is the vitamin D which is used to enrich milk, so that, in most localities, a quart of milk contains 400 I.U. of vitamin D.

In the case of vitamin E, this is called by scientists alpha tocopherol. There are other related tocopherols also named with Greek letters: beta, gamma and delta. But we are concerned only with alpha tocopherol because it is the most active of the group. There are two forms of this—the natural and the synthetic. The natural form is d-alpha tocopherol. The synthetic is called dl-alpha tocopherol.

The confusion over whether to speak of vitamin E in terms of milligrams or International Units arises from the fact that the international standard for alpha tocopherol was set using the synthetic form (dl). One I.U. of dl-alpha tocopherol equals 1 milligram. But in the case of the "natural" vitamin E, 1 milligram equals 1.49 International Units.

The official USA booklet, *Recommended Dietary Allowances*, published in 1974 states that, since food analyses for vitamin E are chemical rather than biological, values should be reported in milligrams of vitamin E per serving of food. But, in terms of human beings, the biological nomenclature should be used—hence International Units for us. In general, labels of d-alpha tocopherol, which is the natural form, are labeled accordingly. A 100 I.U. capsule would be labeled: "Each capsule contains d-alpha tocopherol (or d-alpha tocopherol acetate) equivalent by bioassay to 100 International Units of vitamin E."

In other words, the vitamin E in such a capsule has been tested with living animals and found to be equivalent to the International Unit. So you can be sure, with such labeling, that you are getting precisely one I.U. of vitamin E—no more and no less. But when we print a list of foods and their vitamin E content, this will appear in milligrams.

Vitamin K is one of the craziest, mixed-up vitamins of all. But, since we manufacture this vitamin in our intestines, there is no recommended dietary allowance for it. It exists in two forms—vitamin K1, in plants, chiefly green leafy vegetables, wheat germ and bran, and as vitamin K2 in animal cells: liver, kidney and egg yolk.

Vitamin K is not spoken of in International Units, but in dam units (named after Henrik Dam, discoverer of vitamin K) or ansbacher units. Twenty dam units are equal to 0.0008 milligrams of vitamin K, a fact which need not concern us at all since we do not take this vitamin in supplements and there is no reason for us to be concerned about it or try to learn its various names and ways of measuring it.

All the B vitamins are spoken of in terms of milligrams, except for folic acid and vitamin B12 which occur in such very small amounts that it is easier to speak of them in terms of micrograms (millionths of a gram). Vitamin C is spoken of always in terms of milligrams.

As we have seen, the fat soluble vitamins occur in various forms. The vitamin is made up of different compounds, each of which has its own name. There are many members of the B complex of vitamins. Some of these are officially called vitamins; others are called "vitamin-like substances."

The official B vitamins are these: thiamine (vitamin B1), riboflavin (vitamin B2), niacin (also called nicotinic acid and niacinamide), folic acid, vitamin B6 (pyridoxine), vitamin B12, pantothenic acid, biotin, choline. Vitamin-like substances which are part of the B complex are inositol and para-amino-benzoic acid, (PABA).

Looking over the above information on vitamins, it appears to be a veritable hodge-podge of names and numbers. For goodness sake, why don't the scientists make it all names or all numbers? Why don't they refer to all vitamins either in units or in milligrams? Why are some of them called vitamins and others not called vitamins? Why are there official recommendations for some and not for others?

Scientific work with vitamins is in its infancy. It is going on in many laboratories all over the world, as it has for the past 50 years or so. When Dr. Roger J. Williams of the University of Texas discovered pantothenic acid he gave it that name from a Greek word meaning "available everywhere." When he studied folic acid (which had no name then, but was just a chemical compound) he named it folic acid, because it occurs mostly in leafy green vegetables, or foliage.

Vitamin B12 is a generic name for "all cobalt-containing corrinoids" (this refers to the central structure of the vitamin). Between 1926 and 1955, many scientists were working with various substances in widely scattered laboratories to determine what the substance is in liver which cures pernicious anemia. In 1948 two researchers named it vitamin B12, since it was then thought that there might be vitamins already tentatively named vitamin B10, B11, etc. The chemical name for B12 is cobalamin or cyanocobalamin. (It's a lot easier to deal with the simple number 12, isn't it?)

"The need for this vitamin in human nutrition has not been established" means just what it says. Officially, we know that this is a vitamin. And, by definition, the word vitamin means something that is essential for life. But in the roundabout way of scientific bureaucracy, some committee or other decided that not enough laboratory work had been done to decide finally that this or that vitamin is absolutely necessary for good health. Para-amino-benzoic-acid is one such. Undoubtedly in the future much more research will turn up the many significant facts indicating that this substance is indeed essential to health. But for the present, manufacturers can legally only use the sentence above to indicate "yes, it may be a vitamin, but possibly it may not be."

The labels on food supplements cannot tell you exactly how much of any tablet or capsule to take, since this would be interpreted as prescribing medicine. "Take two aspirin and call me in the morning" is legal for your doctor to tell you over the phone. But only doctors can prescribe exact doses of medicine. Vitamins and minerals are not medicine. They are wholly beneficial, harmless (in reasonable amounts) elements of *food, not drugs*. And nobody but you can or should decide how much of any of these to take. You alone know what your health and diet circumstances are, as well as your way of life.

For example, if you regularly drink large amounts of freshly made raw fruit and vegetable juices, you probably have no need to take a vitamin A supplement. But someone who shuns all fruits and vegetables should certainly take a vitamin A supplement. How could anyone write a recommended dose on a label which would apply to both of you?

Why do you find words like "ferrous gluconate" and "calcium pantothenate" and "pyridoxine hydroxide" instead of just the words "iron" and "pantothenic acid" and "pyridoxine"? Just because, chemically speaking, things are usually combinations not single elements. Table salt is sodium chloride, not just sodium, because that's the way it appears in nature. The word "ferrous" refers to one form of iron. Ferrous gluconate is iron combined with glucose because this kind of iron has been found to be acceptable and easily assimilated by the body. Pantothenic acid combined with a bit of calcium is a convenient form in which to take this B vitamin. So don't be overly concerned about this chemical terminology.

Manufacturers of vitamin-mineral supplements must legally deal with all these facts and apparent inconsistencies when they label their products. They must also include on the label information on which vitamins, minerals and other food factors are recognized as "essential," and which have been given official recommended daily amounts. And they must include other information, somehow crowding it all onto a label which, in the case of a small bottle, may seem a near impossibility. In general, they do a good job.

CHAPTER 7

Might Not Massive Doses (Megadoses) of Vitamins Be Dangerous?

IF THE OFFICIALLY recommended amount of a vitamin is only several milligrams daily, isn't there a chance that doses far larger than that—megadoses as the doctors call them— might be dangerous? Couldn't very large amounts of vitamin C cause kidney stones? Niacin, the B vitamin, has an acid reaction in the stomach for some people. Could it cause ulcers? Of course, nobody should take immense doses of vitamin A and vitamin D over long periods of time, but what about taking all those other B vitamins in large doses along with the niacin?

It seems to us that the people who probably know more about this subject than anyone else are the physicians who regularly give their patients massive doses of vitamins along with whatever other treatment they give. Do these medical men also take the same amounts of vitamins every day? Do they give them to their families? What do they say about the possible dangers?

In March, 1972 a group of such physicians and scientists got together in New York under the auspices of the Huxley Institute for Biosocial Research to discuss problems of aging. Most of us must face these problems eventually. Most of us have such problems in our families already.

Here are some of the statements made by various physicians present, chiefly in regard to the physical and mental problems of aging, senility among them.

Dr. Roger J. Williams of the University of Texas is one of the most distinguished researchers in the field of nutrition and vitamins. Speaking of old folks, Dr. Williams said in part, "A most important part of the environment of an aging person is the food that he or she eats. This provides an internal environment for the cells and tissues. This environment is never perfectly adjusted. That it is often poorly adjusted is due in part to the fact that our staple foods are often trashy and provide in scanty fashion the nutritional essentials which make possible the adequate maintenance and repair of body cells and tissues.

"My work with pantothenic acid (a B vitamin) and longevity was precipitated by the well known observation that worker bees that are fed ordinary food as they develop, develop into worker bees. But the very same larvae, if fed extraordinary food which we call Royal Jelly, develop into queens, fertile queens and live several years, even as long as 8 years. Workers do not live more than a few weeks . . . at one time royal jelly was the richest known source of pantothenic acid. . . . We tried an experiment on the longevity of mice. There were 40 animals in each group. We treated them exactly alike except for the fact that in one group of 40 we gave them extra pantothenic acid in their drinking water. The result was an almost 10 percent increase in the longevity of the mice that got this extra pantothenic acid. I would assume that for some of the mice this did not do any good, but some of them needed larger amounts of pantothenic acid and when they got it they lived longer."

Dr. Abram Hoffer is a distinguished psychiatrist in Canada, who was the first to use large doses of certain vitamins in treating mentally ill patients. He said: "Every time a physician has to treat a patient with a chemical, he has to decide which is more dangerous to that patient—the disease untreated or the chemical he is using for the treatment. This is always the decision we have to face and from this point of view 'optimum' nutrition is that which does the job without producing any harm. . . . You can start with certain levels and see what happens; and gradually increase the level until you get what you want without producing side effects.

"Are there any contra-indications for this regime of large vitamin doses? With niacin (vitamin B3) you may have acidity factors. Rarely there are skin lesions that are not very pleasant. You can have changes in color that you have to deal with. . . .

"Is niacinamide as good as niacin? (Niacinamide is the amide form—a different chemical form—of niacin). It depends on what you are using it for. If you are using it to prevent pellagra, they seem to be equivalent. If you are using it to lower blood cholesterol, the niacinamide will not do it, but niacin will. So in each case you have to decide what it is that you expect from the 'medication' and then you will be able to determine.

"Is there any danger of kidney stones from vitamin C? It has been suggested that large doses of vitamin C might prove to be harmful because it would increase the formation of kidney stones. I have gone over the medical literature very carefully . . . so far there is not a single report in the medical literature where this has been established and in fact many physicians have recommended that vitamin C be used to dissolve kidney stones. . . . I am sure there are at least 50 theoretical dangers but this one doesn't have any data yet to confirm it . . . I have given patients as much as one gram (1,000 milligrams) of vitamin C per hour, day and night, for certain conditions. I have never seen acidosis. It may be I don't know what to look for."

". . . There are two energy yielding chemicals commonly consumed for which self-selection often fails to work advantageously. One is sugar. The other is alcohol. Children who are raised on soft drinks and given a choice will choose more of the same in preference to nourishing food. Adults who commonly consume alcoholic beverages regularly and copiously for long periods of time not infrequently reach the point where they lose interest in nourishing food and have on the contrary a prevailing interest in consuming alcoholic beverages. In each case, the appetite controlling mechanism in the brain goes awry. In children excess sugar consumption leads to general malnutrition. In adults, consuming too much alcohol can lead not only to general malnutrition but to severe damage to the brain. Brains of alcoholics are so badly damaged that their cadavers are unfit for brain dissection by medical students. Alcoholism is a terrific health hazard and elderly people are highly susceptible, particularly if they have had extended drinking experience.

"The brain cells of individuals need a good environment throughout their entire life history—from conception through the prenatal months and into the postnatal years up to old age. The environment of these brain cells is determined largely by the quality of food made available during pregnancy and consumed during youth, middle age and beyond. The environment of these brain cells is also determined in part by the poisons and near poisons that we consume.

"It was shown many years ago, with animals, that if you placed them on a vitamin B3 (niacin) deficiency program and produced black tongue or pellagra, if you kept them on it for a matter of a month or so, you could then bring them back to relative health by giving them the usual vitamin doses of niacin. If, however, you kept that same animal on the same diet for up to six months, he no longer responded to the usual vitamin dosages and now required what we in human terms would call megadoses of niacin, merely to bring him back to health and to maintain his health.

"It was also known by the early researchers in pellagra that when you were dealing with chronic pellagra you might have to give a daily maintenance dose of as much as 600 milligrams per day of niacin... I am suggesting that when human beings are deprived over a period of many years of the proper nutritional supplements, especially vitamins, that in time they are converting themselves into an acquired dependency condition. I think that what senility is, in fact, is merely a prolonged chronic form of malnutrition.

"... You must provide the optimum quantity of nutrients in the right organ at the right time ... in order to stave off senility, not old age but senility—we have to take into account the following factors: an adequate diet, a good diet. Enough high quality protein; a proper balance of fats, a marked reduction in the consumption of refined sugars, especially of sucrose (table sugar), supplements, and here we must use those nutrients which seem to be most relevant: niacinamide which was used by Dr. William Kaufman in 1939—three to four grams a day of niacinamide on 600 cases of arthritis. The results were fantastic. He was able to reverse the arthritic changes which are so often associated with senility. Niacin is a vitamin that lowers cholesterol and fats and is now the subject of a large-scale $55 million experiment by the American government. The results are interesting and it seems they will now decrease the coronary death rate over a four-year period by about 65 percent.

"The next subject is ascorbic acid (vitamin C) ... I can assure you that it is safe, and I myself have taken as much as 10 grams a day. We have given our patients as much as 90 grams a day. We have never yet seen any toxicity. If any person doubts that, I will challenge you to a duel. You eat a spoonful of salt and I will eat a spoonful of vitamin C and see who stops eating first. I think the average dose should be three grams a day. I take four. Pantothenic acid increases the longevity of animals ... Vitamin E should be investigated for its ability to prevent free radical formation." (He is referring here to the ability of vitamin E to prevent rancidity from occurring in body cells.)

"What I am doing is taking at least 30 pills of vitamins a day: four grams of niacin, four grams of vitamin C, 800 units of vitamin E, 250 milligrams of thiamine (vitamin B1), 250 milligrams of pyridoxine (vitamin B6), A and D, calcium and a bit of iron and a mineral supplement. I feel fine."

CHAPTER 8

Vitamins Plus a
Nourishing Diet
Prevent Cataract
in a
Laboratory Experiment

PEOPLE JUST BEGINNING to learn about vitamins often ask, "What vitamin can I take that will cure this or that condition?" as if vitamins were drugs and you could pop one of them at meals for a week or so and cure high blood pressure, or diabetes or heart disease. Or cataract.

It doesn't happen that way. Vitamins are not drugs and you cannot cure some disease of long-standing by simply taking "a vitamin" and doing nothing at all about correcting that non-nourishing diet and unhealthful way of life that had a lot to do with creating the condition in the first place. Nor is it likely to do much good to take two vitamins or three, even if you throw in a few minerals. While one vitamin may make a difference in the way you feel, after the vitamin has had some time to "work", and you may even notice some additional good effects that you had not expected, chances are that you will do much better by taking a full schedule of vitamins combined with the best possible diet and a way of life that is conducive to good health.

The fallacy of demanding that one vitamin cure one disease is highlighted by an experiment performed in the laboratory of one of the world's most distinguished biologists in the field of nutrition—Dr. Roger J.Williams of the University of Texas. All his professional life Dr. Williams has been trying to educate the general public and his professional colleagues as well as government officials to the basic principle that vitamins and minerals are not drugs—that all of them work together as a team, that there is no such thing as one vitamin or one mineral curing a disease. They must all be involved.

Says Dr. Williams in an article in the *Proceedings of the National Academy of Sciences*, October, 1974, "No nutrient by itself should be expected to prevent or cure any disease; nutrients as such always work cooperatively in metabolism as a team... Unlike drugs, single nutrients always act constructively like parts of a complicated machine and are effective only when they participate as members of a team. This does not prevent nutrients from having drug-like actions when used in amounts higher than the physiological levels... When particular vitamins appear to cure specific diseases, it is because they round out the team, transforming a limping incomplete team into one that is complete enough to function with some degree of physiological adequacy... Testing nutrients for their effectiveness is thus entirely different from testing drugs. Unless a nutrient is tested under conditions which allow it to participate in teamwork, the results are likely to be seriously misleading."

Dr. Williams and a colleague set out to test this theory on laboratory rats. It is well known that rats lack an enzyme which is necessary to use properly a sugar which appears in milk—galactose. Since they lack this enzyme, they generally get cataracts when they are fed lots of milk or milk products. The Texas researchers set up an experiment using 18 groups of rats and 18 different diets. All the diets except one (the control diet) contained quite large amounts of galactose—up to 20 percent of the diet. The rest of the diet was arranged so that some of the rats got just the usual chow which adequately nourishes laboratory rats: some diets contained nothing but eggs in addition to the galactose. An all-egg diet has been found by Dr. Williams to constitute a complete and very healthful diet for rats. Some of the diets contained the usual laboratory chow plus vitamins in quite large amounts.

At the end of nine weeks cataracts had formed in the eyes of many of the rats which got the plain chow with no vitamins. Although they were getting the same large amount of galactose (the cataract former), those rats which got, in addition, the vitamin supplements had no cataracts at all. In every case the number of cataracts increased in direct proportion to the lack of nutrients in the diet. Those diets which contained most in the way of vitamins, in addition to the basic good diet, produced no cataracts. Those which contained no extra vitamins did produce cataracts. The diets in between—with fewer vitamins added—produced some cataracts, but not as many as the diets with no added vitamins. The control group of rats which got no cataract-producing galactose—also had no cataracts.

In a second experiment all the rats were fed a diet designed to produce cataracts. They were then fed a good diet plus all the vitamins to see if the cataracts would regress. The results of this experiment were not as clear-cut as those of the first experiment. Of 26 cataracts, 16 showed improvement from 40 to 80 percent. But, in general, the regressions were slow and incomplete, "though improvement in many cases was clearly manifested," says Dr. Williams. It seems that the lens of the eye (where cataracts form) has a slow rate of metabolism—that is, any improvement might be expected to be slow.

Dr. Williams points out that his experiments do not prove that one or another vitamin will prevent cataracts. Nor is it possible to decide which of the vitamins given to the test animals was responsible for preventing the cataracts. There is no way to know if leaving out one or more of the vitamins would have changed the results. There is also no way to know whether the vitamins given are in complete "balance"—that is, whether too much of one vitamin was given, perhaps, or too little of another.

The point is that, however complete the traditional nourishing laboratory diet for rats is, it can always be improved by the addition of vitamins—all the vitamins. It can be improved to such an extent that the mere addition of all these vitamins can prevent cataracts forming even when the rats are given very large amounts of a substance which is almost guaranteed to produce cataracts in rats!

How does this happen? What do the additional vitamins do to perform this near-miracle? We do not know, says Dr. Williams. It is possible that, with the extra nutrients, the animals build enzyme systems to substitute for the one they lack—the one that is necessary to handle galactose, the cataract-causing substance.

What about human beings? Cataract is a frequent accompaniment of diabetes. Can enough of all the vitamins provide enough extra nutritional building materials to overcome the tendency to diabetic cataracts? What about those cataracts that appear in older folks, called senile cataracts? It seems quite possible that here, too, providing the optimum nutrition—not just enough to nourish but lots more than that—may be effective in preventing these cataracts from forming.

Dr. Williams thinks, too, that by treating the cataract with "supernutrition" as he calls it, the moment it is discovered, rather than waiting until it has fully developed, we might be able to prevent it from progressing any farther. And if we afflict the eye with less of the toxic substance which causes the cataract, we may be able to prevent or stop its further growth. In the case of the rats, galactose is the toxic substance. Most human beings have no problems with galactose because they have the enzyme necessary to metabolize it with no difficulty. Those few people born without this enzyme may (probably will) be afflicted with the full range of symptoms which lack of this enzyme produces—failure to thrive in infancy, jaundice, involvement of liver and spleen, mental retardation and formation of cataracts.

It seems obvious that all the many cataracts now being treated or removed from the eyes of diabetics and older folks are not the result of inability to metabolize galactose. We do not know what causes most human cataracts. Some specialists think it may be the result of eating too much sugar, since cataract is common among us Westerners who consume such large amounts of sugar. No matter what it is that causes human cataracts, doesn't it seem possible that they might be prevented by following the design of the experiment described above?

Eat the most highly nourishing diet possible, like the laboratory chow which nourished the rats. Then add vitamins to achieve supernutrition. The best way to achieve the most nourishing diet for human beings is to eliminate sugar from your meals and snacks. Many modern people eat so much sugar and refined white flour products that half of the meals consist of these two foods. There is little that nourishes in either of these foods except for starch, sugar and otherwise empty calories. Laboratory rats die of malnutrition when they are fed diets like this.

Once you have eliminated the twin hazards of refined sugar and refined cereal and bread products, everything else that you eat is nourishing. There's no need to plan outlandish, difficult or expensive meals. Just be sure that you include the high protein foods: meat, fish, poultry, dairy products, all the seed foods like wholegrains, bran, wheat germ, seeds of all kinds, nuts, soybeans, peas, beans, peanuts, all the fruits and vegetables, especially those that have lots of bright yellow and/or green, like carrots, apricots, parsley, broccoli, spinach. Eating this kind of diet—as widely varied as possible—you will get the same highly nourishing food as the laboratory rats had.

Then, according to Dr. Williams' experiments, add to that excellent diet all the known vitamins, some of them in quite large amounts. The accompanying chart shows the amounts of vitamins Dr. Williams used for his animals. No vitamin C is included, since rats make their own vitamin C and do not need to get it in food. You, however, need it very decidedly and you should add comparatively large amounts of it to your supplement program.

To calculate the amounts for human diets, estimate the number of calories you eat every day. It's probably in the neighborhood of about 3,000 for an adult man and about 2,000 for an adult woman. These are the officially recommended number of calories for people who are of average weight and height. The nutrients given in the chart are for every 100 calories of food. If you are eating 3,000 calories multiply the numbers in the chart by 30 to get an estimate of how much you should be taking to achieve what was achieved in the rat experiment.

Nutrients (Per 100 Calories) Furnished by Vitamin Mixture in Diets Which Prevented Cataracts

Vitamin A	1,333 I.U.
Vitamin D3	66.7 I.U.
Vitamin E	40 milligrams
Thiamine	0.83 milligrams
Riboflavin	1.67 milligrams
Niacin	10 milligrams
Pantothenic acid	5.3 milligrams
Pyridoxine	0.8 milligrams
Vitamin B12	3.3 micrograms
Folic acid	3.3 milligrams
Biotin	70 micrograms
Choline	50 milligrams
Inositol	33.3 milligrams

Plus some vitamin K and some fatty acid mixes.

It appears quite possible that the added vitamins may have such an excellent effect on your otherwise very nutritious diet that you will have achieved that "supernutrition" which Dr. Williams believes may be essential to prevent not just cataracts, but also other modern diseases like multiple sclerosis, muscular dystrophy, mental retardation, heart disease, dental disease, allergies, arthritis, premature senility, obesity, mental disease, alcoholism, and perhaps even cancer. It's worth a try, isn't it?

CHAPTER 9

The Special Vitamin Needs of Women on "The Pill"

Medical World News for August 24, 1973 reported on a National Institutes of Health study of medical records which showed that women on The Pill are 9½ times more likely to suffer a stroke than women not taking The Pill. Another study in Boston showed that blood clots are much more frequent in women on The Pill, who were also found to be twice as susceptible to gall bladder disease as women not on The Pill.

We have known for a long time that blood-sugar-regulating apparatus is disordered by The Pill. This could lead to diabetes or low blood sugar. Medical journals recommend that any woman whose family has a history of fatty accumulations in blood which cause hardening of the arteries should not take The Pill because the drug increases levels of certain fats in the blood. Many women suffer depression and discoloration of the skin when they take The Pill.

The list of serious ailments which afflict many women taking contraceptives seems almost endless. But there is apparently little hope of discouraging the use of oral contraceptives. Indeed medical researchers now promise even more mysterious and potentially damaging substances as contraceptives of the future.

The least we can do, as health seekers, is to examine what possible steps women can take to protect themselves against the more ominous threats they face from The Pill. Such information comes to us in *The Journal of Applied Nutrition* for Spring, 1974. An article by B. Pal, Ph. D., Research Associate of the Department of Medicine at the University of Rochester, discusses the metabolic and nutritional effects of oral contraceptives.

He tells us that one hormone commonly used in The Pill causes high blood sugar problems and the other hormone used with it makes this situation worse. In women with an inherited tendency toward diabetes, overt diabetes may develop when the contraceptive is taken, and disappear when it is withdrawn. Quite often, high blood levels of fat are also present in diabetes. Since oral contraceptives create a false pregnancy, the body responds by increasing blood levels of the triglycerides, one kind of bothersome fatty substance. The effects on cholesterol levels are inconsistent. In some women these levels, too, go up. Since raised levels of fats are linked to hardening of the arteries and many circulatory disorders, it is obvious that such side effects as these are highly undesirable, especially in women so young.

In women taking The Pill, blood levels of the B vitamin pyridoxine are below normal. So serious and widespread is this situation that many physicians believe the B vitamin should always be taken in the same tablet as the contraceptive. If not, additional pyridoxine—at least 30 milligrams daily—should be taken. Four of the essential amino acids or forms of protein are also low in women on The Pill. Dr. Pal says these proteins are concerned with the production of pigments, so it's possible this deficiency may explain the discolored skin many women on contraceptives complain of.

Folic acid is another essential B vitamin which is deficient in pill takers. Quite often pregnant women are short on folic acid. So apparently pregnancy causes a drain on this vitamin, lack of which brings on a very serious anemia. Since The Pill induces false pregnancy, this B vitamin may be used up very rapidly while The Pill is being taken. Many scientists concerned in this research believe that folic acid supplements should be given to pregnant women and to women on The Pill. Another complication is that women may become pregnant after they discontinue The Pill and may be in a state of folic acid depletion during this pregnancy—a very serious complication indeed.

Researchers have reported a decrease of 30 percent in vitamin C in the blood of women on The Pill. Part of the reason may be that the copper content of the blood increases during this time and copper causes the destruction of vitamin C. Says Dr. Pal, "the requirement for vitamin C may be well above the normal level during the oral contraceptive use."

Vitamin A is another nutrient affected by The Pill. One of the hormones in this drug impairs the ability of the liver to store vitamin A. Now, vitamin A is fat soluble, meaning that it is *supposed* to be stored in the body, unlike the water soluble vitamins. If its storage in the liver is disrupted, this might mean that a woman who takes The Pill would have to get, every day, the full quota of vitamin A which she needs, rather than depending on stores of the vitamin in her body.

If one or two of the B vitamins are in short supply due to The Pill, it seems likely that all the rest of the B complex are lacking, as well. If vitamin A and fat metabolism are disorganized, this suggests that all is not well with the other fat soluble vitamins—D, E, and K. Is the body storage of these vitamins disrupted, too?

The only certain fact out of this review of scientific findings is that any woman taking oral contraceptives should go out of her way to eat the most highly nourishing diet possible and should certainly take food supplements in ample amounts to make up for the abnormal decrease in certain of these, due to the drug.

How much of each vitamin should she take? This

depends on the individual. Some people require many times more than others just to stay healthy. Dr. Pal suggests 30 milligrams of pyridoxine (vitamin B6) daily. The official recommendation is a daily intake of 2 milligrams. So apparently the woman on The Pill needs 15 times this amount. She would have to get it from a high potency food supplement. On the same basis, should she be taking 15 times more of all the other B vitamins and vitamin C? We do not know, but certainly there is no harm in such a dose since these water soluble vitamins are not stored in the body and cannot accumulate. In the case of vitamin A, the woman on The Pill should make certain she gets, every day, a supplement containing at least the recommended daily amount of this vitamin which is 5,000 units.

The evidence on the way The Pill depletes vitamin stores has been piling up in medical journals year after year. As early as 1970 *The Lancet* published evidence that the depression of which many women on The Pill complain is caused by deficiency of vitamin B6, pyridoxine. Two Wisconsin physicians studied 58 patients who had been taking The Pill for an average of 14 months and who complained of at least three of these mental symptoms: emotional flareups and irritability, depression, fatigue, mild paranoia (they thought other people were persecuting them), difficulty with concentration and sleep disturbances.

Twenty-two of the patients had all five symptoms. Fifty had some of the symptoms before they started on The Pill, but the symptoms became worse on The Pill and new ones developed. The doctors gave them 50 milligrams of pyridoxine to take once daily when their premenstrual symptoms began. Eighteen reported complete cure of all symptoms. Twenty-six reported considerable improvement. Fourteen reported no change.

In those who noticed improvement with pyridoxine, the results were noticed within hours or by the next day at the latest. (This must have seemed like a miracle to women tormented with these troublesome symptoms.) The 14 patients who showed no improvement on 50 milligrams of pyridoxine daily were then given 100 milligrams—and still showed no improvement. No patients complained of any side effects.

One patient was so pleased with the results of the 50 milligrams of pyridoxine that she thought 100 milligrams would be even better. Every one of the 44 patients who improved on this vitamin therapy recommended pyridoxine to at least one friend or neighbor. One patient now has 12 friends taking the vitamin for mental symptoms.

Said these Wisconsin physicians, "These results support our clinical impression that pyridoxine is a valuable treatment for the five symptoms mentioned in patients taking oral contraceptives, and underlines the need for further research and controlled objective studies...the implications for treatment of premenstrual tension and pregnancy depression are obvious."

All 44 patients who improved were asked to discontinue pyridoxine to see if their symptoms returned. All refused to do so, because they were so pleased with the results. And even four patients who decided not to go on taking oral contraceptives because of their fear of side effects, went right on taking pyridoxine.

In November, 1970, another article appeared in *The Lancet* describing tests with 20 women using The Pill which showed that 16 of them had deficiency in vitamin B6. The authors, from New York and New Jersey, point out that pregnant women experience a similar pyridoxine deficiency for several months only, but the long-term use of The Pill can result in a "chronic and sustained derangement in a large segment of an essentially young, healthy population. In view of its ready correctibility by oral pyridoxine," they ask, "might it not be advisable to recommend a vitamin B6 supplement for users of The Pill?" Nobody answered their question, obviously, for few doctors seem to have noticed the pyridoxine deficiency produced by the pill they are giving.

In 1971 *The American Journal of Clinical Nutrition* printed an article by a group of New York physicians who studied 43 women all taking The Pill. They monitored the various changes brought about in the women as their supply of pyridoxine decreased. They point out that various processes involved in the way The Pill acts in regard to pyridoxine can produce defective regulation of blood sugar levels and supply of insulin and can cause concern.

They tell us that the recommended daily allowance of two milligrams of pyridoxine given to the women corrected the deficiency in only 10 percent of them. The rest required 25 milligrams. Because they were studying so few women and it was well known (or should be well known) that different people may have widely different needs for various vitamins, they concluded that all women taking The Pill should be given 30 milligrams of vitamin B6 (or pyridoxine) daily along with The Pill. A totally harmless dose of a totally beneficial vitamin. But still no notice was taken of this suggestion by any official medical group or government health group.

My extensive file on The Pill bulges with more and more medical articles relating newly discovered side effects of The Pill, all embellished with the quotation and disclaimer, "There is no such thing as absolute safety when it comes to contraception—you get nothing for nothing."

The Pill may be a cause of migraine headaches. The Pill may impair one's defense against infections. The Pill may bring vaginal discharges, urinary tract infections, susceptibility to chicken pox and other infections, eczema, loss of sex drive, mouth ulcers, high blood pressure, gall bladder troubles, serious alterations in results of laboratory tests which may throw off diagnoses of illness. Eighteen and a half million women were taking The Pill in 1969, undoubtedly many more than that by now. Periodically some researcher gives out a press release on research on the Male Pill but it's never any more than a press release.

And on March 5, 1975 the *New York Times* said that the development of safer methods of contraception is being seriously hampered because the multi-billion-dollar drug industry does not see any chance of making a pile of money out of a new pill before 1990 and that's too long to wait!

Vitamin A Is...

Fat-soluble, meaning it is stored in the body, so that it is not essential to provide vitamin A every single day.

Responsible for the health of the retina of the eye, the production of visual purple in the eye, which helps us to see at night, the maintenance of skin and linings of all body openings and organs, resistance to infections, bone development, maintenance of the myelin and membranes of our bodies, maintenance of color vision and peripheral (side) vision, maintenance of the adrenal gland and synthesis of certain hormones.

Present in most abundance in liver, kidney, carrots, spinach and all other dark green, leafy vegetables and yellow vegetables and fruits such as apricots, peaches, nectarines, yellow squash, sweet potatoes, butter, egg yolk.

Not to be taken in excess. Taking very large amounts of vitamin A over long periods of time can produce unpleasant and dangerous symptoms, which, in adults, disappear when the vitamin is withdrawn, but which may persist in infants and children.

Destroyed in the body by mineral oil laxatives, by several chemicals, estrogens and other drugs.

Required officially in amounts of 5,000 International Units by adults, somewhat less in children, depending on age.

Available in capsules of not more than 10,000 International Units.

Safe in amounts up to 20,000 units daily.

CHAPTER 10

Vitamin A Is
Powerful Against
Cancer

IN A SURVEY released February 26, 1968, the United States Department of Agriculture disclosed that 20% of the American population was eating a nutritionally poor diet. Almost one-half of the households in each region of the United States that were surveyed failed to meet the recommended allowances for all nutrients as established by the Food and Nutrition Board of the National Academy of Sciences, National Research Council. For vitamin A alone, the USDA found that one-fourth of the people were deficient. Projecting these figures onto the entire American population, it may be that between 40 to 50 million people may lack the amounts of vitamin A which experts believe we should have to be well nourished.

An equally alarming report comes from Canada, where autopsies in five Canadian cities showed that more than 30% of the deceased had less vitamin A in their livers than when they were born. In Montreal alone, 20% of the autopsied bodies had no vitamin A stores at all.

This information, which was reported by Dr. T. Keith Murray at a nutrition congress held in August 1968 in Puerto Rico, further revealed that, of the 500 people who had died, about one-third had less than 40 micrograms of vitamin A per gram of liver.

The ages of the individuals studied ranged from stillborn infants to people 92 years old. Most of the subjects were over 50. People who had died of various diseases seemed, generally, to have less vitamin A stores than those who died in accidents. But there apparently was no relation between the nature of the diseases and the amount of vitamin A that was found.

The average Canadian—like the average American—is thought by health authorities to be getting about five times the officially required amount of vitamin A in his daily diet. How does it happen, then, that body stores of this easily stored fat-soluble vitamin are low or entirely absent?

"It is hard to blame diet alone," Dr. Murray said. "Even allowing for wastage, cooking losses and uneven distribution, it does not seem likely that so many of our population do not get enough vitamin A to maintain their reserves."

The Canadian experts indicate that the condition they found may not necessarily be the result of poor eating habits, but may, instead, come about because of the things in our environment which deplete our stores of vitamin A—which cause us to use it at a faster rate than we can get it from our food.

They recommended further studies on the influence of pesticides, DDT especially. Researchers have shown, Dr. Murray said, that steers fed forage contaminated with DDT have much lower levels of vitamin A in their livers than cattle fed from uncontaminated feed. Giving rats DDT impairs the utilization and storage of this vitamin.

The Canadian researchers then looked into the matter of the drugs the people had taken before they died, but they could find no relation between any given drug or drugs and the store of vitamin A in the liver. They were especially interested in drugs which reduce cholesterol, for cholesterol is a fatty substance and vitamin A is a fat-soluble vitamin. Such drugs might, they thought, interfere with the body's use of vitamin A, since their purpose is to block the action of the fatty substance, cholesterol. They could find no apparent tie between drug-taking and vitamin A storage.

Then they took up the amount and kind of fat in the diet. They studied the level of vitamin E in the diet, since this is apparently related to the way the body uses vitamin A. They looked into the amount of protein these folks had been eating, for the amount of protein in the diet is also linked with the way the body uses vitamin A. On diets low in protein, vitamin A is not used very effectively by the human body. Some of the older people appeared to be eating less than the recommended amounts of protein.

Dr. Murray stated that it is not easy to alter the absorption and utilization pattern of vitamin A, so it must be something as yet undiscovered which is robbing people of the amount of vitamin A which they need. Perhaps, he said, it is some combination of poor diet and something in our environment that does the damage.

"Vitamins appear to play a much more vital role in safeguarding lungs from the ravages of air pollution than has been generally realized," said an article in *Chemical and Engineering News* for June 29, 1970. At a symposium on pollution and lung biochemistry at the Battelle-Northwest Institute, Richland, Washington, a scientist from the Massachusetts Institute of Technology told of his experiments with rats in which he found that vitamins A and E play an important role in protecting lung tissues from harm that may be done by two components of air pollution—ozone and nitrogen dioxide.

These two pollutants are among the most destructive compounds we have loosed on city dwellers by industrial pollution and the exhaust from automobiles that jam our city streets. Certain fatty substances in the lungs are broken down by the pollutants releasing other substances that are highly dangerous. Vitamin E appears to "quench" these substances, rendering them harmless.

Scientists from Battelle-Northwest have been conducting a series of nutrition experiments in which they fed rats a specially prepared diet that was high in polyunsaturates—

the fatty substance which is attacked by the air pollutants. Some of the animals got food that contained no vitamin E. Others ate the same diet, supplemented with vitamin E.

The rats were then exposed to a stream of air containing one part per million of ozone. They soon showed signs of severe stress in breathing, and died. Those which were getting the vitamin E lived twice as long in the ozone polluted atmosphere. In other experiments researchers autopsied the rats after they had been exposed to nitrogen dioxide. The animals that had eaten the diet deficient in vitamin E had far less of the polyunsaturates in their lungs than the rats which had plenty of vitamin E. Apparently the vitamin had preserved the valuable polyunsaturates and prevented their destruction.

Dr. Daniel B. Menzel, who heads the Battelle nutrition and food technology section, believes that vitamin E might perform still another beneficial function in safeguarding vitamin A from being destroyed by the air pollutants. "This in itself would be an important function," says the article, "because it is now becoming increasingly evident that vitamin A is crucial for the healthy metabolism and growth of epithelial cells." These are cells in the skin and linings of body cavities like the lungs, digestive tract, reproductive tract and eliminative tract.

At M.I.T. scientists have been experimenting with vitamin A, giving it to rats, then examining their lung cells. The rats which had plenty of vitamin A showed a healthy condition of the lungs. Those which had a deficiency showed cells that were thick, scaly and hard, instead of being soft and covered with healthful mucus. After identifying a certain compound present in the healthy lungs and absent in the deficient ones, they found, furthermore, that when they gave supplements of vitamin A to the deficient rats, this beneficial compound was formed in their lungs *within 18 hours,* even though they had been eating a deficient diet for a long time.

The researchers went on to say that we know now that vitamin A can prevent the formation of cells that later turn into cancer cells. They don't know exactly how the vitamin does this, but they are investigating the process. And now they are wondering whether massive doses of vitamin A may be able to reverse the growth of certain kinds of cancers. They are working with Dr. Umberto Saffioti who was then at the National Cancer Institute.

It was Dr. Saffioti, incidentally, who reported to the 9th International Cancer Congress that vitamin A can prevent lung cancer. This was discussed in the October 25, 1966 issue of the *New York Times*.

At the time Dr. Saffioti worked out elaborate experiments with hamsters in which he induced lung cancer in the animals by blowing into their lungs some of the same chemical particles that are found in urban air pollution and in cigarette smoke. Hamsters, like human beings, do not develop lung cancer unless they are exposed to some cancer-causing agent, or carcinogen. Dr. Saffiotti was at the time Associate Scientific Director for Carcinogenesis with the National Cancer Institute; he was in the news in the fall of 1969 in connection with whether or not the cyclamates were cancer-causing.

In his research, Dr. Saffiotti noted that the changes which occurred in the cells of the hamsters' lungs are changes that precede cancer. Eventually up to 100% of the animals got lung cancer, depending on how much of the cancer-producing chemical they received. Giving the hamsters vitamin A prevented these changes in lung cells and hence prevented the lung cancers, Dr. Saffiotti noted.

The Times goes on to say that Dr. Saffiotti "stressed that his findings were not an invitation for cigarette smokers or people living in air-polluted areas to try to get vitamin A, or eat a lot of carrots. Too much vitamin A can be harmful to humans."

Let's examine this statement. Obviously the hamsters were not given too much vitamin A to be harmful, but they were given enough to prevent the cancer. So there is every indication that human beings, getting "enough" vitamin A might have the same experience the hamsters did—they might be able to avoid an otherwise inevitable cancer.

Of course, Dr. Saffiotti can't say this and let it appear on the front page of *The New York Times*, because our official government spokesmen have said that all of us, eating the average American diet, are already getting enough vitamin A. They leave it to other specialists to explain why so many Americans are victims of lung cancer and of many other diseases which plenty of vitamin A just might help to prevent.

What we are concerned about is lung cancer. According to the American Cancer Society, the mortality rate for lung cancer in 1968 was 59,367: 48,831 men and 10,536 women. The estimated deaths from lung cancer in 1972 were equally grim: 68,800. This breaks down as 55,800 men and 13,000 women. The death rate from this kind of cancer is increasing more rapidly than that from any other kind of disorder. The agonies of death from lung cancer are unimaginable.

Yet we are told by an authoritative scientist that Americans should not begin to take vitamin A "or eat a lot of carrots," because we might get a bit too much Vitamin A and suffer some unpleasant symptoms which disappear as soon as we discontinue the vitamin A.

Also at the above-mentioned Congress, Sir Alexander Haddow, a British scientist, announced *that as many as 80% of all human cancers may be due to environmental causes*. If this is true, he said, "The implications for prevention are immense and exciting." He believes that scientists will be able to eliminate most cancers, even if they never find out what causes cancer. We're sorry that we cannot agree with Dr. Haddow.

What he is saying, in essence, is that as soon as we have final, irrevocable proof that air pollution, water pollution, chemicals in food, pesticides, drugs, cigarette smoke, radiation, and the hundreds of thousands of other pollutants of our industrial society . . . cause cancer, then all we have to do is to eliminate these hazards and we won't have any more cancer. But what an impossible premise!

VITAMIN A AND CANCER

All men of good will admit today that these environmental hazards pose serious threats to health. But the job of eliminating them from the world we live in is impossibly immense. No government has made even a token start on such a job. Nor is there any assurance that, with the best will in the world, any government will ever succeed in protecting us from the environmental toxins to which our present technological society exposes us.

Two cancer researchers at the National Cancer Institute in Bethesda, Maryland decided to see if large doses of vitamin A might prevent cancers of various kinds in laboratory hamsters. They used several chemicals which are known to produce cancers in the stomach and various parts of the genital organs.

They fed the chemicals to the animals. And by also painting the chemicals on the animals' reproductive organs, they found that they could produce cancer in just about 100% of the animals. Then, using a second group of animals, they added quite a large amount of vitamin A to their diets when they fed the cancer-causing chemicals and added vitamin A to the chemicals which were applied to reproductive organs. They found that the vitamin prevented the stomach cancer from occuring. It also protected the cervix and vagina from cancer, but not the skin around the anus and vagina.

From a hospital in Israel comes word of experiments in which vitamin A was used to retard the growth and inhibit the induction of benign and malignant tumors in laboratory animals. This means that applying the vitamin to the skin of the animal prevented cancer from forming when chemicals known to cause cancer were applied. In animals which were already suffering from cancer, growth of the tumor was slowed.

This protective action took place only in the cervix and vagina of the female animals, not on other parts of the body. The experiments were described in *Cancer* magazine.

Three Swiss physicians reported on a test of vitamin A used against leukoplakia and basal cell carcinoma (cancer) of the skin. Leukoplakia is a pre-cancerous condition of the mouth and throat. The abstract of their article in *Schweizerische Medizinische Wochenschrift*, July 17, 1971, does not indicate how much vitamin A they gave. It involved probably quite large doses, but not large enough to harm the patients.

Of the 24 patients studied "a therapeutic result" was achieved in 11 who had leukoplakia and short-term remissions were observed in two patients with skin cancer. There were no unpleasant side effects, except that several of the patients complained of headaches.

The cancer cells of all patients who were treated showed changes when the vitamin A was given, and the changes depended upon how much of the vitamin was given. We assume this means that when the dosage was decreased, the cells began to look unhealthy again.

Among the many ill effects of the oral contraceptive pill are tumors of the liver. At any rate doctors have reported an association between those who take The Pill and liver cancers. In the March 22, 1975 issue of *The Lancet*, a British physician raises the question of whether this may be due to the fact that contraceptives decrease the amount of vitamin A in the liver. It is known, says Dr. Isabel Gal, that hormones (the Pill is made up of hormones) influence the way the body uses vitamin A. It is also known that vitamin A participates in cell division in certain tissues of the body. Cancer is a disorder of cell division. So, she asks, if a deficiency in this vitamin is caused by The Pill and the woman's diet also contains little vitamin A, is it not possible that this plain lack of vitamin A may be the cause of such tumors? It seems to us quite possible, especially since all nutritional surveys show that many of us are not getting even that amount of vitamin A which will satisfy our basic needs. If, in addition, we are subjected to many environmental factors which deplete our store of vitamin A—and apparently The Pill is one of these—then it would certainly be sensible for anyone taking oral contraceptives to be certain she is getting enough and more than enough vitamin A.

Science, the publication of the American Association for the Advancement of Science, devoted a page in its December 27, 1974 issue to the unchallengeable fact that vitamin A prevents cancer, in both laboratory animals and human beings. A number of papers read at a symposium on the subject in November clearly showed that such is the case. No one knows why or how this occurs, since, it seems, biologists have really very little information on just what vitamin A does in the body and how it does it.

But two scientists from the National Cancer Institute in Washington reported at the symposium that when they applied known cancer-causing substances to parts of the breathing apparatus of animals, much more damage was done to those animals which had been deficient in vitamin A.

Two scientists from Massachusetts Institute of Technology reported that when laboratory rats are given cancer-causing substances which exist in certain fungi that grow on food, there were fewer colon cancers among those rats which got plenty of vitamin A.

Another researcher has found, he said, that in animals who are not at all deficient in vitamin A giving more of the vitamin than they are getting will protect them against cancer of the respiratory tract.

A scientist at the Southern Research Institute at Birmingham, Alabama reported at the symposium that when he applied vitamin A to mice prostate glands he could prevent the cancer that would be expected to follow exposure to certain cancer-causing chemicals. And even if he gave the vitamin A *after* he had exposed the glands to the carcinogens, cancers were prevented.

Another scientist at the same institute tested vitamin A in relation to liver and lung cancer. He found that vitamin A prevented the formation of a cancer-causing substance from a benzene product. Both liver and lungs of the animals were protected.

A scientist at the Oak Ridge National Laboratory

showed that vitamin A can reduce the incidence of lung cancers produced by still another cancer-causing compound. A cancer researcher at the Illinois Institute of Technology reported that giving one form of vitamin A to hamsters prevents cancers that would otherwise be caused by another benzene compound.

And even after the cells have been transformed into precancerous cells, administration of vitamin A can reverse the change and prevent the cancers in some cases, according to a Hoffman-LaRoche scientist who prevented the formation of one kind of cancer in rats which had been exposed to a substance known to cause this kind of cancer. Their cells had already been starting to form cancers when the vitamin was given.

A Swiss scientist reported that he has prevented certain kinds of cancer in both mice and human beings, after they have been exposed to cancer-causing substances. The evidence appears to be quite substantial and authoritative. There seem to be no doubts. And these reports follow many earlier reports telling the same story—vitamin A given either to animals deficient in the vitamin or to those which are getting enough vitamin A, prevents cancer before it can get started or even after it has started.

One of the participants in the Vitamin A and Cancer symposium told the assembled scientists that surveys have shown that at least one-third of all Americans are deficient in vitamin A—that is, they do not get every day even that small amount of the vitamin which is officially stated to be essential for good health, let alone enough more to protect them from whatever cancer-causing chemicals they are exposed to day after day.

CHAPTER 11

Vitamin A, Old Age and Infections

THREE ARTICLES ON vitamin A and its effect on various aspects of cancer therapy assume added importance because they appear in the *Journal of the National Cancer Institute*. This is a Washington-based, government-sponsored organization which should, we believe, be dedicated to the *prevention* of cancer in any conceivable manner. Instead, they deal mostly with research relating to "cures" and laboratory methods.

So it is heartening when one finds anything in their journal which seems to be related to prevention of cancer. Certainly anything pertaining to vitamins would be in this area.

In the first article (March, 1972) six scientists described their discovery that vitamin A deficiency produces the same condition in the respiratory tract of the hamster as a certain cancer-causing chemical produces. In other words, a diagnostician examining such an animal would not be able to tell whether the condition he found was due to simple lack of vitamin A or to exposure to a cancer-causing compound.

In a second article in the same journal, three Texas doctors report on some experimental radiation to control a cancer. They found that, if they were injecting vitamin A at the same time, they could reduce to 15 to 20 percent the radiation needed to stop growth of a certain kind of cancer. Most of the article deals with the methods they used and their thinking in regard to why this protection should take place.

Finally they say, "if the effectiveness of a radiation dose to a human tumor could be increased by 15-20 percent without influencing damage to normal tissues, the results of clinical radiotherapy would greatly improve." Although the circumstances of the tumor were not the same as they would be in a human case of cancer, the authors say, "the use of vitamin A ... with therapy of various animal tumors and normal tissues seems worthy of further studies."

It certainly seems so. Radiation is, of course, a terribly dangerous procedure. It must be controlled in such a way that only the cancerous cells are irradiated. This must be done without harming healthy cells. If the simple, easy, inexpensive administration of vitamin A beforehand could lessen the danger of this treatment 15-20 percent, what in heaven's name are we waiting for? Why isn't vitamin A being used in every cancer-treatment center in the world where radiation is used?

Furthermore, the environmental radioactivity of our world is increasing at a rapid rate. As more and more radioactive substances are used, as nuclear power plants spring up on all sides, releasing their toxic by-products into air and water, isn't it possible that vitamin A could help to protect us against the harm we will certainly face eventually from this increasing contamination?

Finally, an article from the November, 1971 issue of the *International Journal of Vitamin and Nutrition Research* tells the dismal story of how little prepared are some of the most vulnerable people to meet any situation which requires plenty of vitamin A for protection. Old folks are always at a special disadvantage. Cancer takes a high toll in these age brackets. Cells are worn out. Resistance is low. Nutrition is usually very inadequate. Meals are skimpy and planned with little attention to vitamin needs.

So vitamin A supplements in ample amounts would seem to be essential for their good health. Yet every survey done, especially among older people, shows that their meals contain less than recommended amounts of vitamin A, in some cases far less.

The *Journal* article reports on studies of the vitamin A content of food in three old age homes. They happen to be in Switzerland, but old age homes are the same the world around, those in our country included. All of the 38 subjects studied were getting less than 85 percent of the recommended amount of vitamin A which is 5,000 units daily. Four of the people studied were getting less than 1,250 units daily. *In only one home did the diet which was served provide enough vitamin A. In the other two it did not.* In any case, most of the old folks refused to eat considerable amounts of their meals, so they did not get even the less-than-recommended amounts of vitamin A that were offered to them.

The study included vitamin C as well and here the deficiency figures are horrifying. All of the subjects were getting less than 75 percent of the recommended 55-60 milligrams of vitamin C. In one home the average intake of vitamin C reached only 8 milligrams during the entire week. Twelve of these old people ate less than one milligram of vitamin C on certain days!—and they refused up to 87 percent of whatever vitamin C was offered.

Old people suffer from many complaints which are likely to involve nothing more or less than lack of vitamins. They are highly susceptible to infections (lack of vitamin A and vitamin C). They have troubles with eyes and ears, digestive tracts and elimination. Vitamins in ample amounts can help prevent all these. Their bones, joints and muscles ache—a sure symptom of scurvy which is the disease of vitamin C deficiency. And certainly anyone getting as little vitamin C as these folks were getting is on the very edge of scurvy or perhaps has a full-blown case of scurvy which has just not been diagnosed.

And what of the frightful risk of cancer to which these old people are exposed when they are eating not even a tiny fraction of the amount of vitamin A and C which is recommended for perfectly healthy adults? Old age is stress. The diseases of old age are a form of stress. Under stress our bodies need more of all vitamins, but especially vitamin A and C.

How is it possible that dieticians in old folks homes who supposedly know the essential nature of vitamins and minerals, do not offer, as part of the meals they serve, a complete vitamin capsule at every meal, with extra added amounts of the B vitamins and vitamin C which, being water soluble, are needed every single day! And the older you are the more you need, it would seem.

If you are caring for an older person, make sure the meals you serve are well balanced in regard to all the vitamins and make sure the food is in a form the old folks can eat (pureed or chopped, if there is difficulty in chewing). And, as added insurance, insist on a well-balanced, complete vitamin and mineral capsule, with additional amounts of the B vitamins and vitamin C. And don't forget, as well, that circulatory troubles benefit from plenty of vitamin E. An aging circulatory system is especially vulnerable.

Though vitamin A was discovered 60 odd years ago and its chemical nature has been known 40 years and more, there are signs it may have valuable properties not suspected up till now, according to *Medical World News* for December 14, 1973. This is not news to any health seeker, for we have been using this vitamin for many years as a shield against many different kinds of disorders, including infections.

But now it seems that a physician-researcher has tested vitamin A to see if it actually does protect against infections. And—what do you know?— he found that it does! Dr. Benjamin E. Cohen of Massachusetts General Hospital reported on his experiment at a meeting of the American Society of Plastic and Reconstructive Surgeons.

Presumably these surgeons would be interested in such information since, in many kinds of surgery, the "immune response" is involved. This is the ability of the body to protect itself against invaders of any kind—bacteria, or foreign proteins.

Dr. Cohen found that vitamin A strongly stimulated his laboratory animals' "immunue response"—that is, it gave them far more capability to withstand diseases.

The drug cortisone is known to block this immune response. This is one reason why people taking cortisone and related drugs are likely to be much more susceptible to infections than the rest of us. So Dr. Cohen gave cortisone to his laboratory mice along with vitamin A and found that the vitamin almost completely prevented the action of the cortisone, thereby protecting the body from infection.

Then he inoculated germs into the animals to which he had previously given injections of 3,000 units of vitamin A—an immense amount of this vitamin for a creature as small as a mouse. He then injected the mice with a gram-negative bacterium, or a fungus or a gram-positive bacterium. He had another group of "control" animals which got no vitamin A.

In the group of mice infected with gram-negative bacteria the control animals suffered massive invasion of the germs and died of the infection within 24 hours. The mice treated with vitamin A developed severe infection for the first three hours, but by the fifth hour "no more organisms could be cultured from their blood". While the mice which had received no vitamin A were dying, the mice treated with vitamin A were found to have blood "still virtually sterile" so far as the injected germs were concerned.

In the case of the other kind of bacteria and the fungus, the vitamin A treatment greatly prolonged the animals' survival time, although they did die eventually from the disease, as the untreated mice did.

Dr. Cohen suggested that vitamin A should be given to

patients who are being treated with cortisone and related drugs, for it will apparently greatly help to protect them from infections. Other researchers have used vitamin A, he says, to reduce the incidence of digestive tract stress in patients suffering from severe trauma, burns or the aftermath of surgery. Dr. Cohen thinks the vitamin should be used to protect burned patients from infection.

He also thinks, he says, that "vitamin A could play a significant part in cancer therapy if further studies of its use with BCG support preliminary findings with mice" given a certain kind of cancer (BCG is a vaccine). "In our first couple of experiments we looked at the effects of vitamin A with BCG, compared with BCG alone, on susceptibility to tumor inoculum", said Dr. Cohen. "We found that animals receiving both vitamin A and BCG had a lower incidence of tumors than those getting BCG alone."

CHAPTER 12

Vitamin A May
Relieve Acne and
Other Skin Disorders

A UNIVERSITY OF PENNSYLVANIA specialist in dermatology declared in 1974 that acne, the curse of teenagers, is not just very common, but actually afflicts 100 percent of American teenagers. Dr. Albert Kligman said that one should not speak of young people with or without acne. It's just a question of whether they have a mild or acute form. They all have it, he said.

Fifty years ago acne was quite uncommon, almost unknown, in our country. It is still unknown among people we call "primitive"—that is, those few scattered groups of people who are still eating as their ancient ancestors ate down through many generations, back into prehistoric times. This seems to indicate that something in our modern world has produced this unsightly and embarrassing condition. What could it be?

Acne begins when the oily substance sebum is secreted into a skin cell. The sebum dries and becomes horny and infected. A small head of pus appears, crowned by a "blackhead". Doctors call these "comedones". Teenagers call them "pimples". If these are pressed out inexpertly, the infection spreads to neighboring cells which begin to develop "blackheads". The body tries to cover the whole mess with a layer of skin which causes the underlying infection to fester, then drain, leaving a scar. Of course many medical treatments used in the past also leave scars, so that many young people become adults with scarred faces.

Dr. Kligman and his colleagues at the University of Pennsylvania don't speculate on what the causes of acne are. But they do use a vitamin A preparation to treat it. It is called retinoic acid. It is given in the form of a salve—a "potent agent" the doctors call it. Applied to the skin it produces redness and peeling. At first it also produces more "pimples" than before. The discouraged teenager is tempted to give up. But after about ten weeks the peeling and redness disappear and so in many cases do the skin manifestations of acne.

Vitamin A appears to be an appropriate substance for use in a skin condition, for part of its job in the body is to nourish the skin, as well as all the linings of the body— linings of respiratory, digestive and elimination tract, for example. It is also essential for important functions involved in eyesight.

The Pennsylvania doctors tell us that their vitamin A treatment is no quick miracle cure. After about eight weeks, they say, they can estimate whether it will succeed. At the end of 12 weeks, they can be sure. The patient must use the salve until all the skin manifestations of acne have disappeared. If they stop before that, the condition will reappear.

Is it dangerous? Apparently not. Among hundreds of patients who have used the vitamin preparation daily for as long as two or three years, "we have not encountered serious or irreversible local side effects," they say,

Sometimes, in addition, they give massive doses of vitamin A for short periods of time. Vitamin A in large doses taken for long periods of time can produce unpleasant and dangerous symptoms. So the doctors check their patients carefully. They sometimes give 100,000 units of vitamin A daily for one week. Then they may raise it to

400,000 units for a short time, then reduce it gradually and finally withdraw it entirely.

It is not recommended under any circumstances for the patient to experiment on himself with massive doses of vitamin A. It is always wise to get enough of this vitamin in daily meals and to take a supplement to cover any individual needs over what comes with meals.

The form of vitamin A which is used by the Pennsylvania doctors is not something you can buy at the drug store. A doctor must administer it and watch progress, it seems, as well as possibly giving the large doses of vitamin A orally and along with antibiotics, if the inflammation is especially bad.

Two West German physicians have found that vitamin A acid (one form of this vitamin) is effective treatment against acne. They treated 80 patients between the ages of 19 and 25 with vitamin A acid. It was in the form of cream or jelly. The patients had varying degrees of this disfiguring skin disorder—some much more serious than others. The drug, as these doctors call it, was applied only once a day for nine weeks. The occurrence of comedones or pimples was reduced by 90 percent. That is, the acne was almost entirely eliminated. Two thirds of the patients had no problems with the medication. We assume this means that the other one-third had some unfavorable reactions.

All acne could be and should be prevented, and most acne can be treated by taking one precaution which is essential to good health, whether or not one has acne. Stop eating sugar or any foods that contain it. Acne is unknown among primitive people who have no access to sugary foods. It appears in their young people almost as soon as they move to "civilization" and begin to use soft drinks, candy, cakes, desserts of all kinds and sugary snacks. Taking yogurt daily, or the lactobacillus tablet preparations daily, is a great help, along with a no-sugar diet, in preventing acne.

A disfiguring skin condition called *ichthyosis* is yielding to a vitamin A preparation applied to the skin, according to a recent issue of *Medical World News*. The name of this disease means that the skin of the victim looks like fish scales. Some forms of it are hereditary.

Two Wisconsin children, aged 11 and 12, suffered from the condition, and nothing had ever improved it. They had been treated with antibiotics on the skin and taken internally, compresses, emoliments to soften the skin, kerolytics (drugs which cause the outer layers of the skin to slough off) and vitamin A taken by mouth. Nothing helped. Their father also suffered from the skin condition and no treatment had ever helped him.

Dr. William F. Schorr of the Marshfield Clinic, Marshfield, Wisconsin, had been treating the girls unsuccessfully since their birth. Finally, he tried a different form of vitamin A called Retinoic acid. It is made by Johnson and Johnson under the trade name of Retin-A.

The younger girl applied the ointment to half of her abdomen in order that any improvement in the condition could be compared to the other untreated half. Within three weeks the thick, horny, foul-smelling crust on the treated skin was clear. Nothing remained but a mild redness. Both children were then hospitalized for a thorough test. The ointment was applied two to three times daily and both children improved almost at once. The father was given ointment to apply all over his body and there was considerable improvement.

Doctors and patients alike could easily see improvement. But when the doctors examined the skin under the microscope the great change was apparent. Normal skin has overlapping cells so that there is continuous protection to the layers of skin underneath. But in the "alligator" kind of skin which this disease produces, there are masses of heaped up cells separated by deep crevices. In these crevices bacteria lodge. Since no amount of washing will remove them, they produce foul odors which are one of the distressing aspects of the disease.

Skin specimens taken after treatment with Retin-A showed that the deep crevices had disappeared, the skin cells were growing much more naturally and overlapping one another as they should. And the number of bacteria on the skin were considerably reduced. Dr. Schorr stated that the drug is "more than just a salve to produce skin scaling. The normalization of the entire skin parallels the remarkable clinical improvement."

Dr. James E. Fulton of the Department of Dermatology at the University of Miami School of Medicine, agrees. He has treated several patients with this form of vitamin A which he calls, "probably the only useful treatment we now have for ichthyosis."

And Dr. Phillip Frost, co-chief of the skin and cancer unit of the Mt. Sinai Medical Center of Greater Miami has treated about 40 victims of this disease and has found the vitamin A preparation successful in the severe forms of the disease. It seems that it may be necessary for these people to use this preparation for the rest of their lives, but this is surely a small price to pay for relief from such a disfiguring and disagreeable condition.

All the doctors who are using the salve treat it as a drug and are concerned apparently only with curing their patients. But doesn't it seem very possible that such a condition, from birth, must be caused by some gross malfunction of all the body mechanisms that process vitamin A? Perhaps treatment of the mother and father with large doses of vitamin A before the children are conceived might prevent this condition.

And one hopeful word on psoriasis comes to us from the *New York State Journal of Medicine*, Volume 11, January, 1973, page 2584-2587. Twenty-two patients were treated with the same retinoic acid (vitamin A) and found significant improvement. They were also given cortisone at the same time. We are not told what part this may have played in the improvement. In the same journal we learn of a case of severe liver damage caused by treatment of psoriasis by a more familiar drug—methotrexate—which is given for psoriasis.

CHAPTER 13

Chlorophyll, Daylight and Vitamin A

CHLOROPHYLL IS THAT substance in green leaves which captures the sun's energy and manufactures carbohydrates in plant tissues from this energy. Without chlorophyll there could be no life on earth, for all living creatures, including human beings, depend on the food from green plants, chiefly the carbohydrates manufactured by chlorophyll in the green leaves. The process of making chlorophyll is called photosynthesis by scientists. This means creation by light. Only in daylight can this process take place.

Scientists have been studying this rather mysterious process for many years and thought they knew just about everything they needed to know about it. But the other day, according to *The New York Times* for March 15, 1976, they uncovered an astonishing new fact about the whole process that staggered them. It seems there is another compound in the world which can also take the sun's power and convert it into usable energy. This substance is the bacterial form of something called "visual purple" which exists in the human eye. The human retina, to be exact.

Visual purple is essential for sight. And visual purple can be made in your eyes only if enough vitamin A is present! Visual purple is used up helping you see in bright light. It renews itself after dark while you are sleeping. A day in bright sunlight at the beach may use up so much visual purple that you may have trouble with glare driving home after dark. The glare from oncoming vehicles may bother you greatly. And when you get home, it may be hard to find the keyhole or even the path to the door because of lack of visual purple in your eyes.

We suggest that you do not turn on TV after such a trip and subject your eyes to still more light. We suggest you go quietly to bed in as dim a light as possible. And don't read yourself to sleep. The visual purple in your retina will be renewed while you sleep, if you have enough vitamin A available in your blood to help perform this manufacturing process.

The implications of the new finding that visual purple can also convert the sun's energy into energy useful to man are staggering in many ways. Scientists are now talking about using this substance (in its bacterial form) to create energy for many purposes. Perhaps it can be stored in battery cells and used to fuel cars or heat homes. The prospects are almost limitless, it seems. The *Times* says "Whether this discovery turns out to be useful or not, it must still inspire awe as one more indication of how much more splendidly complex the miraculous world of nature is than earlier generations could even imagine."

Now that we have established the elemental importance of visual purple (it ranks with chlorophyll as one of the basic materials essential to life on the planet!) we should make note of some related things. First, visual purple reacts with light. It is apparently destroyed or "used up" by light, so that it must be renewed in darkness. New York researchers have discovered, using rats as subjects, that animals given no vitamin A could manufacture enough visual purple to see well if they were kept in darkness all the time.

Other rats, subjected to some light, then darkness, and deprived of all vitamin A, could not manufacture visual purple, but lost it continuously from their retinas. Presumably if the animals had been kept without vitamin A and with recurring light and darkness, they would eventually have become blind if the experiment had continued long enough.

What does such an experiment imply for human beings? It indicates the great importance of a given amount of darkness—total darkness—every day and the great importance, too, of vitamin A for eye health. If our eyes are similar to those of the animals tested—and it seems most likely that they are—then it appears that we may be doing ourselves grave harm by spending so much time under artificial light and staying up so late.

Up until about 75 years ago, most human beings lived each day by rising with the dawn and going to bed as darkness fell, summer and winter, for there was almost no way to create light after dark. There were candles and open fires and oil lamps and torches, but these gave off very little light. And most people could not afford them for everyday use. When they could afford a candle or an oil lamp they used them for only a few hours for special occasions. So they lived much as the animals live, in regard to the amount of light that entered their eyes during any 24-hour period.

Now consider for a moment how we live today. Most of us are exposed to extremely bright light for perhaps 18 to 20 hours a day, if we stay up late watching television. All of us extend the daylight hours with electric light in winter when dark comes early. We pore over books, papers and close desk-work with brilliant reading lamps to light our way. We walk on streets brilliantly lighted day and night, where spotlights play and electric signs glitter.

Our young people go to "light shows" where they spend hours watching flashing lights of many colors in a dazzling array of electrical splendor which surely would challenge the best eyes in the world to survive this kind of punishment. Our actors, musicians, cameramen and anyone speaking before an audience must expose his or her eyes to spotlights and footlights for long hours while they are working.

What is all this doing to that precious substance in our eyes—visual purple—which is destroyed by light and can be renewed only in total darkness and then only if enough vitamin A is present? Every official survey of the way Americans eat has shown that lack of vitamin A is very common. Many of us are probably not getting enough vitamin A to protect our health. If, in addition, we are getting far too few hours of darkness to renew the visual purple in our retinas, might these two things not be a significant reason for many of our eye problems?

Aside from its function in helping to make visual purple, vitamin A performs many other helpful biological tasks. It helps to maintain a healthy skin and takes care of the welfare of the linings of things—the lining of throat, esophagus, stomach, intestines, reproductive organs, mouth and so on. It helps us to resist infections. It is active in developing bones and teeth and keeping them healthy. It also helps maintain the myelin sheaths of the nerves which are disordered in multiple sclerosis and polio. It helps us to see colors. It is essential for the healthy functioning of the adrenal glands and the hormones they make.

That's quite a lot of work for one vitamin. And scientists say they are still in the dark as to just how most of these functions are performed. The one thing they know surely about vitamin A is its importance in maintaining our supply of visual purple in the retina of the eye.

The story of one student is told in *This Week* magazine for September 12, 1965. For several years he had noticed that his eyesight after dark was getting worse. Driving at night, he could barely see road signs, pedestrians or the edge of the road. When he went to the movies he had to wait for fifteen minutes before his eyes had adjusted to the dark so that he could find a seat. He had also noticed a dry skin and itchy eyes, both symptoms of vitamin A deficiency.

What did he eat? We imagine his diet was fairly typical of many college students who have absolutely no idea of the rules of good nutrition. He had coffee and doughnuts for breakfast, hamburgers, dessert and coffee for lunch, lean meat, white potatoes, white bread, dessert and coffee for dinner. When he ate vegetables, they were either beans, corn or peas. His daily vitamin A intake was about 1,000 units. The official daily requirement is 5,000. He was given 25,000 units of vitamin A in fish liver capsules daily and was told to add to his diet: milk, ice cream, butter, cheese, liver, fresh fruit, spinach, raw carrots, squash, sweet potatoes and prunes.

Within ten days his night blindness was greatly improved; within two months it was completely normal. And his other symptoms of vitamin A deficiency disappeared. Many people on reducing diets may run into the same kind of trouble, if they are attempting to reduce on black coffee, lean meat and salads, with little or no fat. Vitamin A is abundant in cream, butter, eggs, margarine and especially liver. In the case of young people or elderly people, peculiar dietary habits may cause them to skip foods that are rich in vitamin A.

Night blindness is not the only visual difficulty caused by lack of vitamin A. An extremely serious eye condition causing blindness results from long-continued deficiency. Susceptibility to infections, dry skin, digestive troubles and many other unpleasant and unhealthful conditions may mean you are not getting enough vitamin A. Why take chances?

Medical World News reported on March 5, 1971 that massive doses of vitamin A have been used in the treatment of a very serious eye disease, *retinitis pigmentosa*. This condition is defined as hereditary, with slowly progressive blindness.

Two patients with clouded vision from this condition were given 200,000 units of vitamin A by a team of doctors at the National Institute of Arthritis and Metabolic Diseases in Washington. Hours after they took the vitamin, their vision began to clear. Within a day they were seeing well. The effect of this one dose of vitamin A lasted for three months! (Vitamin A is stored in the body). One patient, who started treatment seven years ago now has relatively good vision. The other patient has since died of heart failure.

The eye condition which has hitherto been considered incurable, affects children who are unable to absorb the fat-soluble vitamins. As we have mentioned, vitamins A and E are fat-soluble. We wonder whether the heart failure of one patient may have been due to simple inability to absorb vitamin E! Dr. Peter Goursa, who treated the patients, feels that his success may indicate that vitamin A deficiency is at the root of most types of retinal degeneration.

Dr. Arthur Alexander Knapp of New York City treats retinitis pigmentosa with vitamin D and calcium supplements. He has been using this therapy for 30 years, he says in a letter to the editor of *Medical Tribune* for February 23, 1970. Vitamin D is also a fat-soluble vitamin, so it is easy to see how a victim of this disorder might be short on vitamin D as well as E and A.

CHAPTER 14

How Much Vitamin A Is Too Much?

IN ALMOST EVERY article you read these days on the subject of vitamins, you are reminded that vitamin A can be toxic if consumed in large amounts, you are told you must be very careful about taking vitamin supplements containing vitamin A, since you may poison yourself. Usually the impression is given of hundreds of thousands of people sickening or dying from vitamin A poisoning every year.

It is difficult indeed to dig out any information about these cases of vitamin A poisoning. You can search the medical literature for months and not uncover a single mention of anyone actually treated for vitamin A poisoning, although you will find frequent vague mention of this possibility. A standard book on biology, Geoffrey Bourne's *Biochemistry and Physiology of Bone*, tells us that since 1912 more than 20 cases of vitamin A overdosage have been reported in the entire world!

Since that book was published there have undoubtedly been more, so we were glad to get a copy of a new report, *A Conspectus of Research on Vitamin A Requirements of Man* by two researchers of the Agricultural Research Service of the U.S. Department of Agriculture, Mildred S. Rodriguez and M. Isabel Irwin. These two scientists have combed medical and scientific literature and have uncovered *all* the reported cases of people getting too much vitamin A.

They say on page 919 of their paper, "Fifteen cases of chronic adult hypervitaminosis A (too much vitamin A), 12 of which occurred in the United States, have been reported." One of these people took 100,000 units of vitamin A every day for three and a half years before there was any damage to report. In another case a physician experimented with the vitamin to see how much he could take over a long period of time without trouble. He took 1,000,000 units daily for about three weeks as an experiment! In other cases people took too much vitamin A for as long as eight years before experiencing any bad effects.

What about acute poisoning—that is, enormous doses given in a short time which caused distress? The USDA scientists tell us that there is one report of 98 acute cases in very young children who were given doses of 300,000 to 400,000 units daily. In some of these, distress appeared within days, in others it took almost two years.

Five cases reported from Sweden involve infants given 7,500 to 10,000 units daily. Keep in mind that vitamin dosage is estimated by weight—that is, generally speaking, the more you weigh, the more vitamins you need. Infants need very little compared to adults. So the doses being given to these infants and children were really enormous. Even so, only a few more than 100 cases were reported.

We asked the authors of this report if their study had covered all the cases ever reported in medical literature. They told us, "This covers the literature through 1970."

So we must conclude that there have been, in all of medical history in the whole world no more than 120 to 150 cases of anyone getting too much vitamin A. Practically all of these were children or infants. In very young children there is a possibility of permanent damage from getting too much of the vitamin. For older people symptoms disappear as soon as the massive doses are discontinued.

So how great is the threat of getting too much vitamin A? Every year hundreds of thousands of people are poisoned by aspirin or some other drug which can be bought casually over the counter. Countless others sicken or die from overdoses of sleeping drugs or tranquilizers. Hospitals are full of patients suffering from "iatrogenic disease"—that is, some disorder brought on by some medication their doctor is giving them. Every advertisement for drugs which appears in medical journals must carry a long list of possible harmful side effects—every drug.

And the effects listed are very frightening indeed: nausea, vomiting, tremor, lethargy, coma, rapid heartbeat, confusion, skin eruptions, edema, constipation, menstrual irregularities, increased or decreased sex urge, jaundice, blood diseases, liver disorders, cramps, dizziness, headache, rash, hives, muscle spasm, gastric irritation, blurred vision and hundreds of others! Some of these symptoms may appear even when the drug is given in recommended doses.

But over all of history only about 150 people in the world have taken too much vitamin A over long periods of time and have experienced some slight discomfort which has left them as soon as they stopped taking the vitamin. This is the basis on which we are advised in loud, warning tones to beware of vitamin A.

The harm that can come from vitamin A is due to the fact that this vitamin is fat-soluble—that is, it can be stored by the body, unlike water-soluble vitamins B and C, which are rather rapidly excreted. So there is little or no need to take vitamin A every day. Your body probably still has some stored from last week's vitamin pill. But if you do take it every day, the official guideline says that adults and teenagers need 5,000 units daily. Infants need 1,500 units, young children 2,000 to 3,500 units, depending on age.

It is estimated that "the average American" gets about 7,500 units of vitamin A from food: about 3,500 from vegetables and fruits (the bright yellow and bright green ones); about 2,000 units from fats, oils and dairy products (butter and milk), about 2,000 units from meat, fish and eggs. There is, of course, no "average American." There are instead some 200 million people, all individual in their ways of eating and ways of living, many with disorders which influence their need for vitamin A.

If you suffer from any condition which slows down fat absorption like diarrhea or celiac disease, you will not absorb much vitamin A. If you take mineral oil, vitamin A will be absorbed and eliminated by this laxative. Certain antibiotics also cause loss of vitamin A. Unless you have very well functioning metabolic machinery (this means no diabetes, no liver or gall bladder problems) you are likely to be unable to use the vitamin A in fruits and vegetables. It occurs in the form of carotene which must be re-made into vitamin A inside the body.

We have little information on elements in our environment which destroy vitamin A. It seems likely, however, that DDT may be destructive of the vitamin. All of us have some DDT in our fatty tissues. It seems likely that nitrates and nitrites in our food may destroy the vitamin A in our digestive tracts. Much more research should be done in this field. It is almost impossible to avoid these substances, since they are put into most processed meats, and occur, as well, in many vegetables raised with commercial fertilizers.

Exposure to a number of antagonists of vitamin A may prevent its absorption. Some of these are sodium benzoate (a chemical preservative used in many foods which the FDA has pronounced perfectly safe), bromobenzine, citral (a flavoring agent used in hundreds of foods), estrogen (the female hormone used in The Pill) and thyroxine, the thyroid gland hormone, when it is present in large concentrations, as when it is given as a drug.

Vitamin A as such does not exist in vegetables and fruits. They contain carotene which must be made into vitamin A inside our bodies. Diabetics may have trouble making this conversion of carotene to vitamin A. The carotene may also be lost if fibrous foods like raw carrots are not chewed enough before they are swallowed. The cells of these tough vegetables must be completely broken down before the carotene is liberated. This is one reason why cooking may help absorption of carotene in the case of carrots and tough salad greens.

Vitamin A as such does appear in some foods of animal origin: liver, eggs, butter and cream chiefly. Many people have been told by their doctors to shun such foods because of their cholesterol content. This would deprive them of much of the vitamin A they should normally have.

So how can you tell how much vitamin A you and your family need? And how much will be too much? If you eat liver once a week, this should supply a full week's vitamin A requirement—some 50,000 units. If you're healthy and eat lots of bright green and yellow vegetables and fruits like carrots, spinach, dandelion greens, peaches, apricots and so on, you are getting considerable amounts of vitamin A in these foods.

No one has ever reported any kind of damage in an adult who is taking up to 50,000 units of vitamin A daily in a food supplement in addition to what he gets in food. Many people settle on 25,000 units. If you decide to take vitamin A in this range—5,000 to 25,000 units daily, the only problems with overdosages would occur if you deliberately double or triple this dosage every day. There would be no sense at all to such an action.

If you switch brands, it's wise to read carefully all the information on the new label. If you decided on 25,000 units of vitamin A daily, make certain you will get that in one capsule, or two, or whatever the label indicates. Sometimes the label will tell you that you get such-and-such an amount of the various nutrients in one tablet or capsule. Sometimes you have to take two or three daily to get the same amount. This is probably because there are other nutrients in the same pill, and there is a limit to how much content one pill can contain and still be capable of being swallowed.

As long as you are observing these simple precautions, there is no danger at all that you will get too much vitamin A. With infants and children, adjust the dose accordingly.

And, of course, don't neglect the foods that are rich in vitamin A just because you are taking a vitamin A food supplement. You need green leafy vegetables, liver, carrots and fruit for the many other nutrients they contain, as well as the vitamin A.

And the next time somebody threatens you with dire harm because you are taking a vitamin A supplement, tell them to write to the U.S. Department of Agriculture in Washington and ask how many people have ever suffered harm from taking vitamin A, how much they were taking

Foods Highest in Vitamin A	
Foods	Units of Vitamin A
Carrots, raw, ½ cup	11,000
Sweet potatoes, 1	7,700
Beet greens, ½ cup	6,700
Chard, ½ cup	8,720
Chicory, ½ cup	10,000
Dandelion greens, ½ cup	15,170
Endive, 10 stalks	3,000
Kale, cooked, ½ cup	8,300
Spinach, cooked, ½ cup	11,780
Turnip greens, cooked, ½ cup	10,600
Pumpkin, cooked, ½ cup	3,400
Cantaloupe, ½ small	3,420
Apricots, 6 halves	2,790
Apricots, dry, 8 halves	3,700
Peaches, fresh, 1 large	880
Prunes, dry, 12	1,890
Tomato Juice, 4 oz.	1,050
Liver, beef, fried, 1 serving	53,500
Liver, calf	32,200
Liverwurst, ¼ pound	5,750
Eggs, 2	1,140

and for how long. The evidence is astonishing.

In a recent issue of *Medical Tribune*, Dr. Fred Klenner of Reidsville, North Carolina, who treats his patients with massive doses of vitamins, says, "There is very little chance of damage to humans from ingesting vitamin A. I have one patient with ichthyosis (a skin disease) who has taken 200,000 units of vitamin A daily for over 10 years just to keep his skin within normal texture limits. No toxicity. I have taken from 75,000 units of vitamin A up to 150,000 units daily for the past 25 years. No toxicity.

"I recommend to my patients who drive to take at least 50,000 units of vitamin A daily to improve their night vision. Many traffic deaths could be averted by taking not only vitamin A but also vitamin B1 (200 milligrams) and vitamin C (2 grams) every hundred miles of driving."

The vitamin A content of common foods is listed in the chart. How much does your family get of these foods every day?

Vitamin B Is...

A complex of water-soluble vitamins and vitamin-like substances including thiamine, riboflavin, niacin, pyridoxine, pantothenic acid, biotin, folic acid, vitamin B12, choline, inositol, para-amino-benzoic acid.

Responsible chiefly for the health and maintenance of nerves, eyes, digestion and skin, as well as the processing of carbohydrate, fat and protein, appetite, growth, production of hormones and digestive juices, prevention of anemia, maintenance of sex glands, sebaceous glands, bone marrow, and many more complex body functions.

Present in most abundance in liver, kidney, whole-grains, all seeds, nuts, dairy products, eggs, bran, wheat germ, brewers yeast, lentils, beans, peas, soybeans, leafy green vegetables.

Safe in very large amounts. Because the B vitamins are water soluble they are not stored to any extent in the body, so whatever is not needed is rapidly excreted. However, a certain balance is advisable among the B vitamins, since they are closely related. So it is best to get plenty of all of them in food and supplements, rather than taking large amounts of just one or two.

Destroyed in food preparation by light, steam, long cooking, high temperatures, long storage and so forth. Destroyed by many antagonists in the form of drugs and chemicals, also by alkalinity in the stomach caused by taking antacids.

Required in very small amounts. See individual requirements in the chart on page 19.

Available in low or high potencies, in one-a-day supplements or individual supplements.

CHAPTER 15

Introducing the
B Complex
of Vitamins

VITAMIN A IS easy to understand. It comes in bright yellow and green foods. It's most abundant in fish liver oils. Vitamin C exists in fresh, crisp fruits and vegetables. It's important for many things in our bodies and many of us take it in large doses to saturate our tissues with it.

But what about the B vitamins? How does it happen we always speak of them as a "complex" and what does that mean? How many of them are there and are they all equally important or can we do without some of them? How are they discovered and why do scientists keep telling us that important supplements like brewers yeast and liver may contain more B vitamins than they have yet discovered?

Biochemists call them "the B Complex," because you do not find one of them in food or in a living tissue without the others being somewhere near at hand. They go together. They complement one another. They help one another out. If one of them is a little short, for some reason, another may be able to take up part of the work the first would have done, perhaps substituting for it in some complicated physiological function.

Vitamins do not suddenly appear in a laboratory

labelled "vitamin B1" or "vitamin B2." The biochemist does not pick up a cup of brewers yeast, stir it around a little and decide that the big pieces of yeast must be vitamin B1 and the little pieces vitamin B2. Until about 50 years ago no one knew there were such things as vitamins, although scientists and physicians knew, in general, that there were some substances in certain foods which could prevent certain deficiency diseases. If these substances were destroyed by heat or soaking or exposure to light, the disease would not be prevented, no matter how much of the depleted food was eaten. This was about all the early nutrition scientists had to go on, and they made plenty of mistakes.

Until about 1926 scientists thought that vitamin B was a single element. Then several researchers showed that there were at least two kinds—one that could be destroyed by heat and another which was not destroyed by heat. Soon nutrition scientists in many parts of the world began to isolate different parts of these substances and, of course, called them by whatever name they happened to think appropriate. Vitamin B2 was called riboflavin in the USA and lactoflavine in Europe, because it is abundant in milk. For a long time it was also called Vitamin G.

What is now called pyridoxine has been labeled Factor Y, Factor I, Factor H, adermin and Factor B6. Other B vitamins were discovered and identified in the same way without, at first, much appreciation of the fact that they were all related, all part of one complex of vitamins. A B vitamin has been defined as "an organic substance which acts catalytically in all living cells and which is essential for the nutrition of higher animals."

By "catalytically" we mean that the B vitamins are involved all together in many of the very complex cellular functions inside the body. One B vitamin, biotin, is known to take part in at least 15 or 20 processes which involve many different enzymes. So it is not important for scientists to know only that lack of biotin brings about certain symptoms. They want to know, too, exactly what biotin does to the body to prevent these symptoms. Work is going forward in hundreds of laboratories all over the world, for scientists have only begun to untangle and understand these mysteries. It may be many years before all the complexities are understood, or perhaps they never will be.

But we do know, basically, that the B vitamins are a complex, which means that they are closely related to one another, that they work together and they occur, generally speaking in the same groups of foods. Here are their names and some of their varying functions.

Thiamine, also called vitamin B1, prevents beriberi, a disease which was widespread and took many lives in the East when rice was first milled to eliminate the coating and germ of the rice in which thiamine is concentrated. Polished or refined rice was prettier and easier to cook. No one knew of the terrible health consequences which would follow. Thiamine is essential for proper nerve function. Its deficiency brings neuritis, paralysis, atrophy of muscles, edema or swelling, fatigue, loss of weight and appetite, depression, "pins and needles." Symptoms disappear almost magically when thiamine is given.

Deficiency in *Riboflavin*, also called vitamin B2, can bring a variety of symptoms: inflammation of mouth tissues, sores at the corners of the mouth, visual fatigue, a "sandy" feeling in the eyes, inability to endure bright lights. Seborrhea, a scaly skin disorder, is also a symptom of riboflavin deficiency. Many people today have such symptoms without knowing that they could easily prevent them by getting enough riboflavin. It's hard to get enough of this B vitamin from food if you slight the dairy foods— milk, yogurt and cheese, for it is most plentiful there. Liver, kidney and brewers yeast are other abundant sources.

Niacin, also called vitamin B3, is responsible for the health of skin, nerves and digestive tract—a big order for a substance needed only in milligrams. Pellagra is the deficiency disease when niacin is lacking. It produces three conditions: diarrhea, dermatitis and dementia—death if not treated. Today many psychiatrists and physicians are using niacin in massive doses to treat schizophrenia and other serious mental conditions.

Pyridoxine (Vitamin B6) has been found to be essential for many things that contribute to good health. Lack of pyridoxine causes anemia, skin disorders, nerve disorders including convulsions, mouth disorders and seborrhea. This is another B vitamin which has been found to be helpful in large doses in fighting mental illness and many other conditions. It is most plentiful in all seeds and wholegrains, wheat germ, bran, brewers yeast.

Lack of *Biotin* causes lassitude, lack of appetite, depression, muscle pains, scaling dermatitis, sometimes nausea, anemia, changes in heart rhythm. It occurs most plentifully in all those foods in which other B vitamins are abundant: nuts, wholegrain cereals, liver, eggs, brewers yeast.

Choline is regarded as a B vitamin officially. In animals it protects against abnormalities in pregnancy and lactation. Lack of it brings anemia, heart and circulatory disease and muscle weakness. Many recent experiments have shown that it is important for the body to use fats properly.

Pantothenic acid was discovered by Dr. Roger J. Williams, one of the all-time great nutrition scientists. It is involved in many enzyme systems in the body. Lack of it can bring apathy, depression, instability of heart action, digestive disease, abdominal pains, increased susceptibility to infection, impaired function of the adrenal glands which protect us against all kinds of stress, and certain nerve disorders including "pins and needles" and muscle weakness.

Vitamin B12 prevents pernicious anemia, a kind of anemia that always proved fatal until it was treated with lots of liver which is the best source of vitamin B12. In this extremely serious disease nerves are involved and eventually the spinal cord. This vitamin is not present in fruits, vegetables and grains, so it must come from foods of animal origin only which is important for total vegetarians to remember.

Folic acid is closely related to vitamin B12. Lack of it also produces anemia which can be fatal. Some symptoms of deficiency are: intestinal disturbances, inflammation of mouth tissues and gums, gland disturbances, sprue and various blood disorders. It is plentiful in liver, green leafy vegetables, wheat germ and bran, brewers yeast, beans, lentils and other seed foods.

Para-animo-benzoic acid (PABA) is considered to be a vitamin by some scientists, though not recognized as such officially. It is an excellent protector against too much sun and is used in suntan lotions. It exists in the same foods in which all the B vitamins are found.

Inositol, not officially called a vitamin, is essential, along with choline, to make lecithin, that excellent emulsifier which may help to render cholesterol harmless.

Workers in other countries call several other substances B vitamins—Vitamin B15 and B17. These are substances which occur along with the other B vitamins. Ample demonstration that these are essential for life and health will undoubtedly result in their being classified as vitamins by our official classification experts.

The one lesson to be learned from studying the vitamins is the lesson our food technologists have never learned and apparently are incapable of learning. Nature likes things whole. Nothing worthwhile is achieved in nature with fragments. Removing all the B vitamins from our wholegrain cereals and flour then returning only bits of three of them is probably the worst possible thing we could do, for the imbalances thus created are complex. All the B vitamins work together.

One food may contain a bit more of this or that B vitamin, but, in general, they all exist most abundantly in these kinds of foods: liver and all organ meats, eggs, milk, cheese and yogurt, meat, fish, poultry, green leafy vegetables, wholegrains, seeds, nuts, legumes, wheat germ and bran and brewers yeast. A diet consisting of just these foods is a complete diet, if you add fruits and other vegetables for their vitamin A and C content. These foods are also the richest sources of protein which is what we are made of and which we must have in quantity for good health.

As soon as you begin to dilute such a diet with foods made from white refined flour, refined cereals and white sugar, you lose quantities of B vitamins as well as the precious minerals that accompany them. In nature the B vitamins are responsible for processing carbohydrates. By removing them from carbohydrate-rich foods like cereals and sugar, we invite nutritional disaster. One-half of all food eaten in our country consists of these depleted substances.

The B vitamin complex must be kept and eaten whole as it occurs in the excellent foods listed above. Make them the backbone of your diet. And when you buy a food supplement, make certain it contains all the B vitamins as well as yeast, liver, wheat germ or some other rich source, so that you will also be getting those B vitamins and related substances which have not as yet been discovered.

Here is a story which indicates how the B vitamins can be used by innovative and creative doctors to ease some of the problems of old folks. There are at present in our country about 20 million people over the age of 65. All of us will eventually attain this age, if we're lucky and cherish our health. Why not try to guarantee that life after 65 will be pleasant, rewarding and free from the mental and physical problems that torment so many of today's older folks?

Dr. Abram Hoffer, distinguished Canadian psychiatrist who successfully treats patients with massive doses of several vitamins, in addition to trace minerals and other therapy, tells how he brought his aging mother back to excellent mental and physical health by the simple expedient of suggesting that she take large doses of the B vitamin niacin, because she was suffering from arthritis, incipient blindness and failing memory.

He knew, he said—every doctor knows—that nothing can be done for such complaints of the aged. Senility and disability come and the only thing to do is to ignore it and keep the patient as happy as possible. The niacin could not hurt his mother, he knew, and she would feel her physician son had tried to help.

Six weeks later she wrote him a lively letter saying, "My vision is okay, my arthritis is gone and I feel marvelous!" Today, said Dr. Hoffer, "she is 86. Her mind is just as keen as it ever was and she spends her time writing her memoirs." She had been taking 3 grams a day of niacin—3,000 milligrams.

An article in the *Journal of the American Geriatrics Society* some time ago reported on a British experiment in which 254 elderly patients were tested for their blood levels of the B vitamins and vitamin C. These folks suffered from Parkinson's disease, congestive heart failure, asthma, anemia, hardening of the arteries, bone fractures from falls, bronchitis, high blood pressure, kidney disorders, eye troubles, alcoholism and many other degenerative conditions which are commonplace among older people. Some of the patients were found to have pellagra and scurvy, disorders resulting from lack of B vitamins and vitamin C. All of them were confused.

They were given a concentrate liquid solution of the B vitamins and vitamin C. It contained 20 milligrams of vitamin B1 (thiamine), 2 milligrams of vitamin B2 (riboflavin), 80 milligrams of vitamin B3 (niacin), 2 milligrams of vitamin B6 (pyridoxine), and 40 milligrams of vitamin C. This liquid formula was given three times a day. In some cases twice this much was given three times a day, presumably with meals.

In almost every case the mental confusion disappeared completely and the patients were discharged as normal. One 66-year-old woman with hardening of the arteries and Parkinson's disease was discharged after only two weeks, her mental confusion cleared and the other conditions much improved. In an 88-year-old woman all mental alertness was restored in one month.

An 89-year-old woman suffering from anemia, dehydration and confusion went home mentally well. After two weeks an 81-year-old woman with bronchitis and mental confusion was able to go home in good shape much improved. A 75-year-old woman in "an acute confusional state" and congestive heart failure went home two weeks later. A 68-year-old alcoholic went home, mentally well, after two weeks of treatment.

Two aged women with pellagra were able to go home in two weeks. A 95-year-old woman in great pain if she was touched, and with bruise marks over her entire body, was given one gram of vitamin C (1,000 milligrams) every day for two weeks and went home in good health. A 70-year-old woman had been in a mental hospital for attempted suicide. She had bacterial endocarditis which was treated with antibiotics. She was confused and lethargic and had many bruises as well as painful legs. She was given one gram of vitamin C daily and in three weeks felt so well she wanted to go home.

During the time this triumph of preventive medicine was going on Dr. M. L. Mitra, who conducted the test asked six of the nursing personnel if they would act as "controls." To his great surprise he found that five of them were deficient in vitamins according to blood tests. They had no suspicion there was anything wrong with their health.

Many of the elderly patients had been put on drugs by their physicians. No allowance was made for the vitamin deficiencies that might result. Diuretics are those drugs given frequently for high blood pressure and other circulatory troubles. These drugs cause excessive urination. They naturally wash out of the body any of the water soluble vitamins which are in the digestive tract at the same time. They destroy minerals in the same way.

The doctors giving the drugs had made no allowance for such terrible losses, so understandably such patients were deficient in the B vitamins and vitamin C which are the water soluble ones. It seems likely that the only thing causing the supposedly irreversible confusion in the patients was vitamin deficiency. Until Dr. Mitra's experiment, no one recognized it. No one did anything about it.

We are not even sure that any of these patients, miraculously rescued from so many of the troubles of old age, were given any of the powerful vitamin preparation to take at home, or if they were given any instructions on how to shop for and prepare a reasonably nutritious diet for themselves, so that they would not succumb to mental confusion and other disabling conditions in the future.

Part of the reason for this, we suspect, is that no one appreciates the difficulties older people have in providing themselves with nourishing food. It's expensive, especially protein food, which is essential, far more expensive than cheaper refined carbohydrates. Older folks have great difficulty shopping for food. If they live some distance from a market they must take a bus or a cab or walk a long distance, carrying a heavy shopping bag on their return trip.

For those who live alone there is little incentive to prepare full course meals. It hardly seems worth the trouble. So they subsist on sandwiches or cereal, cakes or canned food which is easy to buy and easy to prepare. In a modern supermarket it is extremely difficult to buy small enough quantities for only one person. Meat is packaged for a family. Cheese comes in pound packages. Potatoes are bagged in five pound bags, and so on. In the average small apartment there is little room for storage, so frequent trips must be made to make small purchases every few days. In many stores where old folks buy prices are higher since management knows these people cannot go to the other end of town to seek out less expensive food.

If you are caring for the older person in your family or if you have reached the "golden years" yourself, you can work wonders with a nourishing diet, rich in high protein foods, with all the refined carbohydrates eliminated and the kind of vitamin supplements outlined in the story above. As Dr. Hoffer admitted, he did not think any treatment could bolster his aging mother's health and clear up the confusion in her mind. He gave her only one B vitamin and worked a near miracle. Undoubtedly by now he is giving her—and other elderly patients—massive doses of all the water soluble vitamins. That is, all the B vitamins and vitamin C. These are the vitamins in which older folks are most likely to be deficient.

But the fat soluble ones are important, too—especially vitamin A and E. Vitamin A protects all the linings of things—the respiratory tract, the digestive tract, the reproductive tract and the skin. Recent research has showed it to be a powerful preventive of some kinds of cancer. Vitamin E has been shown by thousands of innovative physicians to be valuable for preventing the circulatory problems which beset us as we age. The mineral calcium is essential as we grow older to protect the health of bones. Dairy products are the best sources: milk, cheese, yogurt, buttermilk. Calcium supplements are available at the health food store, as are all the vitamin supplements mentioned above.

It is cruel and irresponsible to allow our old folks to degenerate into senility and a hundred related kinds of disability when we have the power to prevent many of them with nothing more than a good diet and an abundance of vitamins and minerals. Old age, with all the troubles it brings, is a form of stress. People under stress need more nutrients than those who are not under stress.

We do not know the name of the liquid supplement which Dr. Mitra gave his patients. And it is probably not available in this country. There is no reason why anyone must take just that special preparation. A vitamin is a vitamin, no matter in what form it appears. He probably gave the preparation in liquid form because this would be easier for the old folks to swallow.

You can, of course, find the same potency of vitamins in many preparations, either in tablet form or liquid. Any of these containing the same ingredients in approximately the same amounts would presumably work the same kind of near-magic.

CHAPTER 16

Thiamine Prevents Many Painful and Debilitating Disorders

THIAMINE, called vitamin B1, is the substance that prevents beriberi. This extremely serious disease has just about disappeared in most parts of the world where cereals have been "enriched"—that is, thiamine has been added to the refined cereals and white flour and white rice which make up such a large part of our diet. In countries where this procedure has not been followed, beriberi still presents a troublesome problem. Thiamine is especially necessary for the health of the nerves and the digestion. Lack of it results in painful neuritis.

Since thiamine is essential for the body to use carbohydrates properly, the more starches and sugars you eat the more thiamine you need. Enrichment of cereal foods provides some thiamine to take care of our requirement when we are eating them. But the tremendous amounts of white sugar eaten in this country, especially by children, make obvious the great continuing and unsatisfied need for thiamine. Most of the sugar-rich foods like candy and soft drinks contain no vitamins of any kind. Yet eating them steadily increases one's need for vitamins, especially thiamine.

The *British Medical Journal* for April 10, 1971 reports on two cases of beriberi which occurred in Blackpool, England. According to *Heinz Handbook of Nutrition*, there may be conditions even in the United States where so little thiamine is included in the diet that beriberi may

Thiamine (Vitamin B1) Content of Some Common Foods

Food	Milligrams
Almonds, 1 cup	0.34
Asparagus, 1 cup	0.23
Avocados, 1 cup	0.16
Beans, Lima, 1 cup	0.22
Beef heart, 3 oz.	0.23
Beef and vegetable stew, 1 cup	0.12
Brazil nuts, 1 cup	1.21
Bread:	
Cracked wheat, 1 lb.	0.53
Cracked wheat, 1 slice	0.03
French, enriched, 1 lb.	1.26
Italian, enriched, 1 lb.	1.31
Rye, 1 lb.	0.81
Rye, 1 slice	0.04
Pumpernickel, 1 lb.	0.04
White, enriched, 1 lb.	1.05
White, enriched, 1 slice	0.06
Whole wheat, 1 lb.	1.17
Whole wheat, 1 slice	0.06
Cashew nuts, 1 cup	0.49
Collards, 1 cup	0.15
Cowpeas (or Black-eyed peas), 1 cup	0.41
Dandelion greens, 1 cup	0.23
Dates, 1 cup	0.16
Flour, whole wheat, 1 cup	0.66
Grapefruit juice, frozen, 1 can	0.29
Grapefruit juice, dehydrated, 1 can	0.41

result. Chronic alcoholics substitute drinks for foods that contain thiamine. And other conditions increase one's demands for this essential B vitamin: pregnancy, breast-feeding, fevers, hyperthyroidism or diseases which interfere with proper absorption or utilization of food (like diarrhea,

Grape juice, 1 cup	0.11
Ham, smoked, 3 oz.	0.46
Ham, boiled, 2 oz.	0.57
Liver, beef, 2 oz.	0.15
Milk, dry, whole, 1 cup	0.30
Milk, dry, nonfat, 1 cup	0.28
Oatmeal, 1 cup	0.22
Orange, 1	0.11
Orange juice, frozen, 1 can	0.63
Orange and grapefruit juice, frozen, 1 can	0.47
Oysters, raw, 1 cup	0.30
Peanuts, roasted, 1 cup	0.47
Peas, green, 1 cup	0.40
Pecans, 1 cup	0.93
Pineapple, raw, 1 cup	0.12
Pineapple, canned, crushed, 1 cup	0.20
Pineapple juice, 1 cup	0.13
Pork chops, 2 to 4 oz.	0.60
Pork roast, 1 slice	0.71
Raisins, 1 cup	0.13
Sausage, Bologna, 8 oz.	0.36
Soup, bean, 1 cup	0.10
Soybeans, 1 serving	1.07
Soybean flour, 100 grams	0.82
Spinach, 1 cup	0.14
Tangerine juice, 1 cup	0.14
Tangerine juice, frozen, 6 oz. can	0.43
Walnuts, black or native, 1 cup	0.28
Walnuts, English, 1 cup	0.33
Watermelon, 1 wedge	0.20
Wheat germ, 1 cup	1.39
Yeast, brewer's, 100 grams	9.69

colitis, etc.) or disorders of the liver.

What are the typical symptoms of a deficiency in thiamine? The earliest are vague: lack of initiative, lack of appetite, depression, irritability, poor memory, tendency to tire easily and to be unable to concentrate. Then there are vague abdominal and heart complaints. (Don't these symptoms sound like those of many older folks you know—perhaps those who live alone and prepare their own meals?)

As the deficiency grows worse, nerves are affected, chiefly in the legs. The victim suffers from neuritis and from a feeling of "pins and needles" in toes, along with a burning sensation. Arms and fingers are generally affected next. The heart suffers injury resulting in shortness of breath and irregularities of heartbeat. There may also be accumulations of fluid, causing puffy swelling in ankles. The only remedy is large amounts of thiamine—injected, if there is evidence that it will not be thoroughly absorbed.

The two British beriberi patients were admitted to a psychiatric ward. The first was an 80-year-old widow who had lived alone since the death of her husband. She was depressed, slept poorly, ate little, was hopeless about the future and thought frequently of suicide. She was underweight, had a rash on her face and on parts of hands and arms exposed to sunlight—this is another symptom of beriberi. Her chest x-ray showed an enlarged heart.

The second patient was only 48. He had suffered from stomach ulcers and had part of his stomach removed. Because of his wife's death seven years before, he also was depressed and apprehensive. He ate little. He could not sleep without barbiturates. His legs were wasted. His ankles showed swelling with fluid.

Both patients were given thiamine by injection and within three weeks depression and swelling had cleared and they had gained weight. They were well physically and mentally and were discharged from the hospital. One can only hope that they were told how easily and inexpensively the symptoms could be prevented—a diet which includes plenty of the foods in which thiamine is abundant plus food supplements containing plenty of all the B vitamins.

The British physician who treated these patients says that the disease may be commoner in England than is generally supposed. He says that vitamin deficiencies in England are usually brought on by other factors— disorders of the digestive tract and the mind, alcoholism, "food faddism" and, among the elderly, social isolation, which leads to loss of appetite and loss of desire to prepare nourishing foods.

He goes on to say "Thiamine deficiency is frequently mis-diagnosed and it is noteworthy that the first patient was initially treated for congestive heart failure. Beriberi would probably be frequently recognized if the possibility were considered in 'at risk' patients, particularly those in psychiatric and geriatric wards. . . ."

In a later issue of *British Medical Journal* (May 1, 1971) a London physician reports still another case. This was a 64-year-old man with a three-week history of shortness of breath and cough. He appeared to have all the symptoms of heart failure. His lungs showed infection. He was given large doses of antibiotics. His ankles were badly swollen and the swelling did not go down. He was given several diuretics, those drugs which cause urination and disappearance of accumulations of water in tissues. There were no results.

Someone thought of beriberi. He was given thiamine by injection. The swelling disappeared. The man lost considerable weight which had been largely unwanted water. He was cured. The physicians then asked about his diet! It seems he was a heavy drinker, ate a very poor diet and had a mild deficiency in iron. All this would indicate that he was not eating nearly enough of foods rich in thiamine, as shown on pages 116-117.

Time and again we are told by health officials that "the average American" gets enough of all the food elements in "the average diet". But as the above stories illustrate there must be many of us who are not eating such a good diet or who have needs for one vitamin or another which are far greater than "the average".

CHAPTER 17

Riboflavin (Vitamin B2)
Is Scarce in Food

OF ALL THE B vitamins, the ones we hear most about these days are thiamine and niacin, mostly because they are often given in quite large doses to treat various manifestations of mental illness and to prevent senility. Another equally important B vitamin, riboflavin, is not so much in the news. But riboflavin is essential for good health. It is not nearly so abundant in food as other B vitamins. And recent evidence we have turned up seems to show that lack of this B vitamin may play an extremely important role in illnesses such as alcoholism.

Riboflavin, called vitamin B2, is very abundant in foods which are labelled "faddist". Lack of riboflavin may produce symptoms in various parts of you: fissures and inflammation at the corners of the mouth, eye disorders resulting in eye fatigue and a "sandy feeling" and great abhorrence of strong light. Certain skin and mouth conditions may also be related to deficiency in riboflavin. One important piece of cancer research has indicated that riboflavin in large quantities in brewers yeast and liver protected laboratory animals from liver cancer.

Riboflavin was formerly called vitamin G and some older nutrition books still speak of it that way. It was not until 1937 that the AMA decided this vitamin should be called riboflavin or vitamin B2. It had already been identified in milk, eggs, liver and whey. The textbooks on vitamins tell us that riboflavin is widely available in natural foods. Then there seem to be so many qualifications having to do with cooking, processing and storing foods, that one might wonder just how much of this vitamin actually remains in the meals we eat daily.

For instance, light is very destructive of riboflavin. Until quite recently, most milk was sold in cities in clear glass milk bottles. If the milkman delivered them just before dawn they were likely to sit on the doorstep, in full light or sunlight, until the cook got up and began to prepare breakfast. It seems likely that there was little riboflavin left in the milk by then.

Some of the riboflavin is lost in milk when it is irradiated to produce vitamin D. Much of today's milk has been treated. Cooking in glass utensils is also destructive of riboflavin, although heat generally is not involved in the destruction. But cooking milk or eggs, fresh green vegetables or liver in a glass utensil or without a lid will result in some loss of the vitamin.

Milk from cows fed on green grass contains more riboflavin than when they are fed on hay, so spring and summer milk will contain more of the vitamin. Boiling foods results in considerable loss of riboflavin and loss from roasting meat may be as high as 26 percent. Cafeteria food is most likely to be short on this vitamin, since the food is generally cooked thoroughly, then allowed to stand on steam tables, exposed to light. Such a procedure destroys other vitamins as well.

What is likely to happen if you are not getting enough riboflavin? In general, the symptoms parallel some of the deficiencies produced by lack of other B vitamins, for, as we point out, the B vitamin group is clearly related and appears, in general, in the same foods.

Lack of riboflavin produces distinctive symptoms in the mouth and skin of both animals and human beings. There may be a sore mouth, with cracks and fissures at the corners of the mouth. The lips may be sore and crusted. The tongue may burn and develop a bright magenta color. There may be patchy areas inside the mouth, the tongue may be fissured and inflamed. Seborrhea is a common symptom of lack of riboflavin. This involves a scaly dermatitis around the nose, the ears, the eyelids and perhaps the chest or back. There may be inflammation of the vagina or dermatitis on the hands, the scrotum, the anus or the vulva.

Eyes are especially susceptible to damage from deprivation of riboflavin. They become extremely sensitive to light. (Is deficiency perhaps the reason why so many folks must wear dark glasses these days?) They also may be inflamed with conjunctivitis, they may feel scratchy or sandy; they may burn, they may tire easily, and, if the deficiency is prolonged, more serious troubles may result in permanent damage to the iris and the cornea.

B vitamins are closely associated with the health of the nerves. Lack of riboflavin may produce very definite nervous symptoms: "Pins and needles" in legs or feet, tremor, difficulties in walking, muscular weakness, vertigo and a condition called "burning feet", which was common among war prisioners suffering from gross deficiencies in the B vitamins.

Other conditions that appear to be related to too little riboflavin in the diet are: anemia, acne rosacea, cataracts, inability to urinate (in animals), difficulties with producing insulin, the hormone which processes carbohydrates, oily skin, ulcers and many more conditions. Riboflavin is essential for the stomach to secrete enough of the digestive juices so that other nutrients can be absorbed.

Most interesting are experiments performed many years ago which clearly demonstrated a relation between prevention of cancer and the amount of riboflavin in the diet. In 1951 experiments were performed with rats at the Sloan-Kettering Institute. They were given a diet of rice plus a chemical known to cause cancer. Then one group of rats got, in addition, a considerable amount of liver. At the end of the experiment these rats had developed no cancers, while the unprotected rats had cancerous livers within 150 days. Cutting down on the liver supplement gave less protection and it had to be continued or the cancer would develop later on. It was later discovered that the chief element in liver which gave this protection was the riboflavin. Brewers yeast produced somewhat the same results.

Such experiments are seldom reported today. Past experiments lie mostly forgotten in the dusty pages of medical journals on library shelves. Today if you write to the well-endowed Cancer Societies and the National Cancer Institute, which is funded from taxpayers' money, you are treated with condescension and told that everyone in this country is well nourished, so lack of any vitamin could not possibly be related to our soaring incidence of cancer, which at present affects at least one-fourth of all Americans at some time during their lives.

At the same time, official nutritional surveys are revealing that perhaps half of all American families are not eating diets which completely nourish them! An additional factor is the individual need for vitamins and minerals, which may vary greatly. Some people may have far greater need for certain food elements than others, so these folks would be least able to get enough of all vitamins from a slightly deficient diet.

There is no evidence that all disturbing eye conditions or all troubles with sore mouth and nerve afflictions are due to nutritional deficiencies of the B vitamins or any other one group of vitamins. Of course, we might add, nobody much has really set out to look for such a relationship, so perhaps it does exist and has not yet been discovered.

The medical profession generally is woefully ignorant of nutritional matters and takes the attitude that if their patients are "eating a good diet" that is all they need to know about this aspect of health. Since most people believe they *are* eating "a good diet", even if it's mostly beer and pretzels, the doctors don't have any very satisfactory material on which to base nutritional treatment of disease, even if they are interested.

Lack of B vitamins is most likely to occur in older people, especially those living alone, who have little interest in preparing nourishing meals, little information on nutrition and almost no resources for shopping for the kind of foods that contain most vitamin B. School children who continually neglect the "protective foods" like milk, cheese, meat, eggs, vegetables are likely candidates, too.

Disorders which prevent the absorption of vitamins may cause deficiencies. Diarrheal conditions are especially destructive of B vitamins. There is evidence that some B vitamins are synthesized in the human intestinal tract. When antibiotics are given by mouth, the valuable bacteria which perform this job are destroyed. The best way to replenish them is to eat lots and lots of yogurt which contains these same bacteria.

We usually think of anemia as having to do with lack of iron in food. And there is a more serious anemia caused by certain very toxic drugs. Pernicious anemia can be prevented and cured by taking vitamin B12 along with certain substances that help the stomach to absorb it. Now we are told that a deficiency in riboflavin can also cause anemia. According to two Baylor University researchers, eight volunteers were put on a diet from which all riboflavin was carefully excluded. Then they were given vitamin supplements to make sure they had enough of all other vitamins and minerals. They rapidly developed anemia resulting in disorders of the blood cells and of the bone marrow where certain blood cells are manufactured. When riboflavin was given again, the anemia was cured.

In the *American Journal of Clinical Nutrition* for August, 1973 four physicians from the New York Medical College Metropolitan Hospital Center describe the lack of riboflavin which they found in chronic alcoholics who were also suffering from other disorders.

It is well known that chronic alcoholics usually suffer from many complications as their illness progresses. In this case, 22 alcoholics (some of whom were also heroin addicts) were studied. They ranged in age from 22 to 69 years. And they were suffering from the following conditions: disorders of the muscular tissue of the heart, seizures, acute and chronic inflammation of the pancreas, acute and chronic hepatitis, alcoholic weakening of many muscles, alcoholic liver disease, infections, bleeding in stomach and intestines, and delirum tremens. Such are the horrors of a life of alcoholism.

Riboflavin (Vitamin B2) Content of Some Common Foods

Food	Milligrams
Almonds, 1 cup	1.31
Apricots, 1 cup	0.24
Asparagus, 1 cup	0.30
Avocados, 1 cup	0.30
Beef, hamburger pattie, 3 oz.	0.18
Beef, heart, 3 oz.	1.05
Beef, steak, 3 oz.	0.16
Beef, corned, 3 oz.	0.20
Bread:	
Cracked wheat, 1 slice	0.02
French, enriched, 1 lb.	0.98
Italian, enriched, 1 lb.	0.93
Rye, 1 slice	0.02
Pumpernickel, 1 lb.	0.63
White, enriched, 1 slice	0.04
Whole wheat, 1 slice	0.05
Broccoli, 1 cup	0.22
Buttermilk, 1 cup	0.44
Cashew nuts, 1 cup	0.46
Chicken, broiled, 3 oz.	0.15
Collards, 1 cup	0.46
Dandelion greens, 1 cup	0.22
Dates, 1 cup	0.17

The doctors examined them for symptoms of riboflavin deficiency. They could find none. But they tested their blood and found that eleven of the patients were sadly deficient in riboflavin. In general, these eleven had far more serious diseases than those whose riboflavin levels appeared to be more normal. Giving the B vitamin brought blood levels up to normal within a week.

So, say the doctors, it is possible to be seriously deficient

Egg, raw, 1	0.15
Egg, scrambled (w/milk and fat)	0.18
Flour, whole wheat, 1 cup	0.14
Kale, 1 cup	0.25
Lamb chop, 4.8 oz.	0.24
Liver, beef, 2 oz.	2.25
Mackerel, 3 oz.	0.23
Milk, whole, 1 cup	0.42
Milk, dry, nonfat, 1 cup	1.44
Mushrooms, 1 cup	0.60
Mustard greens, 1 cup	0.25
Oysters, 1 cup	0.39
Peaches, 1 cup	0.32
Peas, green, 1 cup	0.22
Prunes, cooked, 1 cup	0.18
Pumpkin, 1 cup	0.14
Sausage, Bologna, 8 oz.	0.49
Shad, baked, 3 oz.	0.22
Soybeans, 1 serving	0.31
Soybean flour, 100 grams	0.34
Spinach, 1 cup	0.36
Squash, winter, baked, 1 cup	0.31
Strawberries, raw, 1 cup	0.10
Turnip greens, 1 cup	0.59
Watermelon, 1 wedge	0.22
Wheat germ, 1 cup	0.54
Yeast, brewer's, 100 grams	5.45
Yogurt, 1 cup	0.43

in this B vitamin without showing any of the traditional symptoms of deficiency. Some of these are as follows. The mouth is one of the first parts of the body to indicate too little riboflavin. Cracks and fissures may show up at the corners. Lips may be sore. The tongue may have a burning sensation and may turn bright magenta. Or it may show fissures and inflammation.

Seborrhea is a symptom of riboflavin deficiency. This is an unpleasant skin condition involving scaly, greasy dandruff and scaly patches around the nose, ears, chest or back. The individual who lacks riboflavin cannot stand bright light. His eyes may feel scratchy or "sandy". They may burn. And if deficiency is prolonged, serious and irreparable damage may be done to the iris and cornea.

Like other B vitamins, riboflavin protects the nerves. Deficiency may produce "pins and needles" sensations, tremor, muscular weakness, vertigo. A condition called "burning feet" developed in war prisoners suffering from gross deficiency in this B vitamin. Riboflavin is essential for the stomach to produce enough digestive juices to assure good digestion.

Today cancer is second only to heart attacks in producing deaths among Americans. We know of no recent research on the possibility that B vitamins—especially riboflavin—might be helpful in preventing the ravages of this terrible scourge. Yet it is obvious that many of us are getting far too little riboflavin for good health. This is especially true among teenage girls who are following outlandish diets in an effort to reduce. It is true of older folks who have little interest in eating and few facilities or little money for buying and preparing nourishing food. Too often these and other groups of people tend to live on boxed cereals, cakes, toast and tea.

Most disturbing of all is the fact that some physicians believe sugar addiction may be almost as destructive to the liver as alcoholism. Children who eat candy and soft drinks all day may be especially susceptible to some disorders which we mentioned as typical of chronic alcoholics. These children, too, may be suffering from riboflavin deficiency without any of the usual symptoms developing.

In any case, lots of us get far too little riboflavin to be on the safe side. Just the need to wear sunglasses in bright sunlight may be a warning of lack of riboflavin.

How do you get enough riboflavin? Eat plenty of those foods which are rich in all the B vitamins: liver, meat, eggs, milk, cheese, yogurt, leafy green vegetables like broccoli and spinach, plus seeds and wholegrain breads and cereals. If you can't eat liver, use desiccated liver. Brewers yeast contains far more riboflavin than any other food. Use it every day. Make it a part of everything you bake. Add it to casseroles, blender drinks, meatloaves, salads.

One final note of hope for drinkers. A team of researchers in Philadelphia recently found that some of the harmful effects of smoking and drinking could be lessened in severity by taking vitamin C, thiamine (vitamin B1) and cysteine, an amino acid or form of protein found in most high protein foods. These scientists believe these two substances may help to prevent the heart and other symptoms which develop after years of drinking.

Said Dr. Herbert Sprince of Jefferson Medical College, "I don't want to go on record.... saying that once you've taken some vitamin C and B1, to drink and smoke all you want and it isn't going to hurt you.... I can't do that for one second.

"I can say," he went on, "that this combination offered rats 100 percent protection against lethal doses of acetaldehyde, the first step in the body's metabolism of alcohol and a substance that has been implicated in heart disease."

High protein foods rich in amino acids are meat, eggs, fish, poultry, dairy products, wholegrains, seeds and nuts. So eating a diet in which these foods are abundant will help to ease the dire effects of smoking and drinking. Vitamin C and thiamine are inexpensive and harmless in any amounts. All of us should be getting lots of them. This is obviously even more important for smokers and drinkers.

CHAPTER 18

The New and Exciting Potential of Niacin

NIACIN IS OTHERWISE known as nicotinic acid, nicotina-mide, niacinamide or vitamin B3. Nicotinamide and niacinamide are names for the amide form of this vitamin. There are a few differences between the amide form and the non-amide form which will be explained later.

Niacin is the important factor in preventing pellagra, a disease which was once almost as prevalent as the common cold in certain parts of our country. Pellagra, the disease of niacin deficiency, brings symptoms of the three D's: dementia, diarrhea and dermatitis. And, if not treated, death.

The tongue is red, painful, the mouth burns, digestion is completely upset and severe cases bring on such mental disturbances that hospitalization is required. All these symptoms disappear almost immediately when niacin is given. Diets lacking in niacin can be tolerated if they contain enough of a certain protein, tryptophan. But when this is lacking, too, then pellagra is certain to follow.

Important enough to rate first-page treatment in many newspapers was the announcement of a researcher at the New Jersey Neuropsychiatric Institute that a form of vitamin B3 was effective in treating 1,000 patients with schizophrenia. Furthermore, Dr. Humphrey Osmond said on April 4, 1966 that 75 percent of the patients were cured. "Cured" is quite a significant word to use in regard to schizophrenia, the terrible mental illness that afflicts most of the patients in our mental hospitals. But the word Dr. Osmond used was "cured". He specifically mentioned one patient who had been ill for 29 years and was free of symptoms after only five days of treatment.

Dr. Abram Hoffer of Saskatchewan, Canada, who is working with the New Jersey psychiatrist, has been reporting in medical journals for at least 20 years on his almost miraculous results with many schizophrenic patients. Some of these needed treatment over a period of many years. Dr. Hoffer had been using a different form of the vitamin. Now, apparently, the new compound gets results in less time.

It is not known how niacin brings about these astonishing results. The theory of Drs. Osmond and Hoffer is that schizophrenia is caused by a by-product of the adrenal gland, adreno-chrome, which builds up in the body and produces the hallucinations, the mania, the depression and other frightening disturbances involved in this disorder. Supposedly, different forms of the B vitamin, niacin, have the power of preventing this buildup.

Says Dr. Hoffer, in an article published in *The Lancet*, February 10, 1962, "Niacin has some though not all the qualities of an ideal treatment; it is safe, cheap and easy to administer and it uses a known pharmaceutical substance which can be taken for years on end if necessary.... Why then have these benefits passed almost unheeded? (One reason may be the extraordinary proliferation of the phenothiazine derivatives since 1954. These are tranquilizers). Unlike these, niacin is a simple, well-known vitamin which can be bought cheaply in bulk and cannot be patented, and there has been no campaign to persuade doctors of its usefulness."

So all these years desperate patients suffering from this

almost incurable disease might have benefitted from the use of this vitamin in the large doses in which it must be given to be effective. We hope that psychiatrists will begin to use it and that drug companies will begin to promote its use, as they promote the use of tranquilizers.

Niacin, like other B vitamins, is removed from our grains and cereals when they are refined. Some of it is then replaced in synthetic form. People who eat unenriched breads and cereals are likely to be short on this vitamin, as well as those people who do not make any effort to eat well-balanced diets. Now it seems possible, from the work reported above, that people who become schizophrenic may have enormously high biological needs for this vitamin. Where can they get it, eating modern refined diets and listening to the constant steady propaganda of the FDA that no American ever needs extra vitamin supplements?

Niacin is most plentiful in all seed foods: Whole grains, wheat germ, soy bean products, beans, peas, peanuts and other nuts and seeds like sunflower and sesame seeds. Meat, fish and poultry are good sources of niacin. Liver contains more niacin than any other food we might use in menu-planning. Brewers yeast is the richest source of all. (See the list of foods containing the most niacin on pages 134, 135).

Brewers yeast was used by Dr. Tom Spies to cure cases of pellagra in the South. He found it much more effective than giving the isolated vitamin. And he used to give his pellagra patients as much as one-half cup of brewers yeast a day—with nothing but excellent results.

Drs. Hoffer and Osmond have written a book on schizophrenia and their treatment of it. In it they carefully explain every step in the complicated process that goes wrong in the sick person's body. Then they explain how massive doses of the B vitamin correct this process. They point out that the vitamin is almost completely harmless even in these immense doses, although one form of it sometimes produces an unpleasant flushing sensation.

They point out that other methods of treating schizophrenia are potentially quite harmful and others are almost completely ineffective.

The authors describe many other useful aspects of the treatment of schizophrenics. Smoking realeases adrenalin in the body—something these doctors are trying to control, so smoking is very bad for the mentally ill person. So are reducing pills. Diet should be high in protein and calories. Infections should be treated promptly. Lack of sleep and exhaustion are two extremely important causes of symptoms in schizophrenics.

It seems to us that these two pioneering physicians have started an encouraging new chapter in the treatment of mental illness—the biochemical treatment. As further research reveals more and more about the physical causes of this disorder, we can look forward to a day when mental hospitals will be a thing of the past, when mental illness will be treated as we now treat diabetes and heart trouble. Most of all, we welcome the recognition that such serious disorders as schizophrenia can result from physiological imbalances which can be controlled by diet and vitamins. This is indeed a great step forward in medical thinking.

Dr. Hoffer, formerly director of Psychiatric Research in the Department of Public Health in Saskatchewan, is now in private practice. Dr. Osmond is at Bryce Hospital, Department of Mental Health, Tuscaloosa, Alabama. Their book is *How to Live with Schizophrenia*. It is published by University Books, 120 Enterprise Avenue, Secaucus, New Jersey 07094. The price is $8.95.

On the shiny pages of the prestigious journal *Psychology Today*, April, 1974 is the story of a schizophrenic eleven-year old boy and the treatment he was given which controlled his disease within several months, although his psychiatrist believes he should continue the treatment for several years. The psychiatrist is Harvey M. Ross, M.D. The treatment he gives is the orthomolecular treatment, (megavitamin therapy) along with a diet to combat low blood sugar.

The child's symptoms were very serious. He talked to phantoms he believed were in the room with him. He set fires. He attacked his sisters. He stole. Sometimes he stole candy bars. And sometimes he ate as many as 60 candy bars in one day. Says Dr. Ross, "Mitch's story, with some variations, is all too common." His parents had taken him to several psychiatrists who had not helped. One of these doctors told Mitch's parents he would not recommend megavitamin therapy for it is too dangerous. He did not explain how it might be dangerous—more dangerous than therapy in a mental hospital, for example?

"I totally disagree with this position," says Dr. Ross. "I practice orthomolecular psychiatry. This relatively young school of psychiatry believes that thoughts, emotions and

Niacin (Vitamin B3) Content of Some Common Foods

Food	Milligrams
Almonds, 1 cup	5.0
Apricots, dried, 1 cup	4.9
Avocados, 1 cup	2.4
Beef, 3 oz. portion	3.1
Beef, hamburger pattie, 3 oz.	4.6
Beef, steak, 3 oz.	4.0
Beef, corned, 3 oz.	2.9
Beef, heart, 3 oz.	6.8
Beef and vegetable stew, 1 cup	3.4
Bread:	
Cracked wheat, 1 slice	0.3
French, enriched, 1 lb.	11.3
Italian, enriched, 1 lb.	11.7
Rye, 1 slice	0.3
Pumpernickel, 1 lb.	5.4
White, enriched, 1 slice	0.5
Whole wheat, 1 slice	0.7

actions are affected by the physical condition of the body, that the nervous system cannot be expected to perform its complicated functions unless it is provided with proper chemical milieu and that schizophrenia is the result of chemical imbalance."

After a series of tests Dr. Ross discovered that Mitch is hypoglycemic. That is, his blood sugar regulating mechanism is disordered, so that, when he eats carbohydrates the levels of blood sugar decline, leaving his nervous system too little nourishment. Hence he suffered from the distorted perceptions (hearing, seeing, taste and smell) that torture schizophrenics, making them believe that others are their enemies.

Mitch was put on a diet very low in carbohydrate, high

Chicken, broiled, 3 oz.	10.5
Dates, 1 cup	3.9
Flour, whole wheat, 1 cup	5.2
Ham, smoked, 3 oz.	3.5
Lamb chop, 1	5.4
Liver, beef, 2 oz.	8.4
Mackerel, 3 oz.	6.5
Mushrooms, 1 cup	4.8
Oysters, 1 cup	6.6
Peanuts, roasted, 1 cup	24.6
Peaches, dried, 1 cup	8.4
Peas, green, 1 cup	3.7
Pork chop, 1	3.6
Salmon, 3 oz.	6.8
Sausage, Bologna, 8 oz.	6.0
Shad, 3 oz.	7.3
Soybeans, 1 serving	2.3
Soybean flour, 100 grams	2.6
Swordfish, 3 oz.	9.3
Tuna, 3 oz.	10.9
Veal cutlet, 3 oz.	4.6
Wheat germ, 1 cup	3.1
Yeast, brewer's, 100 grams	36.2

in protein, with small meals and frequent between-meal snacks, also high in protein. After each meal he took massive doses of some of the vitamins which have been found to be most helpful in these cases: 500 milligrams of niacin (vitamin B3), 500 milligrams of vitamin C, 100 milligrams of pyridoxine (vitamin B6), 100 milligrams of pantothenic acid (another B vitamin), 200 international units of vitamin E and a multiple B vitamin tablet to furnish some of the rest of this complex. These are very large doses, especially for a child.

Within a week, his parents noticed a difference in Mitch. He became calmer and more cooperative. Dr. Ross increased his dose of niacin to 1,000 milligrams. When Mitch became nauseated, niacinamide (another form of the B vitamin) was substituted for niacin.

After a month, Mitch was losing some of his overweight and his school work improved. Dr. Ross gave him an amino acid which seems to benefit brain function.

In the orthomolecular treatment of schizophrenia, daily or weekly sessions with the psychiatrist are not essential. It's the helpful chemical reactions of the body which bring about the improvement, not the psychiatrist's words. So Mitch saw Dr. Ross infrequently. Three months later his parents said he was doing much better. His phantoms and imaginary wrongs had disappeared. He was losing unwanted weight steadily. He could concentrate much better. Two symptoms remained—weakness when he did not eat and bed-wetting. The first symptom is common in people with low blood sugar. The second is very common among today's children.

Dr. Ross tells us that about 80 percent of adult schizophrenic patients suffer from low blood sugar which can be treated only with a diet high in protein and very low in carbohydrate, with frequent small meals, so that hunger and weakness do not develop.

The more than 200 psychiatrists who are presently using the orthomolecular therapy (described above) for schizophrenia do not use the orthodox psychiatric methods.

They work within the family framework. They talk to the patient's family in his presence. They work to get the family's help in keeping the patient on his diet and vitamin pills. They give him certain tests designed to discover how his perceptions have been damaged—that is, what distortions are plaguing him where sight, hearing, taste and smell are concerned.

Often it is necessary for the patient to see the doctor only once a month. Progress is slow, but usually certain. There are few overnight successes. The patient who begins orthomolecular therapy early in his illness has the best chance of recovery.

Orthomolecular therapy is helpful not only for schizophrenics. Alcoholics and drug addicts have also been helped. *Alcoholics Anonymous* reports that the high protein, low carbohydrate diet plus vitamins helps alcoholics to stay sober. Large doses of niacin are used to offset violent reactions to LSD. The diet and vitamins are now being used to treat autistic children, hyperactive children, minimal brain damage in children and learning disability.

"We do not believe that our biochemical model explains all mental illness," says Dr. Ross. But this group of professional men does believe that physical condition may have a great deal to do with mental health in this field. At the very least, other psychiatrists should be willing to give this new therapy a chance, to use it themselves along with their usual approaches to therapy.

If you know of a sufferer from schizophrenia or some of the childhood disorders listed above, get in touch with the Huxley Institute for Biosocial Research, 1114 First Avenue, New York City, 10021. They have much material available on this method of treatment.

Here is a letter received by the Huxley Institute:

"Our son Bruce suffered a breakdown when he was fourteen. We entered him in a local hospital for psychiatric treatment, believing that the doctors there had the knowledge and concern to make our son well. However, his only treatment was tranquilizers which made him dopey and sleepy all the time; instead of attempting to cure Bruce, the doctors seemed content to maintain him at a level where he was so drugged that life itself was just a blur. After three weeks he was released with the recommendation to continue weekly psychiatric sessions, but after about a year of these expensive sessions, Bruce was no better.

"Then luckily I heard of the Huxley Institute/American Schizophrenia Association from an article in *Look Magazine* and wrote to them for any help they could offer. They recommended the book *How to Live with Schizophrenia* by Dr. Abram Hoffer and Dr. Humphrey Osmond, which discusses the biochemical causes and cures of mental illness. After reading the book, I started Bruce on the megavitamin treatment, and he began to improve immediately. Can you imagine how I felt, after watching my son suffer for so long, and the rest of my family with him, only to find that the psychiatrists who were supposed to be helping us had put us all through a terrible, painful, almost hopeless year with their useless drugs, when the answer to making our son well was one they have never offered?

"When I went to Bruce's psychiatrist and informed him how well our son was doing on the megavitamin therapy, he made a remark that I'm sure many of us have heard time and time again: 'If you give him sugar pills, it would be just as effective.' But how very wrong he is, how very wrong are all the others who agree with him! Bruce is 20 now, and perfectly normal. He graduated from high school with honors, was valedictorian, a straight A student, and won three scholarships. He is now a senior at the University of California, is on the Dean's honor roll, and has lots of friends, which he was never able to cultivate before his breakdown.

"Mere words cannot express my gratitude to the Institute for showing me the way to make my son well, but I have to keep asking myself, Why did I have to accidently stumble over a magazine article to find out about orthomolecular medicine, why didn't my psychiatrist know about it, and if he did, why wasn't he open-minded enough to try therapy when anyone's eyes could see that his 'tried and true' treatment methods were doing no good at all? The Huxley Institute is doing its best to reach psychiatrists, social workers, therapists, patients and their families all over the country, at every level of society, to convince them that there is another way to treat the mentally ill other than drugging them into insensibility and hope that they recover with enough talk therapy. But it takes money to publish articles, money to run orthomolecular conferences and train orthomolecular physicians, money to provide referral services and to continue educating the public to the necessity of including orthomolecular psychiatry as one of the basic treatments for the mentally ill."

The treatment this grateful mother is talking about is a treatment for mental illness based on the premise that this is a physical illness which can be corrected by a highly nutritious diet plus massive doses of vitamins and minerals. This kind of treatment is being used by increasing numbers of psychiatrists around the world.

There are three phases to the treatment. Cases that are not so serious may need only one treatment which is given at home and consists only of the B vitamins and vitamin C, with other vitamins given if needed. These are massive doses. The book gives complete details on just how they are taken and when. The doctors may also give tranquilizers or other related drugs just to make the patient more comfortable.

The patient with phase two condition is treated in a hospital with several other therapies added to his vitamin regimen. The phase three treatment continues with the phase two treatment and several added therapies for as long as necessary.

Sleep and diet are extremely important to the health of schizophrenics. The prescribed diet is high in protein and contains almost no refined carbohydrates or "junk foods" as these authors call them.

Recently an amino acid, tryptophan was found to be conducive to sleep in people who suffer from chronic insomnia. Tryptophan is a form of protein, found in all foods with considerable protein content. It is essential for human health. That is, we cannot make this protein in our bodies, but must get it in food.

Tryptophan breaks down into niacin, the B vitamin, once it is inside the body. So we suggest to our insomniac readers that they might be able to conquer their sleeplessness by taking niacin instead of the rather rare and somewhat difficult to obtain amino acid.

We wrote to Dr. Abram Hoffer, the Canadian psychiatrist who is working miracles in treating mental illness with niacin and other vitamins, given in large doses. We asked him if he had used niacin to induce sleep in insomniac patients.

He answered us thus, "I have heard something about the use of tryptophan for the cure of insomnia and it is quite possible that some cases may be very affected by it. Tryptophan has two final pathways (in the body): one winding up in niacin or NAD and the other winding up with serotonin. If the insomnia is due to lack of serotonin, then increasing the tryptophan will increase that and will cure that particular type of insomnia and in this case nicotinic acid (niacin) would not help. If, however, the insomnia is due to a lack of niacin then of course niacin would be preferable to the tryptophan.

"I have in fact seen a large number of people who, upon taking vitamin B3 (niacin), have been able to sleep. In fact, recently I saw a woman who had not slept for years who, after a few months of treatment with nicotinic acid (niacin) is sleeping normally. However, I have not done any specific studies with niacin for the treatment of insomnia.

In an entirely different area of health is work with niacin in an effort to prevent heart attacks.

Four Edinburgh physicians are experimenting with a form of vitamin B3 to see whether it may prove to be a beneficial aid in treatment of certain heart attacks which might otherwise prove fatal. They report on their work in the October 13, 1973 issue of *The Lancet*.

Drs. M. J. Rowe, B. J. Kirby, M. A. Dolder and M. F. Oliver of the Royal Infirmary in Edinburgh tell us that in patients who have had a myocardial infarction (that is a heart attack in which one part of the heart loses its blood supply) the patient always has raised levels of free fatty acids in his blood. In the case of serious disorders of the rhythm the same thing is true.

The raised levels of fatty acids in the blood come from body fat tissue, say the authors. It is known that nicotinic acid (another name for niacin or vitamin B3) controls this release of fats. So, these physicians theorized if they could give enough of the vitamin they might be able to control the amount of fat being released into the blood, hence improve the condition of the heart.

First they tested the vitamin with healthy volunteers. They tested the amount of fatty acids in their blood, then gave them 200 milligrams of the B vitamin and tested their blood again every 15 minutes for the next two hours, then one hour later and two hours later.

The levels of fatty substances in blood began to fall within 15 minutes after the vitamin was given. The level fell steadily for two hours then rose again to the pretreatment level within four hours.

Then the researchers did the same test on five men who had suffered a myocardial infarct, testing their blood continuously from the time they gave them the B vitamin. The levels of fatty substances in the blood fell 50 percent from their former level. In another test of six patients with acute myocardial infarction they gave the vitamin and tested fatty levels in the blood. "In all the patients on the drug there was a steep fall in plasma free fatty acids in the first hour, reaching a nadir during the first two hours," they say. The greatest decrease was 54 percent in one patient. In a third group of heart patients the same thing occurred, with the greatest decrease being 58 percent. In every case the levels of fats rose again after the vitamin was discontinued.

The authors tell us they have had the same effects in animal experiments. They caution that the "drug", as they call this B vitamin, must be given every two hours to maintain the fall in fatty substances and must be given in large doses—in this case, 200 milligrams. They say they are studying the effects of the vitamin on disorders of heart rhythm.

But treating disease is not our chief interest. We are interested in *preventing* diseases before they occur. Since niacin or vitamin B3 is involved with regulating the amount of fatty acids in the blood, doesn't it seem wise to make certain you are getting enough of this vitamin every day so that you may be able to avoid any of these serious complications which can bring on life-threatening crises?

Niacin occurs in seed foods—that is, wholegrains, peas, beans, lentils and other legumes and pulses, nuts, peanuts, peanut butter. It is also abundant in meat and fish, especially liver, one serving of which may contain up to 17 milligrams of this B vitamin. Officially we are told that adults need about 15 milligrams daily. How often does your family eat bran which contains up to 9 milligrams of niacin? How often does your family eat wheat germ—with 5 milligrams of niacin per serving? Brewers yeast is another good source of this B vitamin. It can be added unobtrusively to almost any suitable food and should certainly be added to any baked goods you make.

It is well to keep in mind that, although "enriched" bread has had niacin added to it, to replace that which was removed in the refining, other bakery products like rolls, doughnuts, pastries, pasta, pizza and so on are probably made from unenriched flour, so that their niacin content may be very low or non-existent. Corn products are rather lacking in this vitamin, so don't limit your cereal and bread eating to corn-based foods.

It seems to us that the epidemic of heart and artery disorders which are at present the chief cause of death in this country have many causes and we should try our best to eliminate all these causes in our own lives. As the above experiment shows, one of the causes of heart attacks may be an excess of fatty acids in the blood which getting enough vitamin B3 might have prevented.

So do not slight foods rich in niacin. See to it that all your cereal foods are whole-grain, get to like wheat germ and bran and eat them every day, and be certain to include in your meals plenty of seafood and meat—especially the organ meats like liver. Check your food supplements. Is there enough niacin there to make up for any excess which your own physiological make-up and way of life may necessitate?

CHAPTER 19

A B Vitamin
Treats Arthritis

ALWAYS ON THE lookout for any new material pertaining to arthritis, that might be helpful, we came upon a note referring to a book long out of print of which a few copies had been found which were for sale for $35, so rare and valuable they were. We sent for a copy and found it was well worth the price. Its author, William Kaufman, Ph.D., M.D., wrote the book for other physicians, so it is not easy reading for the layman. It deals with an astonishing story of many arthritis patients treated and greatly improved in most cases by a B vitamin given in large doses every few hours every day to saturate the tissues. Dr. Kaufman believed that arthritis is a disease of vitamin deficiency.

Here are case histories of several patients out of the hundreds Dr. Kaufman treated and reported on in this book back in the 1940's.

An accountant, sixty years old—arthritis. He was given 160 milligrams of a B vitamin to take every two hours for eight doses daily (1,200 milligrams in 24 hours). In 315 days of such therapy his arthritis improved from a rating of "severe" to "slight."

A 39-year-old woman came into Dr. Kaufman's office complaining of moderate arthritis, transient low back pain, right shoulder stiff discomfort, persistent stiffness of joints.

She had had a "nervous breakdown" several years earlier when her husband died. She had had "the usual" menopause symptoms. She was given 150 milligrams of a B vitamin to take every three hours for six daily doses. Within one month her joint troubles had greatly improved. On the advice of a friend, she decided to take less of the B vitamin. Her condition worsened again. When she went back to the original dose, it improved.

A 61-year-old engineer came to Dr. Kaufman's office with severe persistent headaches, from which he could get no relief. In the past two years they had become much worse. His joints grated, especially in the neck. He was stiff in the morning when first awake, also when the weather was bad. His shoulders had been painful with intermittent stiffness and pain in finger joints. He was given a certain B vitamin in doses of 160 milligrams at regular intervals to equal 975 milligrams per day. His headaches improved gradually. Within 190 days his arthritic condition improved from "severe" to "slight". He was also given large doses of vitamin C along with smaller doses of riboflavin and thiamine.

An attorney of 45 came into Dr. Kaufman's office with severe joint dysfunction, was given 1,800 milligrams of a certain B vitamin every 24 hours, along with other B vitamins and vitamin C. Within 178 days of therapy his condition was greatly improved.

The vitamin which was given in large doses in every case was niacinamide—the amide from of the B vitamin niacin or vitamin B3. The name of the book is *The Common Form of Joint Dysfunction: Its Incidence and Treatment.*

Dr. Kaufman, determined to conquer arthritis for at least some of his patients, developed elaborate devices for measuring what he called "joint dysfunction"—that is, anything which impaired the patient's ability to move about—any dysfunction in arms, legs, wrists, back and so on. By measuring the patient's grasp, reach and other extensions of joints, he was able to classify their ailment according to the numbers on the mechanism he had invented. As time went on, the same patient was asked to perform the same motions, so that improvement or lack of it could be measured and noted. Dr. Kaufman was not content merely to ask the patient, "How are your joints today?" He could actually physically measure improvement or lack of it.

The stories in this book are almost unbelievable, especially in view of the fact that it was written more than 25 years ago when vitamins were almost never spoken of in terms of preventive medicine and when the idea of using vitamins in massive doses had not even been considered by most researchers or physicians. Dr. Kaufman was an innovator—years and years ahead of his time.

Also of interest is the fact that he made no other changes in his patients' lives except for the vitamins he gave them. There is no mention of revising their diets, asking them to exercise more or make any other changes in their way of life. So the record appears to be just a record of what one vitamin—niacinamide—along with several others in smaller doses, can do to improve the condition of patients with painful, stiff joints. It seems to us that far better or perhaps quicker results might have occurred had the patients been placed on diets in which all refined carbohydrates were restricted and emphasis was laid on high protein foods and whole, unprocessed foods. But Dr. Kaufman confined his treatment to vitamins alone.

He did not use just niacinamide. In most cases he also gave quite large doses of vitamin C, thiamine (vitamin B1), and pyridoxine (vitamin B6) and riboflavin (B2). He tailored the dosage of niacinamide according to the individual patient's needs. If there appeared to be little or no improvement, he increased the dosage. If improvement appeared to have stopped at a "plateau", he increased the dosage. He cautioned his patients to continue with the recommended dosage even if they became discouraged with slow progress. Improvement with this completely harmless therapy appears to take quite a long time, although in several cases described in the book almost miraculous improvement occurred in a matter of months in people who had suffered for years from arthritis.

He mentions several things which complicate treatment. These are things we might have neglected to notice ourselves. But a very detailed history sometimes turned up significant items in regard to the possible causes of the complaint.

Sometimes it was allergy. Some of his patients knew they were allergic to certain foods: wheat, chocolate, eggs, etc. When they carefully avoided these foods their improvement was assured. If they transgressed and ate even small amounts of the offending food, their condition always worsened.

Another drawback to continued improvement usually had to do with repetitive work done every day by the patient in an uncomfortable or awkward position. This is almost bound to create joint problems which will not yield to any treatment. Anyone working with tools or machinery, twisting a foot around the leg of a chair while sitting, holding the phone in an awkward position for long conversation, maintaining poor posture year after year, wearing uncomfortable shoes or high heels or socks that are too short. Dr. Kaufman describes a woman whose joint pains occurred only on certain days. It developed that these were the days when she ironed. She habitually held the iron in a tight grip and pressed hard on the ironing board, as well as pulling tightly on the object she was ironing. Correcting these improper methods of work greatly alleviated her joint pains.

Another complicating factor in arthritis, says Dr. Kaufman, is sodium retention. Many women complain of this several days before their menstrual period: bloating, weight gain, irritability, discomfort, insomnia caused by the body retaining sodium or salt. Some people appear to retain salt more readily than others. And of course some people eat far more salt than others. We have no need for salt. The modern American diet contains enough salt for good health without adding any in cooking or at the table.

So specialists in kidney, heart and circulatory problems are recommending that you throw away your salt shaker.

Finally, Dr. Kaufman believes there is a kind of psychosomatic arthritis. People living under constant stress or under unbearable conditions which seemingly cannot be changed may develop joint symptoms which are not actually physical but are brought about by life circumstances, whether they are imagined or real.

Dr. Kaufman's conclusions are these: "During the first month of adequate therapy with niacinamide (alone or in combination with other vitamins) a patient with joint dysfunction (with or without rheumatic or hypertrophic arthritis) will have a rise in the Joint Range Index of at least 6-12 points, and thereafter will have a rise of at least ½ to 1 point per month of adequate niacinamide therapy, provided he eats the average American diet containing adequate calories and sufficient protein, and provided he does not mechanically injure his joints excessively. This improvement in joint mobility occurs regardless of the age or sex of the patient and regardless of whatever other health problems he may have. Subsequently, with continuously adequate niacinamide therapy, the Joint Range Index of 96-100 (no joint dysfunction) is reached and maintenance doses of niacinamide are required to keep the Index at this level." The only exception to this rule, he says, is the patient whose joints are ankylosed—that is, immovably fixed in one position. Such patients cannot ever achieve perfect range of movement, says Dr. Kaufman.

The patient must go on taking niacinamide. If he stops, the symptoms gradually recur. If, after he has achieved the best possible dosage *for him*, he reduces the dosage, he will regress to whatever degree of improvement such a dosage can produce for him individually. Dr. Kaufman says his patients derive other benefits from the vitamin treatment. Digestive complaints may disappear. They may feel more alert, more vigorous. They may tire less easily. Liver tenderness and enlargement may disappear. Muscle strength seems to improve.

"In the last stages of rheumatic arthritis there may be so much retrogressive tissue alteration in non-articular as well as articular tissue, that complete functional and structural recovery may not be possible, even with prolonged niacinamide therapy," says Dr. Kaufman. He tells us, too, that he does not know how or why niacinamide acts to improve the condition of painful, stiff joints. He hopes that more research will be done on this. He does believe, however, that "the evolution of the common form of joint dysfunction can be prevented by adequate niacinamide supplementation of an adequate diet throughout the lifetime of an individual."

Other investigators in earlier years have turned up much valuable evidence that vitamin C is essential, in large amounts, to prevent and treat arthritis. Indeed, there seems to be great similarity between the joint symptoms of scurvy, the disease of vitamin C deficiency, and arthritis. In each case the collagen is disordered. This is the substance of which we are made, especially joints. Vitamin C is essential for the manufacture of collagen. In its absence, as in scurvy, collagen simply wastes away until the poor scurvy victim cannot walk or endure the pain of moving his joints. Is it not possible that modern arthritis may be caused in part at least by all the demands made on our vitamin C stores by all the poisons in our environment, along with the fact that many of us simply don't get enough vitamin C to meet our needs?

Practically all researchers on arthritis stress the need for an adequate diet with plenty of protein and elimination of sugar and all foods that contain it. Past researches have turned up the fact that arthritics tend to eat lots of sugar. Many are victims of low blood sugar which is corrected by a diet in which sugar is eliminated and protein is stressed. Early investigations turned up the fact that children who developed rheumatic heart conditions did not like or did not eat eggs when they were young. Perhaps the bounty of high quality protein plus the vitamins and minerals of eggs are far more important than we know in preventing the aches and disability of arthritis.

We do not know why this fine, well-documented book by Dr. Kaufman was not followed up by many more investigations of the power of the B vitamin niacinamide against arthritis. Perhaps some modern physician may take up the fight where Dr. Kaufman left off. We hope so. Meanwhile there seems to be no reason not to apply his findings in your own life. He reported absolutely no harmful side effects from these very large doses of niacinamide. This vitamin is also being used in very large doses in treating schizophrenia with almost no reports of side effects in doses much larger than those used by Dr. Kaufman.

Finally we remind you that Dr. Kaufman's book is out of print. You cannot buy it at a bookstore. If you wish to try to get a copy for your physician, write to Mrs. Charlotte Kaufman, 540 Brooklawn Avenue, Bridgeport, Conn. 06604 to ask if any of these books are still available. The title of the book is *The Common Form of Joint Dysfunction: Its Incidence and Treatment*.

CHAPTER 20

There's a Lack
of Pyridoxine
in Our Meals

PYRIDOXINE, vitamin B6, was not listed as essential until quite recently in the official chart of *Recommended Dietary Allowances*.

Symptoms of deficiency are somewhat like those of other B vitamins: the skin and the nerves suffer most. A number of years ago a crisis in infant nutrition arose when certain commercial baby formulas were processed in such a way that their pyridoxine was destroyed. Some of the babies eating the food had convulsions.

Mystified physicians who reported the cases and found they were all related to this one food, discovered eventually that the way the formula was processed destroyed all the pyridoxine in it. They injected the vitamin into the children and the convulsions stopped immediately, although in some cases permanent brain damage remained.

The doctors and scientists who studied these cases could not understand why some children who took the faulty formula were affected while others were not. They finally came to the only possible conclusion—that some individuals need much more of this important vitamin than others. Those whose needs were less somehow managed to get along on whatever pyridoxine remained in their tissues after birth, while the affected children could not survive healthfully even for a few days without getting the vitamin in their food.

The formula was withdrawn from the market and supposedly this threat to newborn children is over. But an article in the February 6, 1965 issue of the *Journal of the American Medical Association* may prove otherwise. A Utah physician reports in this article on two babies who had convulsions several hours after birth. One of them died. The other was given massive doses of sedatives and other drugs and became rapidly worse.

An injection of 100 milligrams of pyridoxine quieted the convulsions and brought the baby back to normal. But several times after this, the child required larger doses of the vitamin and finally she was put on a daily dose. Says the author, "Daily maintenence therapy of 4 to 10 milligrams, administered orally, is necessary to maintain the child symptom free". No one knows how long the child will have to take these amounts of the vitamin. One such child is now eight years old, the doctor tells us, and still needs the vitamin to prevent convulsions.

The Utah physician then tells us that in several families more than one child has been so affected. This seems to indicate, beyond a doubt, that the need for large amounts of this B vitamin is inherited. If the obstetrician knows about cases like this he can give the child pyridoxine immediately and thus prevent permanent damage. If he does not, the convulsions may progress to fatality or may so damage the child's brain that recovery is impossible.

The AMA Journal article recommends that all infants with convulsions be given an immediate large dose of pyridoxine. If the convulsions are caused by deficiency, they will stop. So every infant who is thus afflicted at birth should have the benefit of this injection, in case pyridoxine deficiency is responsible.

This is a most significant article from the point of view of the health-seeker. If a greater than average need for only one B vitamin can have such terrible results when not enough of the vitamin is given, isn't it possible that many other disorders—especially those that seem to be inherited—may be caused by a greater than average need for other nutrients? We can look forward to a day when biochemists may have shown that such plagues as cancer, heart disease, diabetes, multiple sclerosis, Parkinson's Disease, muscular dystrophy and many others can be prevented at birth by tests and by supplements which provide more of this or that nutrient than the average person needs.

Until that day, keep in mind the lesson this experience has taught us. No two people have the same requirements for vitamins or minerals. Yours may be twice that of some member of your family, or it may be fifty times greater. The new baby in your family may get along perfectly well on the things the average baby is given to eat. Or he may have been born needing excessive amounts of almost any vitamin or mineral, or even amino acid (these are forms of protein).

Notice that the babies described in the medical article were not taking a formula deficient in pyridoxine. They were getting food that is perfectly satisfactory for the normal baby. But these afflicted children inherited a need for so much more pyridoxine that they took a chance on death or permanent disability if their physician did not give them massive doses of the B vitamin.

Parkinson's Disease is an affliction of the nerves which appears usually in middleaged individuals. A drug (Levodopa) was recently developed which seems to improve greatly the Parkinson symptoms, but at the same time produces very unpleasant side effects in the form of involuntary movements which the patient cannot control.

Doctors using this drug have known for some time that the B vitamin pyridoxine appears to be related in some mysterious way to the effects the drug has on the patient. In the June 28, 1971 issue of *The Journal of the American Medical Association*, two New York physicians tell of their experiences with one patient in whom they could control the Parkinson symptoms with Levodopa, but abnormal uncontrollable movements then appeared. When they gave the B vitamin pyridoxine these movements were controlled, but the Parkinson symptoms appeared again.

By careful dosage they discovered that adding pyridoxine to the patient's medication was the equivalent of doubling the dose of Levodopa, the drug. They tried dosage with other patients and found that the same was true, except that the intensity of the effect of the B vitamin differed with different patients. The doctors feel certain that this discovery will aid in future work with Parkinson patients. They can, by juggling dosages of the drug and the vitamin, produce improvement with few side effects, they hope.

We hope that other investigators working in the field of Parkinson's Disease will untangle this mystery soon and will perhaps make a more important discovery—that Parkinson's Disease may have its origins in lack of B vitamins. One cannot help but feel that, when a vitamin given in massive dose has such a profound effect on such a serious disorder, the origin of the disease must be related somehow to deficiency in this vitamin.

"A number of diseases occur in man whose principal therapeutic requirement is supplementation of the diet with pyridoxine," says a Canadian researcher writing in the *American Journal of Diseases of Children* for January 1967. In other words, many different conditions of ill health can be improved or cured merely by giving the individual plenty of vitamin B6, pyridoxine.

Dr. Charles R. Scriver goes on to list such conditions. People who do not properly absorb their food are likely to be lacking in pyridoxine, he says. This may be either because their digestive tracts do not absorb the vitamin or because it may not be transported correctly through cells and tissues. Or, he says, it may be destroyed by certain types of drugs. One which is known to destroy the vitamin is isoniazid, used in the treatment of tuberculosis. In some cases, pyridoxine may be lost through the kidneys. Certain disorders may inactivate the enzymes which make the vitamin available for the body. There may be increased demand for the vitamin due to pregnancy or fever. Or the individual may just not get enough vitamin B6 in his food.

Nutrition Reviews for December 1966 reported on the relation of vitamin B6 to the health of the pituitary gland. This is the master gland of the body, responsible for triggering other glands into many activities essential for life and health.

The British journal, *The Lancet* , for February 11, 1967, reported on a young girl who had a chronic condition in which a certain amino acid or protein was excreted in her urine. There were three such patients in two families, seeming to indicate that the condition might be inherited. Giving pyridoxine in extremely large doses prevented the condition and returned the child to good health. Related to the urine condition was a blood condition in which blood cells had a peculiar abnormal stickiness.

Another article relating pyridoxine to a blood condition appeared in the *New England Journal of Medicine* for April 7, 1966. A young man with serious anemia was found to have excessively low levels of fats and cholesterol in his blood. One hundred milligrams of the B vitamin pyridoxine was given intramuscularly twice a day. The anemia was cured and the level of fatty substances in the blood became normal.

But the patient had to continue to take the B vitamin every day. On the three occasions when it was discontinued, the anemia returned within one or two months. The authors believe that doctors treating such anemias should be on the lookout for other blood abnormalities that may accompany it. Interestingly enough, the young patient's parents were both alcoholic and he himself drank excessively.

Medical World News for January 15, 1965 reported that a Pennsylvania physician has found that children not getting enough pyridoxine "may become irritable, develop oversensitive hearing, and even suffer convulsions."

Prompt detection and proper nutritional management is crucial, he said. He gives daily doses of 2 to 10 milligrams to such infants. The official recommendation for infants is four-tenths of a milligram daily.

Giving pyridoxine, vitamin B6, in cases of chronic gastritis associated with too little digestive juices has helped to improve the digestion of 18 patients, according to a Soviet physician, reported in *Medical World News* for October 8, 1965.

Dr. M. S. Lamanskaya tested the vitamin in 30 patients and got improvement in 18. Some of these had too little hydrochloric acid in the digestive tract, some had the normal amount and some had too much.

If you are worried about kidney stones, pyridoxine and magnesium are your two best protective agents against the formation of stones. Dr. Abram Hoffer reminds us in the October, 1975 issue of the *Huxley Institute—SCF Newsletter* that pyridoxine is involved in the body's conversion of oxalate to glycine, the next step in metabolizing it. Oxalic acid is the substance in some foods which renders calcium unavailable to the body. That is, if you were to eat nothing but spinach, let's say, you might become quite deficient in calcium because spinach contains considerable oxalic acid.

But we don't eat diets consisting of nothing but foods rich in oxalic acid. We eat a variety of foods. And pyridoxine is in many foods, in any well planned diet. So we suffer no harm from the oxalic acid in spinach or the other vegetables that contain it.

As you can see from the information above, it's lack of pyridoxine and/or the mineral magnesium which brings on kidney stones.

Pyridoxine (vitamin B6) is a part of the body's processing material for fats, carbohydrates and protein. It participates in the enzyme activity which allows us to assimilate these food elements. So we could not conceivably get along without it. It is especially important in relation to the amino acid tryptophan. In diets where vitamin B3 (niacin) is lacking, an amino acid, tryptophan, is converted into niacin in the body to prevent the vitamin deficiency disease of pellagra. This operation can take place only when there is enough pyridoxine present. So this is another important function of this vitamin.

It participates, too, in manufacturing certain body hormones such as histamine and adrenalin. Adrenalin is the hormone which is called up when you are under stress and need all the energy you can summon. So getting enough pyridoxine will help in this emergency. Pyridoxine is also important for the body's manufacture of certain blood elements which prevent anemia. So you must have it, if you would be safe from that debilitating disease.

Says Dr. Hoffer, "Since there is no definite vitamin B6 (pyridoxine) deficiency disease as there is for vitamin C (scurvy), physicians have not been trained to look for evidence of pyridoxine deficiency. The daily B6 intake recommending up to two milligrams per day has no meaning since it ignores wide-ranging differences between people. The need varies with the state of health, with the amount of protein consumed (more protein consumed requires more vitamin B6). Many scientists are worried about the adequacy of our food with respect to B6."

He then quotes a noted nutrition expert, Dr. Nevin Scrimshaw, who said in 1967, "Early malnutrition which stunts growth has also clearly and repeatedly been shown in experimental animals to reduce subsequent learning ability, memory and behavior. To the extent this is true for young children as well, the generations on whom social and economic progress will depend in the remainder of this century are being maimed now in body frame, in nervous systems and in mind."

So a deficiency in vitamin B6 (pyridoxine) can bring on the following effects:

1. Convulsions in babies.
2. You can get painful neuritis from lack of pyridoxine. A number of drugs destroy the vitamin (isoniazid, penicillamine, etc.).

3. You can get anemia from lack of pyridoxine.

4. You can get kidney stones.

Dr. Hoffer tells us of experiments in which animals made deficient in pyridoxine were given magnesium and the expected kidney stones did not materialize. "Out of 36 (human) patients who were chronic oxalate stone formers, 200 milligrams of magnesium oxide and 10 milligrams per day of vitamin B6 over five years prevented recurrence or greatly decreased it in 30."

There are people who need far more pyridoxine than the rest of us. Dr. hoffer believes that as many as five percent of any "normal" population and up to 75 percent of a severely ill psychiatric population have this problem. They need more pyridoxine than they can get in the average diet.

"As well as being mentally ill," he says, "these patients may have constipation and abdominal pains, unexplained fever and chills, morning nausea, especially if pregnant, hypoglycemia (low blood sugar), impotence or lack of menstruation, and neurological symptoms such as amnesia, tremor, spasms and seizures. The treatment consists of optimum amounts of B6 and zinc." About one-third of all schizophrenics suffer from this need for very large amounts of the vitamin.

The Pill, the oral contraceptive, is destructive of pyridoxine. So widespread is this complaint that many scientists believe that the vitamin should be included in every oral contraceptive so that the user will have the benefit of the vitamin whether she gets it at meals or not.

Executive Health (Volume XII, Number 2) for November, 1975 tells us that in mentally retarded children suffering from convulsive seizures these were controlled when pyridoxine was given. Radiologists have found that pyridoxine can prevent the nausea that accompanies x-ray treatment. Obstetricians use it to control the morning sickness of pregnancy. In a group of women and girls suffering from acne the week before menstruation begins, 72 percent of those taking 50 milligrams of pyridoxine daily for one week before and during their periods, found that the acne was controlled.

We are told that the amount of fat in American diets has a lot to do with our soaring figures on heart disease and deaths from heart attacks. Since pyridoxine is one of the vitamins involved with processing fats in the body, might it help to prevent heart troubles? It seems so. Scientists have shown that monkeys getting high-fat, high-cholesterol diets do not get artery troubles if they are getting as much as five milligrams of pyridoxine a day. This means that human beings should be getting about 25 milligrams daily if they want the same protection. But here again, we have individual needs which may be higher.

Executive Health tells us that in one study of 800 mentally disturbed children the need for pyridoxine varied from five milligrams a day to 400 milligrams, which is eighty times more. Dr. Bernard Rimland of California, treating disturbed children, has given them a formula of the following vitamins daily: 2 to 3 grams of vitamin C and niacinamide, 150 to 400 milligrams of pyridoxine, 200 milligrams of pantothenic acid (another B vitamin) plus a high potency B complex tablet which would include all the smaller amounts of all the other B vitamins. Detailed records of the children's behavior showed that most of them improved—more than 50 percent. Doubling the dose of pyridoxine brought improvement in some of those who had not improved on the earlier dose.

Kidney stones and bladder stones made up chiefly of calcium oxalate or a mixture of calcium oxalate and calcium phosphate "present a stubborn and curious puzzle to the urologist," says a review in the January, 1976 issue of *Nutrition Reviews*. There just doesn't seem to be much reason why certain individuals should suffer from these painful disorders, since they appear to be otherwise healthy and the amount of calcium in their blood appears to be "normal."

Symptoms of both kinds of stones are: pain and frequent, bloody urination. Small stones may pass out through the ureter. Larger stones which may block the flow of urine must be removed by surgery or some other method. Up to now, specialists have generally believed that bladder stones are caused by chronic inflammation of the bladder, enlargement of the male prostate gland, contraction of the neck of the bladder, a diverticulum or pouch in the wall of the bladder or kidney stones which have moved down into the bladder.

Now we are told in *Nutrition Reviews* that stones may be caused by deficiency in an important mineral and an equally important vitamin. The mineral is magnesium. The vitamin is vitamin B6 or pyridoxine. A lengthy experiment involving some 150 people seems to show great improvement in the tendency to form such stones when people who are susceptible are given the two nutrients over a long period of time.

The experiment was accomplished by getting the aid of a large number of urologists who agreed to give the two nutrients to a given number of patients who could be expected to form a given number of stones in the time of the experiment—five years. About 150 patients were involved. Certain qualifications were set. Only patients who had formed at least one stone in the previous five years were accepted. They must also be free from urinary infection, have normal kidney function, normal levels of calcium and phosphorus in the blood and be free from other diseases which sometimes accompany stone formation—peptic ulcer, for example.

The volunteers were given a magnesium supplement consisting of 100 milligrams three times a day. By this we assume they took the tablets with meals. They were also given 10 milligrams of the B vitamin pyridoxine daily. No other change was made in diet or treatment.

The reduction in stone formation was dramatic. The group as a whole had formed an average of 1.3 stones before they began treatment. Taking the food supplements for five years resulted in an average of only one-tenth of a stone during the five years the test continued. Furthermore, *the only stones formed were limited to 17 of the 150 subjects*.

The others had no stones at all during this five-year period. None of them suffered any side effects.

The *Nutrition Reviews* writer professes amazement at these results. What could they mean? he asks. Is it possible that the person who regularly forms kidney or bladder stones has a marginal deficiency in magnesium and/or pyridoxine either because he doesn't get enough at mealtime or because he just happens to need more than the average person? We would say, gentlemen, that both of these circumstances may certainly be the reason for formation of stones. Magnesium and pyridoxine are both found most abundantly in wholegrain cereals and breads as well as other seed foods. When white flour is made, most of the magnesium and pyridoxine are discarded and never replaced in the flour. Why should not modern human beings be short on both nutrients?

But, says the *Reviews* writer, these people did not seem to be suffering from a magnesium deficiency. And, what is more, people who are known to be suffering from a magnesium deficiency, as a result of lack of absorption, prolonged diarrhea, excessive alcohol intake or protein malnutrition, do not generally form stones.

In the case of pyridoxine, there seems to be even less evidence of a deficiency. In fact, it seems that the pyridoxine may not be necessary to the success of such a trial. An earlier experiment showed that magnesium supplements alone stopped the formation of stones in the people tested.

The article goes on to tell us that in laboratory rats on a diet low in magnesium bladder stones are *always* found. Calcium oxalate stones are *always* found in laboratory rats on a diet low in pyridoxine. A strongly alkaline urine and a reduced excretion of magnesium will produce stones.

A diet low in magnesium, but high in phosphorus and moderate in calcium tends to cause stone formation in kidneys and heart. This kind of diet is probably widespread in our country, for meat is high in phosphorus, which tends to overbalance the lack of magnesium (found mostly in cereal foods and bread). When all the breads and cereals you eat have had their magnesium removed, the balance between the two minerals would be thrown out of kilter.

The question of why some otherwise healthy people tend to form stones while others do not, and why the addition of magnesium and pyridoxine should stop the stone formation remains a mystery, says *Nutrition Reviews*. But there is valuable evidence that this is so. Since the therapy is completely harmless this study "should encourage its wider application," says the magazine.

Nutrition Reviews is published by the Nutrition Foundation, a trade organization of the giant food industry. It is the official position of this industry that the American food supply is totally adequate in all respects and

---

Pyridoxine Content of Some Common Foods

(We list micrograms per serving of 100 grams, which is a bit more than 3 ounces. Remember that foods like blackstrap molasses and brewer's yeast are used in much smaller amounts than this. Even so, their pyridoxine content is remarkable.)

	Micrograms
Bananas	320
Barley	320-560
Beef	230-320
Cabbage	120-290
Cod	340
Corn, yellow	360-570
Cottonseed meal	1,310
Eggs	22-48
Ham	330-580
Heart, beef	200-290
Kidney, beef	350-990
Lamb	250-370
Liver, beef	600-710

---

that it is totally impossible for any American eating "the average American diet" to be deficient in any nutrient. So one would expect that their publication would be unable to explain how two simple, essential nutrients, given in rather large amounts, might correct a long-standing disorder as serious as stone formation.

In a recent book, *Vitamin B6, The Doctor's Report*, written by Dr. John M. Ellis, the relationship of magnesium and pyridoxine is clearly shown. Dr. Ellis relates stories of his patients who suffered from a variety of disorders which yielded to magnesium and pyridoxine supplements.

One is perfectly safe in taking far more pyridoxine than the 10 milligrams these doctors gave their patients. Many

Malt extract	540
Milk, whole	54-110
Milk, dry	330-820
Milk, dry, skim	550
Molasses, blackstrap	2,000-2,490
Peanuts	300
Peas, dry	160-330
Pork	330-680
Potatoes	160-250
Rice, white	340-450
Rice, brown	1,030
Salmon, canned	450
Salmon, fresh	590
Sardines, canned	280
Soybeans	710-1,200
Tomatoes, canned	710
Tuna, canned	440
Veal	280-410
Wheat bran	1,380-1,570
Wheat germ	850-1,600
White flour	380-600
Yams	320
Yeast, brewer's	4,000-5,700

specialists are now requesting that this B vitamin be included in all contraceptive pills, since it appears that women taking these pills are bound to be short on pyridoxine. Many other conditions of ill health are seemingly related to shortage of pyridoxine, due largely, one must believe, to its almost total absence from those foods which make up half the meals of many people—white sugar and white flour and everything made from them.

If you eat a really well planned diet you are getting considerable pyridoxine. Best sources are: all kinds of liver, herring, salmon, walnuts, peanuts, wheat germ, bran, brown rice, brewers yeast and blackstrap molasses. Medium good sources are meat, especially organ meats like kidney and heart, fish, eggs, wholegrains, legumes (peas, beans, soybeans, lentils) and leafy green vegetables like kale, brussels sprouts, spinach and so on.

Keep in mind that you cannot depend on bakery bread as a source of pyridoxine. This is one of the B vitamins which disappears when white flour is made. It is never returned in the "enrichment" program. So it is missing from white flour. Most commercial bread is made largely from white flour (even the wholegrain and pumpernickel kinds) so you will get almost no pyridoxine from such bread. Make your own bread from real wholegrains available at the health food store or buy real wholegrain bread which is sold there.

Wheat germ and bran are other excellent sources which you should use to enrich every food you prepare for the table. Add them while you are cooking. Drop some into the white sauce, the soup, the meatloaf. Sprinkle them on top of whatever cereal you are eating, stir them into the oatmeal. At all costs, make certain you are getting enough pyridoxine, for the sake of your nerves, your heart, your digestion, your skin.

CHAPTER 21

Biotin, Another
B Vitamin

BIOTIN IS ONE of the lesser known B vitamins, a nutritional substance which is almost completely ignored by the official experts who decide how much of each of these nutrients we need in every day's food.

The official booklet. *Recommended Dietary Allowances,* says about biotin, "Daily needs are provided by diets containing 150-300 micrograms of biotin. This amount is provided by the average American diet." Glancing at the list of dietary sources of biotin, one wonders.

According to an article in *Chemical and Engineering News*, September 23, 1968, Cornell University scientists have discovered that biotin performs a physiological function which they had not known about before. Researchers had long suspected that the B vitamin was present in a certain enzyme (a chemical substance which manufactures an amino acid or form of protein). In this case, the amino acid is arginine, which is essential for human health.

The process by which this takes place is almost unbelievably complicated. The chemical formula for the process takes up the entire lower half of the page in the chemical magazine. However, the finding is important for biochemists to know. And it is important for health seekers to know. For it indicates, once again, that we are just beginning to unravel the extremely complex skeins of knowledge about things nutritional. There is not now and never can be a time when we can state, "Now we know all there is to know about such-and-such a vitamin." There will always be something new to discover.

In this case, only a great deal of future work will determine how important this discovery is for human health in general. For instance, the genes which control our inherited characteristics do so through enzymes. If one or another of these enzymes is absent or partially lacking in a new-born baby, there may be very serious, even fatal, consequences. So the presence of a B vitamin in an enzyme is an important discovery.

Just what does biotin do? We are not quite sure of all its functions. But it is involved in the bio-synthesis (that is, the creation in the body) of various substances essential for health. Among these are the unsaturated fats, those substances which are believed to play an important part in keeping us safe from circulatory disorders.

It is believed that the normal human intestine contains bacteria which manufacture some biotin so that it is not necessary to get all of it that we need from food. But, of course, there are many people in whom these bacteria have been destroyed wholly or partially by various digestive disorders and by taking antibiotics which destroy bacteria wholesale—the harmful and the beneficial alike. So it would certainly be wise to get plenty of biotin with everyday meals, especially if you have, during your lifetime, taken large doses of antibiotics by mouth.

The Lancet reported in its July 3, 1971 issue on a 5-month old infant brought to the hospital in serious condition. He suffered from persistent vomiting and an extensive skin rash. The rash had been present for some time and had been spreading in spite of several drugs with which the physician tried to overcome it. He tended to vomit easily, from birth. His breathing was abnormal. He appeared to have acidosis. His urine had a peculiar odor.

BIOTIN

The doctors decided he was having trouble digesting protein. So they stopped all foods and fed him intravenously. Then they began a series of elaborate tests. Just the description of the tests and their results occupies almost a page of *The Lancet*. Although the words mean little to the average layman, the doctors found that the presence of certain substances in the child's urine suggested that the activity of a certain enzyme was impaired. Biotin works with this enzyme in the complex chemistry of the body. They decided to give the child biotin.

But first they would put him back on protein food, and when his condition was "stable" they would give him massive doses of biotin. But the protein food brought near disaster. The baby went into shock; the vomiting began again. The doctors decided to give the biotin at once. They did. "The effects both clinically and biochemically were impressive," they say. The vomiting stopped. The child's breathing became normal. His blood chemistry righted itself within a day. The skin rash disappeared and did not return. The baby became a happy, responsive, well child once again.

The doctors are sure, they tell us, that the child was born with impaired ability to deal with certain processes of digestion. The biotin corrected this situation. The doctors do not know, they say, whether biotin will always cure such a condition in all children or whether it just happened this way this time.

A very interesting thing about biotin is that it is destroyed or inactivated by a protein that occurs in raw egg white. This was discovered when scientists studied animals kept on a diet of nothing but raw egg white. The animals soon became ill and were restored to health only when ample amounts of biotin were included in their meals.

It is most unusual for a human being to become wholly deficient in biotin. After all, not many of us confine our meals to nothing but raw egg white. But a total deficiency of biotin has been induced in volunteers by feeding them a diet from which all the biotin has been removed, then giving them large amounts of raw egg white. The consequences are immediately noticeable: a scaly dermatitis, a gray pallor, extreme fatigue, lack of appetite, muscle pains, insomnia, slight anemia and some heart problems.

How about using raw egg white daily? We don't recommend it. As we said above, it seems most unlikely that taking one, or even two raw eggs every day, in an eggnog, for instance, would cause any difficulty. On the other hand, many people who are given eggnogs are very sick people who don't eat much else. So it might be possible to induce at least a slight deficiency in biotin. It seems best,

Biotin Content of Some Common Foods

(We give the microgram content of a serving, which is a bit more than 3 ounces.)

Micrograms

Bananas	4
Beans, dried limas	10
Beef	4
Cauliflower	17
Corn	6
Eggs, whole (2)	25
Filberts	16
Halibut	8
Hazel nuts	14
Liver, beef	100
Milk (1 cup)	5
Mushrooms	16
Oysters	9
Peanuts	39
Pork	7
Salmon	5
Strawberries	4
Wheat, whole	5
Yeast, brewer's (3 tablespoons)	75

therefore, to use only the egg yolk when you are making eggnogs, if you plan to make them an important part of your daily meals.

Biotin is one of the B vitamins removed almost entirely from cereals and flours when they are refined to make our modern processed foods. Biotin is never restored, as are several of the other B vitamins. So anyone who relies extensively on refined cereals for the daily supply of biotin will undoubtedly suffer deficiency. It just isn't there. It *is* present, in goodly quantity, in whole grain products and, of course, in wheat germ. Brewers yeast supplies more biotin than any other food except liver.

Should you make a special effort to get this B vitamin? We think you should, especially if your meals do not include every day a plentitude of those foods which are rich in the vitamin or if you have taken antibiotics by mouth recently. Officially, it is believed you need about 150 to 200 micrograms of this vitamin daily. Check the list at left to see if your diet qualifies. If not, add a goodly portion of brewers yeast to your breakfast cereal or beverage, switch over to entirely whole grain breads and cereals, eat liver several times a week, or take a bedtime snack of a half-cup of wheat germ with milk.

CHAPTER 22

Vitamin B12,
The Red Crystal
Vitamin

AN ENGROSSING MYSTERY STORY, as good as any turned out for Perry Mason, concerns the early scientific explorations in regard to cobalt and its relationship to health and disease. The story is told in *Nutrition Reviews* for March, 1975 by Dr. E.J. Underwood, who is one of the great authorities in the field of minerals and trace minerals, and author of *Trace Elements in Human and Animal Nutrition*.

Cobalt is a trace mineral, a silver-white metallic element which occurs usually along with silicon, which is used to give a certain blue color to ceramics. Not much information that would lead one to suspect that human beings just can't get along without cobalt—an amount of cobalt so small that it seems infinitesimal. But there it is. We must have that tiny bit of cobalt.

The need of animals for cobalt was established in the mystery story which Dr. Underwood tells entertainingly. Australian sheep and cattle began to fall prey to a mysterious illness about 50 years ago. It was called "coast disease" or "wasting disease." The animals wasted away and died, destroyed by a kind of anemia which could not be cured except by giving them huge amounts of crude iron salts and ores. Well, it's iron deficiency anemia, said the experts.

But Dr. Underwood and a colleague thought it was strange that so much of the crude iron ore should be necessary to cure simple anemia. So they prepared an extract of the ores with all the iron removed. And it cured the animals' disease! So obviously the cure must be something else in the ore that was missing from the animals' diets—some trace mineral perhaps. And it was—cobalt, which was present in small amounts in the crude iron ore.

But somebody then discovered that giving whole liver to animals also cured the wasting disease. Ah ha, said the experts, it's the cobalt in the liver that does this trick. They removed the cobalt from the liver and gave it to the sick animals as pure cobalt and got no results. "This led to the suggestion," says Dr. Underwood, "that the potency of liver was due to the presence of a stored factor and that cobalt functions through the production of this factor within the body" of the animals in question. In other words, the animals had to have the cobalt in order to produce something else that they stored in their livers. And it was that "something else" which cured the animals.

It took eleven years for workers in laboratories in many parts of the world to discover that the "something else" was vitamin B12 which is the only vitamin that contains a trace mineral. That trace mineral is cobalt. You cannot make vitamin B12 without it. But you need only a tiny amount of cobalt. In the case of ruminant animals (cattle and sheep), the cobalt is necessary so that they can manufacture their own vitamin B12 in their very complicated digestive systems. So actually involved here are three things—cobalt and the intestinal bacteria of the cattle and sheep which together can produce the vitamin B12 without which the animals will die. They must have both the cobalt and the well-functioning intestinal bacteria to produce the vitamin.

But human beings cannot manufacture vitamin B12 in their intestines for they have an entirely different kind of intestinal mechanism. So they must get their vitamin B12 in the form of a vitamin. And it must, of course, contain cobalt. It doesn't matter at all whether the food we eat every day contains any cobalt as such. But it must contain some vitamin B12 or we will not survive. According to Dr. Henry Schroeder, another specialist in mineral nutrition, only one microgram (one-millionth of a gram) of vitamin B12 "can make the difference between life and death from pernicious anemia." But we must have that one-millionth of a gram. Pernicious anemia is fatal without it.

Fruits, vegetables and cereals contain almost none of their cobalt in the form of vitamin B12. This suggests that it is potentially dangerous to eat a diet of completely vegetarian foods, since fruits and vegetables are the only foods, along with seeds, that one could eat. We must depend on food of animal origin for most of our vitamin B12. Consider, for instance, that an excellent food like wholegrain bread contains only 0.2 micrograms of vitamin B12. That is two-tenths of one-millionth of one gram. Carrots rich in vitamin A contain only 0.1 micrograms of vitamin B12. Beef contains up to 4.5 micrograms per serving and liver contains as much as 120 micrograms per serving. Beef kidney as much as 55 micrograms. Fish may contain up to one and a half micrograms. We counsel vegetarians to include some food of animal origin in their meals—dairy products and eggs, for example.

If there is cobalt in the food we eat, we absorb it and, says Dr. Underwood, "why man and the rat should absorb far more cobalt than they can possibly use is unknown, unless a function for this element exists, in addition to its role in vitamin B12, which has yet to be discovered."

This is an extremely important statement, for it suggests that nutrition experts are only at the beginning of their discoveries in relation to food elements and health, especially where trace elements are concerned. They do not know, and may not know for many years, if ever, just what we use cobalt for in our bodies aside from that which is essential for life in the form of vitamin B12.

There seems to be no chance of any of us getting too much cobalt, although a peculiar incident several years ago demonstrated that, under certain circumstances cobalt could cause severe heart failure in people who drank lots of beer! This story involves another masterpiece of sleuthing by scientific detectives in their laboratories. They discovered that, in localities where the heart failures were occurring, cobalt was being used to improve the foaming of the beer.

But even drinking 24 pints of beer daily would give a dedicated beer drinker about eight milligrams of cobalt, an amount well below what is potentially toxic. Up to three hundred milligrams daily have been given for various conditions by doctors without any toxicity. "It seems that high cobalt and high alcohol intakes are both necessary," says Dr. Underwood, "to induce the distinctive cardiomyopathy, plus a third factor which may be low dietary protein or thiamine deficiency (a B vitamin)."

So once again we marvel at the astounding complexity of everything involved in nutrition. Cobalt is harmless in almost any practical amounts unless you happen to get it in combination with alcohol. And then it may not affect you adversely unless you happen also to be eating too little high protein foods and too few foods that contain thiamine. It seems to us there's a good lesson here. Our food today contains up to 10,000 chemicals added either purposely (as the cobalt was added to beer) or accidentally as in the case of chemicals which migrate from plastic wrapping into food. Nobody, literally, has any idea of what life-threatening situations might arise as a result of getting one or several, let alone 10,000 of such chemicals every day in combination with other factors to which one innocently exposes one's self.

The beer-drinkers did not know they were drinking cobalt with their beer. And we do not know what mixture of additives we may be getting in any new product that appears on the supermarket shelves, let alone any of the old products we've been using for years. The reasons why such additives may damage one person and not another are evident in the above story. The person who is damaged may be getting too little protein or too few B vitamins to withstand the effects of the chemical additive. The cocktail, the cigarette or the rich dessert he has for dinner may be the very thing that could trigger some harmful activity like the heart attacks which sickened the beer drinkers.

The lesson is—make every mouthful of food count for good nutrition. Don't eat or drink anything that does not contribute its share of nutrients. Protein is the food element most likely to be lacking. You will certainly get enough carbohydrate and fat in any fairly representative American diet. But you must watch protein to be certain you get enough of it. The foods high in protein are, generally speaking the ones which contain the most B vitamins and vitamin E. These are all foods of animal origin: meat, poultry, fish, eggs, dairy products plus seed foods which include wholegrain cereals, breads, nuts, peanuts and all seeds like sunflower and squash seeds. Fruit and vegetables are valuable mostly for their vitamin A and C content as well as many minerals.

There are some nearly miraculous stories about the power of a serving of liver or a few tablets of desiccated liver to improve health. In most cases it may be the vitamin B12 (including cobalt) content of the liver which brings this increased well-being. It may be the large amounts of iron which liver contains in combination with the vitamin B12. It may be the other B vitamins in liver for it is a powerhouse of B vitamins, containing more of most of them than any other food. It may be the vitamin A in liver—as much as 75,000 units in a single serving. It may be the vitamin C which contributes up to 36 milligrams per serving.

Most probably it is the combination of all these high quality nutrients plus (remember Dr. Underwood's statement about cobalt?) all those nutrients which liver may contain that have not as yet been investigated in laboratories which may play extremely important roles in good health.

Keep all these things in mind when you go shopping. Make sure your family gets liver at least once a week. Serve it to them disguised in any way, if they refuse to eat it broiled, baked or fried. Add onions or bacon. Make it into a dip or a chopped liver sandwich with plenty of seasonings. Slip it into meatloaf or hamburgers without mentioning it to the family. But get it into them.

The alternative is desiccated liver which is liver with nothing removed but the water it naturally contains. It is available in tasteless tablets, capsules or powder at your health food store. And don't forget that the one other important element in this detective story is the intestinal bacteria of the Australian cattle involved in the first part of the mystery. Scientists have as yet only the vaguest notion of all the things that go on inside our own digestive systems, in which our own intestinal bacteria are concerned.

Vitamin B12 is one of the most recently discovered and studied of all the B vitamins. "The fifth of May is still celebrated as 'red crystal day' in my laboratory—the date in 1948 when the first microscopic crystals appeared of vitamin B12 isolated from liver. This newest vitamin still excites great interest among scientists," says British scientist Dr. E. Lester Smith in an article in *New Scientist* for June 11, 1964. Dr. Smith, one of the world's foremost authorities on vitamin B12 goes on to give us some facts on this most remarkable curative agent. It seems that there is a certain substance called the "intrinsic factor," present in the normal stomach, which allows the healthy person to absorb vitamin B12 from food. When this substance is lacking, the individual cannot absorb vitamin B12, so he develops pernicious anemia. This is the reason why injections of the vitamin may be required for a cure. Taking it by mouth would not accomplish a cure since it would not be absorbed in these patients. We are told, however, that huge doses of the vitamin permit some of it to be absorbed even in persons whose stomachs apparently lack the important "intrinsic factor."

Gastroenterology reported in 1962 that laboratory rats

on a diet deficient in iron soon lost their ability to absorb vitamin B12. It is true, too, that people suffering from some chronic condition that does not permit them to absorb their food properly will almost inevitably be lacking in vitamin B12. This means sufferers from diarrhea, dysentery, sprue, and people who have had part of their digestive tract removed.

The nervous and mental symptoms accompanying vitamin B12 deficiency have become so common that medical journals are quite concerned about them. Says a letter to the editor of the British *Lancet*, October 9, 1965 "It is now generally recognized that vitamin B12 deficiency may be present with a wide variety of psychiatric (that is, mental illness) manifestations and without anemia or gross neurological disturbances for months or years." This London physician went on to recommend that all patients admitted to mental hospitals be tested for vitamin B12 deficiency, even if they showed no signs of anemia.

Two groups of people especially susceptible to this deficiency are those who have been treated with certain drugs. It is possible, says this expert, that patients may have none of the classic signs of anemia, yet still be deficient enough in vitamin B12 to have symptoms of mental illness. It is, of course, perfectly possible to be deficient in vitamin B12 simply because you do not eat foods that contain it.

The *Journal of the American Medical Association*, October 11, 1965, stated in an editorial, "Although vitamin B12 deficiency is now well recognized and both the (blood) and (nerve) symptoms respond to treatment with cyano-cobalamin (vitamin B12), patients with this deficiency are still common."

There are many stories in medical journals and books of other uses made of vitamin B12 in the treatment of disease. It has been used with some success in treating neuralgias and neuritis. It has been used for bursitis. One doctor reports excellent results using vitamin B12 for psoriasis. He used 30 injection of 1,000 micrograms each before results were obtained.

He reported on this experiment in the *British Medical Journal* for January 12, 1963. In all these cases, the vitamin is being used as a drug—that is, in amounts which have little relation to the amounts you might get in food. We have no explanation for why the vitamin produces these results. Indeed, some critics say the improvement was not the result of the vitamin, for any injection would have produced improvement. We do not know.

How much vitamin B12 do you need every day and how can you be sure you are getting it? Officially, Americans are told they should have from one microgram (for infants) up to six micrograms daily (for an adult man). Pernicious anemia victims sometimes receive injections of 100 micrograms every day, although injected doses of as much as 30,000 micrograms have been given without any

---

Vitamin B12 Content of Some Common Foods

(We give the number of micrograms in 100 grams, the average serving)

	Micrograms
Beef, kidney	18-55
Beef, liver	31-120
Beef, round	3.4-4.5
Bread, whole wheat	0.2-0.4
Cheese, American	0.6
Cheese, Swiss	0.9
Egg, 1 whole	0.3
Fish, haddock	0.6
Fish, sole	1.3
Ham	0.9-1.6
Milk, whole	0.3-0.5
Milk, powdered	1-2.6
Soybean meal	0.2

unpleasant reactions.

Adelle Davis, in *Let's Get Well* says she believes that strict vegetarians who eat no food at all of animal origin should probably take 50 micrograms of vitamin B12 each week "while their stomach secretions are still normal." She also suggests that, of vegetable foods, only yeast, wheat germ and soy bean contain appreciable traces of vitamin B12—another good reason for making these foods the basis of a vegetarian diet, as well as including them in ample quantities in any kind of a diet.

The chart on page 177 shows you the amount of vitamin B12 in some common foods.

CHAPTER 23

Folic Acid
Is Found Chiefly
in Foliage

SOME YEARS AGO a physician experimented on himself to find out whether the B vitamin folic acid can be manufactured in the human intestine or whether it must be obtained in food. Dr. Victor Herbert, then at Boston City Hospital put himself on a diet from which all folic acid was removed. He did this by boiling all his food three times. The heat and moisture involved in this process virtually destroyed not only all the folic acid but most other vitamins as well.

Then he took plenty of all other vitamins in a capsule so that any nutritional difficulties he encountered would be certain to arise from folic acid deficiency. They began very soon. After three weeks the level of folic acid in his blood was low. At the end of seven weeks the first signs of abnormality in his blood appeared. After he had been on the deficient diet for 16 weeks, he became sleepless, forgetful and increasingly irritable. He lost weight. By the 19th week his bone marrow showed unmistakable changes in the cells, indicating absence of folic acid.

He took some folic acid in a tablet. Within 48 hours his bone marrow tests returned to normal, his mental symptoms cleared up. He believes that this test proves that human beings must get folic acid in their meals or they will eventually develop the perhaps fatal anemia that characterizes this deficiency. Not many of us boil our food three times in an effort to induce a deficiency of folic acid. But, as you think over the diets of your friends and neighbors, perhaps you have observed some which qualify as diets very low in folic acid. The vitamin is easily destroyed by both boiling and sunlight.

Other symptoms of the anemia which occurs when folic acid is lacking are these: weakness, loss of appetite, diminished vigor. Also digestive disturbance—flatulence, impaired absorption of food, and diarrhea. Skin and tissues of the mouth, gums, tongue and eyes are pale. Eventually there is breathlessness, fatigue and, because of the reduced number of oxygen-carrying red blood cells, heart damage and eventual death. A little dose of folic acid can end all these symptoms very quickly.

Alcoholics suffer from deficiency in folic acid. In some startling experiments, Dr. Herbert and a colleague tested alcoholic patients by giving them a few drinks in the hospital. First they cured the anemia of the alcoholics, then they gave them daily doses of alcoholic drinks. Within 10 days the bone marrow symptoms of folic acid deficiency appeared again.

The physicians gave folic acid. It did no good, so long as the men went on drinking. By discontinuing the alcohol or by giving very large doses of folic acid the physicians could prevent the anemia from returning. They finally got to the point where they could tell exactly how much alcohol every day would result in severe impairment of bone marrow. They believe that one reason alcoholics improve in a hospital is that alcohol is unavailable and folic acid is available in the hospital diet.

Arthritis patients have been found to be lacking in folic acid. Diets that are not nourishing, increased need for folic acid because of the arthritis, or possibly increased demand because of the aspirin taken by the patient may be reasons for this. No one knows. Patients with many kinds of skin disorders are also found to be deficient in folic acid.

But pregnant women are most likely to show this deficiency. Apparently the unborn child uses up whatever folic acid is available in the mother, and the health of the mother suffers. We are told that studies of folic acid lack in pregnancy may explain many cases of "spontaneous" abortions, miscarriages and hemorrhaging in pregnancy. No one is certain whether the deficiency in folic acid is only one part of a disturbed state of health or whether it is the folic acid deficiency that directly triggers the health disasters.

One London physician stated that about 60 percent of all pregnant women are unable to meet the demands for folic acid in pregnancy. He based his conclusions on studies of 154 pregnant women. Those who were also deficient in iron suffered the most. The iron deficiency sometimes concealed the lack of folic acid. Sometimes giving folic acid prevented both deficiencies. The pregnant women's anemias responded quickly to injections of folic acid given every other day for six doses.

By 1969 the *Journal of the American Medical Association* was printing articles on folic acid deficiency in women on The Pill. By 1973 the *Journal* reported megaloblastic changes in women on The Pill in the lining of the cervix, similar to those found in folic acid deficiency. Nineteen percent of 115 women taking The Pill had these symptoms—of "severe" folic acid deficiency. Such changes were not observed in other women on The Pill. Examining the blood of these women did not disclose any apparent deficiency. It seemed to be localized in the tissues of the cervical area.

The authors of the *Journal* article point out that changes such as they found in the cervix of their patients are sometimes mistaken by doctors for pre-cancerous changes. But just giving folic acid repaired the damage in a short time. Seventeen to 21 percent of their patients had low levels of folic acid in their blood, but, they say, women who do not have these typical stigmata also have low levels of folic acid in their blood.

They say that there are strong associations between folic acid and sex hormones. It's possible, they say, that oral contraceptives act to cause the body to use up its store of folic acid more rapidly and this is why so many women taking The Pill are short on this important B vitamin. Women who get serious anemia from the folic acid lack following The Pill may be extreme instances of a body condition which is apparently much more prevalent when it is localized in the cervix.

The Lancet for April 14, 1973 tells us that infants have far greater need for folic acid than adults. Premature babies are thought to need about 10 times more folic acid than adults. So early childhood is a time when folic acid deficiencies are very likely to show up, says the *Lancet* editorial. Premature babies tend to develop megaloblastic anemia when they are from 6 to 8 weeks old. Perhaps they should be getting this B vitamin routinely, say the authors.

Other children are also at risk from this kind of deficiency. Babies who develop digestive problems, pneumonia or some other infection, those who have iron deficiency anemia, or scurvy or conditions of malnutrition are more apt to suffer, too, from folic acid lack. They point out that an exclusive diet of goat's milk may produce such a condition since goat's milk has less folic acid than cow's milk. Children on special diets, those with diseases that reduce their appetites or their absorption of food or diseases which increase their need for folic acid—all these may show evidence of deficiency.

Here are some conditions that produce such deficiency: sickle-cell anemia, thalassemia major, hereditary spherocytosis, and celiac disease. Testing for folic acid deficiency is a good test for celiac disease. Epileptics taking anticonvulsant drugs are also at high risk when it comes to folic acid. Heart disease in children may produce folic acid deficiency. Congenital or rheumatic heart disease are two of such conditions in which deficiency is often found.

Apparently low levels of folic acid may harm the brain, so it is wise to discover the deficiency early and give the vitamin, say the authors.

The amount of folic acid you can get in a food supplement is limited by the FDA because of a peculiar quirk in its relationship to vitamin B12. Lack of either of these vitamins produces a similar kind of anemia. The anemia caused by lack of vitamin B12 produces some serious nerve symptoms which are not caused by lack of folic acid. So if the doctor apparently cures the anemia by giving folic acid, a deficiency in vitamin B12 may still continue and destroy nerve tissues before it is discovered. It seems obvious that the best way to prevent this is to supply supplements which contain both vitamins. But the easy, practical way is never the way doctors and the FDA decide to do things.

So the only answer is to make sure you are getting enough of both vitamins along with all the other vitamins of the B complex or group. Foods richest in folic acid are these: Liver, first and foremost. It contains three or four times more folic acid than any other food. Give it to your family at least once a week, oftener if possible. If they refuse to eat it, devise original ways of preparing or camouflaging it so they will enjoy it. Or give them desiccated liver tablets.

The second most abundant source of folic acid is yeast— brewer's yeast. In many of the experiments described in literature about folic acid, yeast extract was given as the sole source of folic acid and successfully prevented deficiency. Get your brewer's yeast at the health food store.

Other good sources are wheat bran, wholegrain cereals and green leafy vegetables of all kinds. Best among these are the dark green ones—spinach, kale, escarole, turnip greens, watercress and so on. Asparagus and cucumbers, cauliflower, cabbage, broccoli and beans of all kinds are good sources. Cottage cheese contains folic acid.

Breast feeding, surely the best way to feed infants, can easily prevent folic acid deficiency in the baby only if the mother's diet has provided enough folic acid. One mother was reported who lost three breast-fed babies to megalo-blastic anemia. The fourth developed anemia at 14 weeks. The mother was given plenty of folic acid during her next four pregnancies and had four more healthy children.

It is especially distressing to find, in the *Journal of the American Medical Association* for October 5, 1970, an article by a Florida physician who says that folic acid deficiency has been found among women taking oral

Folic Acid Content of Some Common Foods

(We list micrograms per serving of 100 grams)

	Micrograms
Almonds	46
Apricots, fresh	3.6
Apricots, dried	4.7
Asparagus	89-140
Avocados	4-57
Barley	50
Beans, Lima, fresh	10-56
Beans, Lima, dry	100
Beans, Navy, dry	130
Beef, round steak	7-17
Beef, liver	290
Beef, kidney	58
Blackberries	6-18
Bread, rye	20
Bread, wheat	27
Bread, white	15
Broccoli	34
Brussels sprouts	27
Buttermilk	11
Cabbage	6-42
Cauliflower	29
Cheese, cheddar	15
Cheese, cottage	21-46

contraceptives. It appears that the drug shuts off some mechanism which is essential for them to absorb the vitamin from food. Dr. Richard R. Streiff tells us of seven women who came to his clinic with anemia. They had been taking no drugs except contraceptives which they had been taking regularly for at least 1½ years. They had been eating good diets, he says, but their bone marrow showed evidence of megaloblastic anemia, which is the condition

Coconut	28
Corn, sweet	9-70
Dates	25
Egg, 1 whole	5.1
Egg, yolk	13
Endive	27-63
Flour, enriched white	8.1
Flour, rye	18
Flour, whole wheat	38
Ham, smoked	7.8
Kale	50.9
Lentils, dry	99
Lettuce	4-54
Liver, beef	290
Liver, chicken	380
Liver, lamb	280
Liver, pork	220
Mushrooms	14-29
Oats	23-66
Peanuts	57
Peas	5-35
Potatoes	2-130
Rice, brown	22
Spinach	49-110
Tangerines	7.4
Turnip greens	83
Watercress	48
Wheat	27-51
Zucchini	11

associated with serious lack of folic acid.

By complicated tests, this doctor discovered that the folic acid given these women in a dietary supplement was absorbed. But that form of the vitamin which appeared in food had to be processed by some body mechanism which apparently did not work when the women were taking oral contraceptives.

In another story (*Journal of American Medical Association*, November 30, 1970), we are told of the families of three physicians (all quite affluent) where the young daughters of the family suffered from lack of folic acid and were anemic. In every case the family was large and their eating habits were irregular, since the father had very irregular hours. Says the author, "Small families usually consume prepared meals together whereas large families often eat food which they select as individuals or in small groups. Frequently this unsupervised diet . . . contains much carbohydrate, with few leafy vegetables and little protein. Since carbohydrate foods usually contain only small amounts of iron and folic acid, members of large families without organized eating habits may develop iron and folic acid deficiency." If doctors cannot discover and correct such deficiency in their own families and ferret out the reasons for it, how can they be expected to perform such a service for their patients?

In the *New England Journal of Medicine* for June 9, 1966, a Connecticut physician writes to complain about the fact that folic acid is usually not in nutritional supplements given to pregnant women. He tells of three women at his clinic suffering from the megaloblastic anemia which is typical of folic acid deficiency. One of them died. She had not sought the aid of a doctor during her pregnancy. Possibly a doctor would have discovered the deficiency and could have saved her life.

The importance of liver and wholegrain cereals and breads is once again highlighted here. White bread contains 15 micrograms of folic acid compared to 27 for cracked wheat and 100 for a like amount of bran. A serving of liver contains 290 micrograms of folic acid compared to only 5 for a hamburger.

One physician from the University of California is quoted in *New Scientist* for September 11, 1969 as saying he believes that folic acid deficiency is the commonest vitamin deficiency in the world, affecting especially elderly people and pregnant women. Don't slight this vitamin! Plan menus with plenty of wholegrain cereals, dark green leafy vegetables (raw or cooked), and liver.

CHAPTER 24

Pantothenic Acid

ROGER J. WILLIAMS, Ph.D., could be called the father of modern vitamin therapy. In his laboratory at the University of Texas, he has done more work than any other biologist on many vitamins, especially two of the B vitamins. He named both of them—pantothenic acid and folic acid.

Forty years ago, discovering a hitherto unidentified substance in yeast, Dr. Williams tested it and found that it qualified as a B vitamin. He named it pantothenic acid, meaning "available everywhere" that is, in all food and all cells. And at first it seemed that this B vitamin was so plentiful in food that no such thing as a deficiency could ever exist.

But Dr. Williams was not content with just discovering and naming the vitamin. He went on with a lifetime of experiments, observations and theorizing until he accumulated a vast body of information about this vitamin. He covers much of this in a new book, *Physician's Handbook of Nutritional Science*. He tells us this B vitamin is part of an enzyme system which is essential for all living organisms as well as many plants.

Says Dr. Williams, "These maintenance chemicals (like pantothenic acid) are never found ready-packaged in ideal proportions for us or for any other organisms. Living with our nutritional environment and adapting to it is an exacting task worthy of our serious attention...in line with nature's plan we must strive and use our intelligence if we are to get a really good assortment for ourselves and our children."

In a well-designed test Dr. Williams discovered the effect of pantothenic acid on the production of normal young among his laboratory rats. Giving them 30 to 35 micrograms of this vitamin a day resulted in 38 percent of normal births; giving 40 to 45 micrograms per day produced 72 percent normal births; giving 50 micrograms per day produced 95.5 percent normal births in the experimental animals. Now he believes that 100 micrograms of the B vitamin would probably produce much better results. In our country where the incidence of children who are defective at birth is way out of line with our income and health expenditures, these early observations on pantothenic acid are vitally significant.

Chickens suffer from "chick dermatitis" which Dr. Williams quickly cured with pantothenic acid. The unhealthy skin and feathers came back to health almost miraculously. This suggests, does it not, that human beings might greatly improve their own hair and skin by getting enough and more than enough of this B vitamin. "The skin," says Dr. Williams, "partly because circulation does not supply it with copious nutrition, is notoriously sensitive to nutritional lacks. In the oral cavity—the tongue, lips and gums—we find a favorite region where nutritionists look to detect evidence of malnutrition."

Dr. Williams tells two engrossing stories later in his book, both concerned with pantothenic acid. One concerns a retired army nurse who took added pantothenic acid for no special reason except that she thought it might benefit her. She delightedly reported to Dr. Williams that the extra vitamin had darkened her graying hair and had remarkably improved her failing memory. Her career as a nurse had ended because of this failing memory. She could not remember what days or hours she was to be on duty. Later, after retirement, she was in an accident and had to give testimony in court. Her memory of every detail of this event was so good that the judge complimented her for her excellent remembrance, resulting in such concise testimony. This, she said, must be due to pantothenic acid.

Another friend of Dr. Williams always experienced allergic symptoms when crossing a Western desert in a car. One day, just to experiment, he took an additional 20 milligrams of the B vitamin. He has done so ever since and has no more allergic symptoms. Dr. Williams reports that a drug company experimenting with pantothenic acid, could not produce these same results in all allergic people, so they dropped their investigation and nothing further came of it. It seems to us that anyone suffering from allergy has nothing to lose and perhaps much to gain by taking added pantothenic acid just to see if it may affect the allergy helpfully.

Another friend conquered lifelong constipation with added pantothenic acid, he reported to Dr. Williams. And every time he stopped taking the vitamin the constipation returned. Dr. Williams does not use this as the basis for a "miracle cure." Instead he says, wisely, "It does not require a long leap of the imagination to conclude that probably in many other individuals similar benefits could be derived if the nutritional environment could be improved in other ways."

One other story which Dr. Williams says he thought so "outlandish" that he could not believe it, but he knows that it did happen—a man with malodorous feet began to take a comprehensive supplement and shortly found that all foot odor had disappeared, to such an extent that he could now wear the same socks for four days without washing, and with no perceptible odor. "Of course," says Dr. Williams, "we know that body odors are the product of metabolism and if nutritional adjustments can alter the metabolism, there is no reason to suppose that body odors could not also be substantially altered."

Dr. Williams discovered that the richest source of pantothenic acid in nature is royal jelly which is the food fed to the bee larva to change it into a queen bee. Without royal jelly the larva would develop into a sterile worker bee living a short busy life. With the royal jelly she becomes a queen who lives for several years and produces many thousands of fertile eggs. Could the pantothenic acid in royal jelly be responsible for all this?

Feeding hens extra pantothenic acid improved the hatchability of their eggs. Giving it to rats and mice increased the size of their litters. Dr. Williams believes that giving pantothenic acid to pregnant women would improve the health of their offspring and lessen the incidence of birth deformities, or mentally retarded children. This theory has never been tested.

Dr. Williams reviews the work of a British physician who gave royal jelly and pantothenic acid to a number of arthritic patients and got excellent results in alleviating their painful symptoms. Dr. Williams believes that long-term, carefully controlled trials of this vitamin for this purpose should be made.

He does not talk in terms of miracle foods. He states that pantothenic acid is found in every cell. So not getting enough of it might influence the course of many different kinds of disorders. The following ailments have been reported in the presence of pantothenic acid deficiency: dermatitis and keratitis (skin conditions), ulcers in the digestive tract, intussusceptions (the collapse of parts of the intestine), anemia, white hair, depigmentation of tooth enamel, sterility, congenital malformations, defects in the contractibility of the bowel, failure to produce antibodies (which protect from infections), hemorrhages in the adrenal glands, spinal cord disorders, dehydration, fatty liver, troubles with the thymus gland, kidney damage, heart damage, sudden death without warning, bone marrow deficiency, lack of white blood corpuscles, spinal curvatures, degeneration of the myelin sheaths of the nerves, uncoordinated gait, decreased longevity, allergies, headache, loss of memory and decreased resistance to stress.

This is quite an impressive list of disorders. Each

statement is carefully documented. "A careful consideration of these facts . . . leads us to recognize pantothenic acid
deficiency as leading to not only a systemic disease but to a
generalized cytopathy (disease of cells) capable of
damaging and incapacitating any and every structure in the
entire body," says Dr. Williams. This kind of disorder is
different from any he has ever seen described, he says.

He points out that the deficiency might take a quite
different course in each individual, since we are all different
in make-up and some of us may need far far more of any
nutrient than others need. "No two individuals would be
expected to suffer the same damage."

Most children get a bad start these days by being fed
formula rather than breast milk. In human milk the ratio
between the pantothenic acid content and the thiamine
(vitamin B1) content is about twice that of cow's milk. So
most of our babies start out with less pantothenic acid than
they would get from breast milk. It has always been
assumed, says Dr. Williams, that we get enough pantothenic acid, even though some of us may need as little as five
milligrams a day and others 25 or more milligrams for best
performance. In animals mild deficiencies may occur when
the animals appear to be healthy.

What about longevity? Dr. Williams fed two groups of
mice in his laboratory on commercial chow. To one group
he gave in their water some pantothenic acid. These mice
lived almost 20 percent longer than the first group in spite
of the fact that the commercial chow was very well planned
to contain "ample" pantothenic acid. Adding still more
brought about this quite considerable lengthening of life. "I
would be willing to wager," says Dr. Williams, "that if a
similar experiment were done with human beings the
results would be comparable . . . human beings are probably unusually susceptible to pantothenic acid deficiency."

Dr. Williams is not a physician, so he cannot conduct
large-scale tests on human beings. The best he can do is to
suggest such tests to the physician readers of this book. One
can only hope that many physicians do read it and take his

message to heart. The book is short, direct and written with the elegant clarity and wisdom which are the hallmarks of this great biologist. Dr. Williams is easily 50 years ahead of his time. It is our privilege to learn of his theories and profit by them now in our lifetime.

There is no official dietary allowance for pantothenic acid, since the scientists who decide these things think most of us get enough in "the average diet." They state that 10 milligrams daily is "probably enough for an adult." Dr. Williams believes that we should be taking at least 15 milligrams in a daily supplement along with whatever we get at meals.

Foods supplying the most pantothenic acid are these: Animal organ meats, chiefly liver, brain, heart and kidney; eggs; wheat germ, bran, dried peas, peanuts, brewers yeast, royal jelly. Foods that supply a bit less of this B vitamin: salmon, clams, mackerel, walnuts, broccoli, soybeans, oats, lima beans, cauliflower, peas, avocado, carrots, kale, dried lentils, spinach, rice, meat of all kinds, mushrooms, wheat and cheese. Foods which are lowest in this B vitamin are: fruits, onion, cabbage, lettuce, peppers, potatoes, turnips, watercress, almonds, oysters, lobster, shrimp, milk and honey.

Pantothenic acid is important in the body's use of cholesterol and other fatty substances. It is involved in so many processes that deficiency produces widely varied symptoms: apathy, depression, instability of heart action, abdominal pains, increased susceptibility to infections, impaired function of the adrenal glands which help one to respond to stress, nerve disorders which may produce muscle weakness and "pins and needles" in hands and legs. This B vitamin is present in many foods, but all that part of one's diet consisting of white flour and white sugar products is bound to be deficient in this important vitamin, for it just does not exist in these foods. It has been removed in the processing.

An answer and a treatment for the enigma of rheumatism or arthritis may be discovered soon in the work of three London scientists who have, they believe, related the disease to a lack of pantothenic acid in the blood.

Every vitamin, mineral and other food substance becomes involved in extremely complicated chemical changes while it is being digested and made into energy or cell structure in the body. During this process, the London researchers theorize, something is missing which the arthritic individual requires in order to use this B vitamin effectively.

They tested the blood of normal people and arthritics for its pantothenic acid content. In a healthy person they found that the level is about 107 micrograms in a given measure, where in arthritics it averages only 68.7 micrograms. In fact, they found, says *Medical World News* for October 7, 1966, that any patient with less than 95 micrograms showed some symptoms of arthritis. And the lower the level of B vitamin, the more severe the symptoms.

In other tests, they found that several other substances which are closely involved with pantothenic acid in digestion were also at abnormally low levels in arthritics. They injected into their patients these substances that were missing. They gave daily injections of pantothenic acid for one month. There were no results. No improvement.

But the doctors were not so easily discouraged. They were sure some other substance must be missing, too. "We had one clue as to what this might be," said one of the scientists. "The richest natural source of pantothenic acid is royal jelly, the larval food of the queen bee." Royal Jelly is also the richest source of another substance with the complicated name of 10-hydroxy-delta 2-descenoic acid.

The physicians injected pantothenic acid along with royal jelly into 20 of their rheumatoid arthritic patients. In 14 there was improvement of their symptoms. They were able to move more easily and other symptoms characteristic of the disease disappeared, so long as the patients continued to take the injections. Later, the doctors found a cheaper substitute for the very expensive and rare substance in royal jelly. And they found they could get results by giving this substance along with pantothenic acid, by mouth rather than injection.

Working with osteoarthritc patients, they added a substance called cysteine to the pantothenic acid and got excellent results with these patients, too. How much did they give? They had no guidelines to go by. So they experimented until they found the dosage that produced results.

Sometimes results were slow in coming. There seemed to be no improvement at all for the first four to eight weeks. But, says one of the doctors, "Just when the patient is deciding that the cure is no good, the symptoms disappear overnight."

The treatment must be maintained indefinitely or the symptoms return. But this leaves the arthritic in no worse conditon than the diabetic who must take insulin indefinitely. If he could prevent the agonizing symptoms of this extremely painful disease, he should surely be willing to swallow a few pills every day from now on.

For a long time health seekers have been sure there is something extremely valuable in royal jelly, which is the food fed to the queen bee larva which causes her to hatch as queen rather than a worker bee—an entirely different kind of bee. Scientists in many countries are studying royal jelly constantly, analyzing it and breaking it down into its parts, then testing these on animals. Now, because of the fine work of these three British researchers, we know that royal jelly contains a substance which, given along with pantothenic acid, will help the rheumatoid arthritis patient to use this vitamin correctly and hence to recover from symptoms of illness. And we know that osteoarthritis patients can gain relief of symptoms by taking the B vitamin along with another substance which apparently helps the body to use it.

We do not know whether this inability to use a B vitamin is inherited or occurs because of some other reason—years of poorly chosen diet, for instance. Or perhaps a much greater than average need for the vitamin over many years. Nor do we know how soon American doctors will begin to use this form of treatment for their arthritis patients, who, at present, are generally told just to take aspirin for relief of their pain.

What we do know is that, once again, natural foods and vitamins have been shown to be curative, apparently because a disease is triggered by the body's misuse of a certain important nutrient. We can hope that eventually scientists will finally unravel all the complex threads of the various steps in digestion, assimilation and absorption, so that we can prevent conditions like this before they arise.

A Japanese medical journal reported early in 1966 an investigation of the diet in one region in Japan where the people eat "washed" rice as a staple. It was found that the blood of these people is lacking in pantothenic acid. Apparently, this vitamin washes away when the rice is processed. Looking further, the researchers discovered that these folks had higher blood pressure than people in other parts of Japan where this B vitamin is not lacking in diet. Could it be that pantothenic acid is important in maintaining correct blood pressure? The Japanese doctors believe so.

In the December 8, 1971 issue of *Medical Tribune*, a biochemist from the University of Pittsburgh, speaking at a symposium on "Nutrition and the Future of Man" said that two B vitamins are essential for the production and transportation in the human body of antibodies—that is those materials which protect us from infections.

The two vitamins are pyridoxine and pantothenic acid. In any individual who does not have enough of these vitamins in his body, the production of antibodies will be decreased. They will not circulate in the blood to accomplish their biological purpose which is to destroy harmful bacteria.

In addition, lack of pyridoxine tends to make one sensitive to various allergy-producing substances. When animals lack pyridoxine their bodies are inefficient in manufacturing protein and nucleic acids, both of which are essential to life.

When animals lack pantothenic acid, there seems to be deficiency in the way the body transports proteins from where they are created inside cells to the outside where they are needed.

Dr. Williams' new book, *Nutrition Against Disease*, talks of "supernutrition"—getting more than one appears to need of all the vitamins and minerals for "superhealth."

This book is a wise, helpful account of many ways in which an abundance of highly nutritious foods and food supplements might improve health, prevent countless disorders, bring indeed a state of well-being never before experienced by living things on the planet.

For Dr. Williams says that no plant or animal in nature actually has optimum nutrition. It is always possible to improve it using the knowledge we have at present. For human beings the benefits that might be won from using this knowledge are almost limitless, for no human being either is getting all that he might need in the way of vitamins, minerals, proteins, essential fats and so on. If doctors could be persuaded to use "supernutrition" as their foremost weapon for preventing disease, we might wipe out world-wide plagues, prevent the birth of damaged and mentally deficient children and bring a whole new concept of health and well-being to the world.

Dr. Williams is perfectly aware of the fact that doctors at present know almost nothing about nutrition and are severely criticized by the orthodox medical establishment if they advocate nutritional measures to treat or prevent disease. He tells us it is up to the layman to change this attitude. He is certain we can do it, if we have the right facts to defend our case. His new book gives the facts.

Dr. Williams talks about heart attacks, obesity, alcoholism, dental troubles, arthritis, mental disease, cancer in relation to the prevention of these plagues by supernutrition. He discusses the ailments of old age and asks if we need to endure these when they might be prevented by supernutrition. He is careful to point out that this cannot be accomplished if we continue to speak of nutrition in terms of "the average man." There is no such individual.

Many years ago, Dr. Williams coined the phrase "biochemical individuality" meaning that each of us has his own inherited nutritional needs which may vary widely from those of members of his own family, let alone people not in the family. He foresees a day when experts will be able to measure quickly and inexpensively every nutritional need of every individual, then outline diets and supplements which will meet these needs individually.

Dr. Williams is one of the giants of nutritional science. He discovered pantothenic acid and named folic acid. He has worked at the University of Texas and the Clayton Foundation Biochemical Institute for many, many years. He is perhaps responsible for more original work in the field of vitamin research than any other scientist. He is apparently afraid of nothing. Recently he gave the press the story of how he fed laboratory rats on baker's bread and produced nutritional disaster, while other rats, fed a highly nutritious bread, flourished. He pointed out there is just no reason for not making bread as nutritious as possible.

He says much of the same kind of thing in a chapter called "What the Food Industries Can Do." The milling and baking industries should have been conducting experiments like his for many years, he says. How can the situation be remedied? Says Dr. Williams, "If medical scientists and the general public were aware that the nutritional environment of our body cells and tissues hinges on what we eat—every mouthful contributes—and that this environment determines the degree of health we possess, then the public would be continually complaining about the poor nutritional quality of the flour and bread and the industry would be forced to act..." A call to arms for all of us! Take up your pen or pick up the phone and complain to your baker!

What kind of diet does such a giant in the nutritional

field recommend? A diet high in protein. Dr. Williams reminds us that the protein in body cells is wearing out continually and must be replaced. He thinks that eggs are among our most desirable foods and has no patience with diets that forbid them. He urges that we use milk and cheese, not only for their excellent protein, but also their calcium and B vitamins. Fruits and vegetables contain B vitamins, iron and many minerals and trace minerals.

Since our nutrition scientists have not yet arrived at any idea of how much we need of most trace minerals, we must get them in appropriate foods. Bright green and bright yellow vegetables are good sources. Flour and cereal foods should be wholegrain. Dr. Williams deplores emphatically the idea that "enrichment" of cereals by putting back three B vitamins means anything at all. All vitamins are equally important and the body must have all of them in ample amounts for any of them to be effective, he says.

In addition, no one knows, he says, whether many of our present-day illnesses are caused by inherited need for more than average amounts of one or more nutrients. This is why apparent miracles can be worked with massive doses of one or several vitamins. The ailing individual actually needs that much of the vitamin to be healthy.

This is a wise book. It is the concentrated essence of the nutritional philosophy of many years of dedicated scientific work by a man whose scientific and moral integrity shines on every page. There are 81 pages of references for statements made. It is impossible to fault or question any bit of information in this book, just as it is impossible to call this distinguished scientist a crank or a faddist. You can safely use the information in his book to convince even the most confirmed skeptic of the power of nutrition against disease and the superpower of supernutrition.

Dr. Williams' other books are *The Human Frontier; Nutrition and Alcoholism* (out of print); *Free and Unequal; Biochemical Individuality; Alcoholism, The Nutritional Approach; Nutrition in a Nutshell* (available in paperback); and *You are Extraordinary*.

Why do we stress the "togetherness" of the B vitamins? Because they work so closely together and because modern treatment of food has shattered this close harmony and is forcing us to get along with possibly serious deficiencies in some of these vitamins, while we may be getting enough or nearly enough of others.

When bread flour and cereals are refined, the germ is removed. Since the B vitamins are concentrated there, all of these vitamins are removed, along with important minerals that work with the vitamins in body processes. Only three of the vitamins are returned, in synthetic form, to "enrich" this lifeless, starchy flour: thiamine, riboflavin and niacin. The others are ignored. In the complexity of modern diets, how can we ever discover what immense damage may be done to human health because of the imbalance of vitamins that results from this kind of manipulation in foods we eat every day at every meal!

The only sensible way to make sure that your family is not becoming deficient in one or another of these important food elements is to eat foods that are rich in all of them. There are some foods available at your supermarket: eggs, fish, milk, meat (especially the organ meats), green leafy vegetables, legumes like peas and beans, and nuts. Do not trust any refined cereal or flour to provide the B vitamins you need—no matter how "enriched" it may be. Remember that only a few of the vitamins have been restored.

All other foods which are rich in the whole family of B vitamins are the foods you can usually buy only in your health food store. We have listed some of these in the charts in this book. Some are especially high in one vitamin or another: blackstrap molasses is rich in pyridoxine, soybeans are rich in pantothenic acid, desiccated liver is the richest source of vitamin B12, ground sunflower seed contains huge amounts of niacin. Wheat germ and brewers yeast contain more of all the B vitamins than any other foods.

Pantothenic Acid Content of Some Common Foods

(We give the milligram content of one serving, about 100 grams)

Food	Milligrams
Brains (all kinds)	2.6
Broccoli	1.17
Bulgur	0.660
Cabbage juice	1.1
Cashews	1.3
Cauliflower	1
Chicken	1
Chickpeas	1.25
Cottonseed flour	4.320
Eggs, whole	1.6
Filberts	1.146
Flounder	0.850
Heart	3
Kale	1
Kidneys	4
Lentils	1.3
Liver	8
Liverwurst	2.7
Mushrooms	2.2
Oatmeal	1.4
Peanuts	2.8
Peas, dry	2
Rice, Brown	1.1
Salmon	1.3
Sesame seed flour	2.7
Soybeans	1.7
Sunflower seeds	1.4
Turkey	2.67
Walnuts	0.900
Wheat bran	2.9
Wheat germ	1.2
Whey, dried	4
Yeast, brewer's	12

Don't cheat your family of B vitamins. If one or more of them has trouble with a "sweet tooth" he or she is more in need of B vitamins than the rest of you. See to it that there are plenty of foods rich in all the B vitamins at hand for every meal and easily available between meals.

Plan your meals around these nutritious foods and accustom your family to their taste. Pack them in lunches. Provide them for bedtime snacks, insist on your family getting their share of B vitamins. What's involved? See above. The health of skin, nerves, personalities, digestion. Isn't it worth it?

CHAPTER 25

Inositol

IN THE EARLIER days of vitamin research inositol was called a B vitamin and investigated as such. Today it is not mentioned in the official booklet which sets standards for the amounts of the different vitamins and minerals which are considered officially to be essential to human life. So perhaps we might say that inositol is a substance which appears with all the other B vitamins in those foods in which the B group is abundant, and let it go at that.

But one aspect of the physiology of this vitamin-like substance worries us to such an extent that we are unwilling to dismiss it quite so easily. *Vitamins in Medicine*, the classic book on vitamins by Franklin Bicknell and Frederick Prescott, tells us that lindane, one of the common pesticides, is believed to kill insects by destroying the inositol in their bodies.

In *Silent Spring*, Rachel Carson recites the list of grievances any sensible person should have against lindane. She says, "We can hang strips impregnated with the chemical lindane in our closets and garment bags or place them in our bureau drawers for a half-year's freedom from worry over moth damage. The advertisements contain no suggestion that lindane is dangerous. Neither do the ads for an electronic device that dispenses lindane fumes—we are told that it is safe and odorless. Yet the truth of the matter is that the American Medical Association considers lindane vaporizers so dangerous that it conducted an extended campaign against them in its *Journal*."

Miss Carson tells us that lindane is stored in the brain and liver and may induce profound and long-lasting effects on the central nervous system. Plants treated with lindane become monstrously deformed with swellings on their roots. Their cells grew in size, being swollen with chromosomes which doubled in number. The doubling continued in future divisions until further cell division became mechanically impossible. She tells us that a Mayo Clinic expert reports that patients admitted with diseases of the blood-forming organs (leukemia and related conditions), almost without exception, have had a history of exposure to various toxic chemicals, among them the pesticide lindane.

Scientists have known since 1948 that lindane destroys inositol in living tissues. Doesn't it seem almost impossible to believe that they could have continued to allow us to use this pesticide all these years without one single warning of its potential for harm?

' There is no way for you to know how many times you have been exposed to lindane even if you yourself never use pesticides of any kind. In the days when lindane vaporizers appeared in almost every public place all of us got a dose of this poison. Does the rising rate of many assorted diseases have anything to do with this exposure? There is no way of knowing. Toxic substances are all around us in our modern technological society. Since the publication of *Silent Spring* we are a bit more careful about pesticides. Government regulations are a bit more strict.

Inositol is closely related in function to the B vitamins choline and biotin. Bicknell and Prescott tell us that rats deprived of inositol lose their hair. Other animals develop severe digestive troubles when the inositol is removed from their food. Adelle Davis tells us (*Let's Get Well*) that both choline and inositol are necessary for the body to manufacture lecithin, that substance which helps to control the fate of cholesterol in our bodies. Patients recovering from heart attacks who were given large amounts of choline and inositol showed rapid decrease of the fatty substances in their blood. Within two months the cholesterol levels had dropped to normal.

In 1950 experiments with rabbits given cholesterol showed that when inositol was given along with the fatty substance, the blood levels of cholesterol did not soar as they might be expected to do in a rabbit whose natural diet does not contain cholesterol.

Dr. Walter Eddy in his book *Vitaminology* mentions a curious fact about the possible relation of inositol deficiency and drinking too much coffee. When laboratory animals were given large amounts of caffeine, a paralysis occurred which could be cured by giving them inositol. So possibly caffeine may have some destructive effect on this vitamin-like substance—something to keep in mind when you are debating whether to go on drinking coffee or switch to one of the caffeine-free kinds or one of the fine herb teas at your health food store!

Inositol is available in food along with other members of the B complex of vitamins—meats, fish, poultry, organ meats, leafy green vegetables, seeds and wholegrain cereals, nuts, wheat germ, brewers yeast, also in many fruits and vegetables. It is noteworthy that, among the organ meats, inositol is very abundant in heart muscle. It is axiomatic that those organs in which vitamins or minerals are stored have special need for those nutrients.

So it seems that inositol may be very important for a healthy heart. That's nothing to be ignored these days when heart disease is our leading cause of death. Get plenty of inositol in those foods in which it occurs. You can also obtain it in natural food supplements where it occurs along with other important and essential members of the B complex of vitamins.

CHAPTER 26

Choline

FOR MANY YEARS nutrition scientists have been calling choline a B vitamin. The official booklet *Recommended Dietary Allowances* lists it among the B vitamins, but does not make any recommendations for how much we should get every day since, says the book, "choline is generally considered to be an essential nutrient in the diet. Choline deficiency has not been demonstrated in man, however, at any stage of life, and whether or not it is an essential dietary nutrient for man is unknown."

We do know, however, that it exists, along with other members of the B vitamin complex, in foods in which this complex is plentiful. We know, too, that choline is essential in the diet of many animals and birds, where it protects them against abnormalities in pregnancy and lactation, anemia, cardiovascular disease and muscular weakness.

Under all the right conditions, choline can be manufactured by the human digestive tract, apparently, if there is enough of all the elements necessary to make it. These include an amino acid or form of protein, methionine, plus folic acid and vitamin B12 and a number of other ingredients. Of course, some condition of ill-health might make this process impossible. And, too, some common American diets will certainly not provide enough of all these essential ingredients.

What are some of the functions of this vitamin in the

human body? As long ago as 1950 scientists discovered that rats, completely deprived of choline, developed high blood pressure. Adding choline to the diet lowered the pressure at once. Other scientists discovered that by keeping rats on a diet in which there was just enough choline to keep them alive, they could produce cancer in about two-thirds of all the rats involved. In 1951 Brown University scientists deprived rats of both protein and choline and produced liver cancer in animals which were not bred to be susceptible to this disease.

Choline was used by a California group of researchers to prevent complications from artery hardening in human beings. After about three years, fatalities from circulatory disorders were far lower in the group which had been taking choline every day.

In *Vitamins in Medicine* (Bicknell and Prescott), we are told that choline is essential for the correct use of fatty food by the body. Liver damage is prevented. Choline is essential for the proper use of cholesterol by the body. This is the fatty substance we have been warned against in recent years as a threat to circulatory health. Perhaps we have somehow lost the ability to manufacture choline internally, or perhaps we have somehow managed to pervert and disorder the elements in our processed food so thoroughly that we have destroyed those things in our food which our bodies need to manufacture choline. There seems to be little hope of turning up this kind of evidence in today's diet surveys where individual peculiarities in eating are hidden in the "averages" which are reported.

Let's say you're on a typical reducing diet. You're taking black coffee and grapefruit for breakfast, a dab of cottage cheese for lunch, and a bit of meat and salad without dressing for dinner. Choline appears, along with the other B vitamins, in food which is almost wholly absent from such a deficient diet. The less protein you eat, the less methionine you will have. You will recall this is the form of protein which is essential for the body to manufacture choline.

Adelle Davis, in her book, *Let's Get Well*, has given us much information about choline, for she has done a thorough job of studying all the medical and scientific literature available. She tells us of the protection given to the liver by choline and vitamin E, when a high fat diet is eaten by laboratory animals. In diets deficient in both choline and protein (diets which contain lots of alcohol, for example) the liver can be badly damaged.

Perhaps most important is the effect of lack of choline on cholesterol levels in the blood. Lecithin is a substance which the body manufactures *when there is enough choline present along with another B vitamin inositol*. The lecithin apparently keeps cholesterol in such an emulsified state that it does not settle on artery walls or collect as gall bladder stones. Eggs are especially rich in lecithin, as well as methionine—so eggs remain one of our most valuable foods, even for people with hardening of the arteries and heart problems.

Says Miss Davis, "When patients recovering from heart attacks received daily 2,000 and 750 milligrams of choline and inositol respectively, the size of the cholesterol particles and the amount of fat in the blood quickly decreased; two months later the blood cholesterol had dropped to normal. Blood lecithin has also increased and cholesterol been reduced after choline has been given."

She tells us that deficiencies in choline may be responsible for high blood pressure in people suffering from diabetes, over-weight, nephritis or heart disease. She points out that alcohol causes the need for choline to increase, and that alcohol causes a rapid rise in fatty substances in the blood. Speaking of reducing diets, she reminds us that the major function of lecithin is to burn fat, so all the ingredients from which the body manufactures lecithin must be present in any successful reducing diet. These are choline, pyridoxine, inositol, plus one of the unsaturated fats and the mineral magnesium. Such research indicates, she says, that "it is not entirely the amount of food eaten that causes obesity, but the lack of nutrients required to convert fat into energy." And choline is one of these.

How can you be sure you are getting enough choline? You can be sure if you are getting enough of all those foods in which the entire B complex of vitamins is most abundant: meat, fish, poultry, eggs, wholegrains, green leafy vegetables, seeds of all kinds. The best sources of B vitamins in foods and food supplements are: wheat bran, wheat germ, brewers yeast.

We cannot end a discussion of choline without talking about lecithin, too. Lecithin (pronounced less-i-thin) is that emulsifying substance which apparently breaks cholesterol down into tiny droplets so that it cannot damage the inside walls of arteries. As we have seen, choline is one of the ingredients of lecithin. So by using lecithin as a supplement you can increase your intake of choline as well as guaranteeing a better metabolism of fats in your body chemistry.

The richest natural sources of lecithin are eggs and soybeans. So, apparently, eggs, which are rich in cholesterol, are also filled with the substance which renders it harmless to arteries. Soybeans are vegetable foods, so they contain no cholesterol. They contain so much lecithin that they are usually the source for the food supplements you can get at your health food store: lecithin flakes, granules, liquid lecithin and so on. You can use these in any appropriate dish: a teaspoon or so in an omelet, or salad dressing, soup or stew.

And, finally, be sure you are taking daily a B complex vitamin preparation which contains choline. With circulatory troubles as prevalent as they are, the health-seeker should do everything possible to protect himself against deficiencies which may contribute to this disease.

CHAPTER 27

Para-Amino-
Benzoic-Acid,
or PABA

THE B VITAMIN with the tongue-twister name, *Para-amino-benzoic* acid, is not listed as a vitamin in the official handbook *Recommended Dietary Allowances*. But its use in human nutrition has been long and interesting. Mostly it has been associated with skin welfare and graying hair. Nobody is quite sure why, or how it acts in the body.

We call it PABA for short. Drs. Bicknell and Prescott in their massive book, *The Vitamins in Medicine*, tell us that PABA is unique in that it is a vitamin within a vitamin. It seems that it is part of folic acid. When sulfanilamide, the antibiotic, first came into use in the 1940's, it was found that its chemical formula is very much like that of PABA. So when people or experimental animals were given the drug internally, the PABA in their intestines counteracted it, so that it became ineffective.

Early in research work with PABA, scientists discovered that, when they withheld it from the diet of laboratory animals, their hair became white. It was believed that PABA was essential for the synthesis of folic acid, another B vitamin, in the intestinal tract and the lack of folic acid was the real reason for the white hair.

At any rate, people with prematurely white hair wanted to know if lack of PABA was the reason for their loss of pigment and if they might be able to restore the color if they took PABA. One researcher claimed that he could restore lost hair color by giving massive doses of PABA over long periods of time.

Adelle Davis, in *Let's Get Well*, tells us that she has seen many instances of gray hair which returned to its original color temporarily, but it quickly became gray again "unless one continues to eat yogurt, liver, yeast and wheat germ. Persons who take 5 milligrams of folic acid and 300 milligrams of PABA and pantothenic acid daily with some B vitamins from natural sources can usually prevent hair from graying and often restore its color."

The other field in which PABA has been recently shown to be almost a wonder drug is in the prevention of damage from sunburn. Way back in the 1940's scientists were finding they could prevent serious burns from the sun and from sunlamps by putting a PABA lotion on the exposed skin. And sure enough, it worked. We have no idea why it took so long for scientists to rediscover this important fact. That's the way things work out in the field of vitamin research. For years we got along with sunburn lotions which accomplished little or nothing.

In Spring of 1969 we began to get enthusiastic reports from scientists that they found PABA to be a "superior" sunscreen agent. The scientists from the University of Pennsylvania told the Society of Cosmetic Chemists that they were getting far better results using PABA lotion than any of the commonly available suntan lotions could give.

Then several Boston doctors developed another formula which they claimed would screen out the ultraviolet rays of the sun "to provide protection from sunburn, skin cancer and aging of the skin." The formula was effective whether you used it at the seashore, the desert or the mountains. They mixed the vitamin with ethyl alcohol and tested it on prisoners in Arizona under the hot, dry sunshine there. The formulas used and all the scientific information about the tests appeared in the *New England Journal of Medicine* for June 26, 1969.

Bicknell and Prescott describe many more experimental uses of PABA in diseases where skin problems are involved. It has been used in massive doses to treat lymphoblastoma cutis, lupus erythematosus, scleroderma, pemphigus, and dermatitis herpetiformis. No one knows what causes any of these conditions or why PABA was effective in relieving them. But pictures in the book show clear improvement in the skin condition so long as the vitamin was being taken, and in massive doses.

Adelle Davis tells us that PABA has also been used to treat vitiligo, the skin condition where pigment is lost, leaving large patches of entirely white skin. She tells us that pantothenic acid has also been used in massive doses to bring the color back to these unsightly patches of skin. PABA applied in an ointment has produced good results.

Says Miss Davis, "I once told a 30-year-old woman with severe vitiligo that liver would probably help her more than any other food. A week later she joyously returned to show me that not a trace of it remained, but she had eaten ¼ pound of raw liver, frozen, diced and covered with catsup, at each meal. Several other persons have had the condition clear up slowly on a more appetizing diet."

The best sources of the vitamin PABA are those same foods in which all the other B vitamins are most abundant: meat (especially organ meats like liver), seeds of all kinds and unrefined cereals of all kinds, nuts, leafy green vegetables, brewers yeast, wheat bran, wheat germ. Be sure to get enough of it.

Vitamin C Is...

Water-soluble, meaning it cannot be stored for a long time in the body, but should be available in food or supplements every day.

Responsible for the health and maintenance of collagen in teeth, bones, cartilage, connective tissues, skin and the small blood vessels called capillaries, the healing of wounds, broken bones and burns, the detoxification of poisons (in the process of which the vitamin is destroyed) the maintenance of white blood corpuscles which fight infection, absorption of iron from the digestive tract, maintenance of the adrenal glands which protect us from stress.

Present in most abundance in fresh raw fruits and vegetables, chiefly the citrus fruits, strawberries, pineapple, guava, acerola cherries, rose hips, all members of the cabbage family, tomatoes, parsley, peppers, also liver.

Safe in very large amounts. Any vitamin C not needed is excreted harmlessly.

Destroyed by many chemicals, poisons, and other substances in today's world such as tobacco smoke.

Required officially in amounts such as 45 milligrams daily for adults. Since individual needs may vary greatly and since individual exposure to poisons may vary greatly, one person's needs may not approximate those of another. All living organisms except human beings and several birds and animals make their own vitamin C in their livers. They manufacture very large amounts, especially when under stress.

Available in low or high potencies in individual supplements or one-a-day supplements.

CHAPTER 28

Linus Pauling Thinks Cancer May Be a Disease of Vitamin C Deficiency

"BECAUSE IT STRIKES young and old alike, because its origins are still so much a mystery and because it is rapidly on the increase, cancer is the number one health threat confronting our society today," according to an article in the Summer, 1976 issue of the *National Resources Defense Council Newsletter*. "It will kill 370,000 Americans this year (as opposed to about 21,000 in 1918), strike 675,000 others, and cause a loss of over 1,700,000 man-years of potential working life."

And Professor Linus Pauling, probably the greatest biologist alive today and perhaps the greatest of all time, believes that cancer may turn out to be a disease of vitamin C deficiency. He made the announcement in June, 1976 on English radio. Dr. Pauling has been working for years with vitamin C in regard to many aspects of life and disease. He is in contact with other scientists and physicians in various parts of the world who are doing work along these lines.

He backed up his claim by referring to the work of a Scots physician which seems to show that large doses of vitamin C increase the average survival times of terminal cancer patients four-fold. And said Pauling, "vitamin C can sometimes produce quite dramatic remissions in advanced human cancer."

Pauling says that the first barrier to the malignant growth of a cancer is the ground substance between cells. Vitamin C is essential for maintaining the structural integrity of this material, hence the vitamin must be one of the body's best weapons for fighting cancer. Dr. Pauling believes that the best treatment for cancer is a judicious combination of medical methods that will eradicate the cancer mass: radiation therapy, surgery, chemotherapy, immunotherapy, plus "supportive measures prescribed in the short term to correct biochemical deficiencies, and in the long term to enhance natural resistance to any residual disease."

Cancer patients are known to be seriously depleted of vitamin C, said Pauling. Short term treatment should include vitamin C to correct this deficiency just as it includes supplemental iron to correct accompanying anemia. In the long-term view, said Pauling, vitamin C provides "a simple, safe, practical method of enhancing host resistance to malignant disease."

One of the tests on which Pauling based his theory is the one conducted in a Scottish hospital by a surgeon who gave 10 grams of vitamin C daily—that's 10,000 milligrams—to terminal cancer patients who were "untreatable by any conventional method of therapy at the time of entry into supplemental ascorbate (vitamin C) as their only definitive form of medication." In other words, everything that could be done for these patients by orthodox medicine had already been done. Vitamin C was the only medication given them in their last weeks.

Pauling reported that there were many instances of relief of symptoms—reduced pain which permitted their doctor to discontinue sedatives. Their appetites returned. They had a renewed sense of well being. It seems that doctors are not especially interested in medicines that just make the patient feel better and many doctors apparently believe that vitamin C does indeed increase the general feeling of well being in many ill people. So, they asked, if that's all the vitamin does—what else is new?

What's new, said Pauling, is that results of the experiment seemed to indicate that these patients lived significantly longer than normal clinical expectations, considering how gravely ill they were. The Scots surgeon then got out records of 1,000 other cancer patients in the same hospital and compared them with the records of 100 patients to whom he had given vitamin C. He carefully matched each of his patients with 10 of those whose records were in hospital files. Matched patients must be the same age, same kind of tumor, same sex and, in the case of the 1,000 past patients, must have had no vitamin C treatment.

The results of this comparison showed clearly that the patients who got the vitamin C lived on the average four times longer than the original 10 patients to whom they were compared. Of the 100 patients treated with vitamin C, 15 survived longer than a year, compared to only 4 of the controls. Six terminal patients treated with Vitamin C lived more than two years, compared to only 2 of the controls. Three of those treated with vitamin C lived for three years. None of those not so treated lived longer than 2½ years.

Of the five who survived more than one year, five are still alive including two who have lived for more than four years. Said the surgeon, "they should have died long ago." He said, too, that 8-10 percent of the patients who were "clearly dying of cancer and as a result of receiving nothing but ascorbic acid (vitamin C) show quite definite evidence of tumor regression and recovery. This is infinitely better than spontaneous regression. I have only seen three spontaneous regressions in my working lifetime."

Critics of this study say that next to nothing can be told by case histories from the files of a hospital. One doctor does not mean the same thing another doctor means when he says "untreatable cancer". And maybe these test patients were just getting better care than those 1,000 past patients to whom they were compared. The surgeon admitted that his assistant had visited the patients once every two weeks to be sure they were taking their vitamin C. He admits that this is therapeutic, but, he says, "I don't think she could have made the tumors regress."

One of the critics, Dr. Kurt Hellman of the Imperial Cancer Research Fund in London, admitted that vitamin C probably could be helpful in cancer treatment. He himself has authored a book on cancer which speculated on the possibilities of vitamin C in cancer treatment. He admits that vitamin C "is supportive and not toxic." Many cancer patients are old and poorly nourished, he said, so giving them vitamin C could be valuable for that reason alone. So he thinks the idea could "be valuable."

The Scots surgeon says it is difficult to arrange comparisons of this kind on patients in a general hospital. So he may not be able to pursue his ideas further. Then, too, he said, "other researchers have been so conditioned by the thought that we have enough vitamin C in our diet that the surgeon might have trouble selling the idea to other researchers." Everyone involved admits that vitamin C treatment is harmless.

The British publication (*New Scientist*, July 1, 1976) commenting on Pauling's statement, mentioned a conference at the New York Academy of Science last year at which the conference in general recommended a daily intake of 500 milligrams of vitamin C.

Once you get into discussion of this highly controversial vitamin, lots of dissenting opinions come to the surface. Some experts feel that large doses of vitamin C might cause kidney stones, although, as we have pointed out, there is no single such case recorded. And there is plenty of evidence that vitamin C may prevent kidney and bladder stones, as well as other serious bladder conditions, including cancer.

Once you get into the question of preventing colds, one scientist who has apparently never tried the vitamin himself announced recently that up to 1,000 milligrams of vitamin C daily will prevent colds, but more than that, he says, decreases the effectiveness of the vitamin. And the same may be true of cancer, says this researcher, Professor Cedric Wilson. Vitamin C must certainly be involved in the body's attempt to "build a wall" around the cancer to prevent it from spreading to other parts of the body. But, he says, by the same token cancer tissue contains more vitamin C than healthy body tissue surrounding it. Therefore, he believes the tumor is bagging most of the vitamin C for its own growth and not leaving enough healthy tissues to maintain themselves. He seems to think that giving more vitamin C will just cause the tumor to grow more. It seems evident that patients of the Scots surgeon did not have that experience.

It is interesting that Dr. Wilson also believes that colds, allergies, rheumatic arthritis, cancer and other diseases decrease the amount of vitamin C available in the body, so therefore we should take large doses of the vitamin "to restore tissue health." Just what the health food movement has been saying all along!

Pauling believes that the material between cells must be kept healthy in order to prevent cancer. These cells are normally restrained from proliferating and running wild by a complex mechanism involving a substance called physiological hyaluronidase (PHI). Vitamin C is necessary for the production of this substance. It is destroyed in the process of building PHI. Given an adequate quantity of vitamin C, says Pauling, the body could presumably manufacture enough of this important substance to prevent cancer.

The effect of such a treatment would be to "disarm" the cancer cells. They would remain there, but further growth would stop. Perhaps ulcers would heal, pain, hemorrhaging, weakness, emaciation, malnutrition and all other distressing symptoms might be controlled. This explanation derives from what happens in scurvy, the disease of vitamin C deficiency. The substance between the cells breaks down, leading to tissue disruption, ulceration and hemorrhage—"identical to the local changes that occur in the immediate vicinity of neoplastic (cancerous) cells," says Pauling.

Why should we, the general public, permit any more guessing, discussion, haggling or arguing about this important life and death matter? Everyone involved in this cancer debate agrees that vitamin C in large doses cannot do any harm. For goodness sake, why not use it then, no matter what else is being done—first to prevent cancer, and as part of the treatment of cancer—any cancer, any treatment. Presumably part of cancer treatment is nursing care plus all the hideously expensive facilities of our finest hospitals, as well as the expensive services of our finest cancer specialists. Why in the world should we continue to debate a simple, ridiculously inexpensive adjunct to treatment, like vitamin C, which might, just might, cure the cancer and prevent its return? What earthly reason is there not to at least try it?

CHAPTER 29

Using Vitamin C in
a Doctor's Practice

DR. FRED R. KLENNER practices in Reidsville, North Carolina. His reports on vitamin therapy for almost anything are not published in the slick, expensive professional journals put out by universities and research centers. He does not report on farfetched experiments on rats which continue for three or four days.

Instead his testimony burgeons with stories of patients who crowd his office to receive massive doses of vitamins and recommendations for healthful diet. There is no experimenting for two or three days. Dr. Klenner's patients take their vitamins for life and, he reports, remain healthy so long as they do.

In an issue of the *Journal of Applied Nutrition* he tells some of the following stories, all having to do with massive doses of vitamin C, otherwise known as ascorbic acid. He uses it fearlessly. He reports no ill effects. He gets improvement in just about any condition he treats.

He has used vitamin C for many patients with after-effects of severe virus infections. In 1953 he had a patient with virus pneumonia, unconscious, with a fever of more than 106 degrees. He gave her 140 grams of vitamin C intravenously over a period of 72 hours. By that time she was almost well. He believes that stubborn after-effects of virus infections are the cause of "crib deaths" that take the lives of so many apparently healthy infants. "Physicians must recognize the inherent danger of the lingering head or chest cold and appreciate the importance of early massive vitamin C therapy", says Klenner.

Dr. Klenner tells us there is a tragic lack of vitamin C in the blood of burn patients. He treats them by enclosing the burned parts in a heated cradle-like arrangement so that nothing touches the skin. No dressings. He uses a 3 percent vitamin C spray over the entire area, alternated with vitamin A and D ointment over the burn. He gives massive doses of vitamin C by mouth. During long periods of massive vitamin C dosage he also gives calcium gluconate to check any tendency to form oxalic acid which is destructive of the vitamin.

Klenner says we are all victims of carbon monoxide, which is one of the most harmful elements in air pollution, especially car exhausts. For carbon monoxide poisoning he gives massive doses of vitamin C which seems able to separate the carbon monoxide from the red blood cell which it is in the process of destroying.

All the conditions listed above are conditions of stress. Animals under stress manufacture in their bodies many times more vitamin C than they otherwise would. Human beings cannot manufacture their own vitamin C. Does it not seem likely that much more of it during stress might protect them, too, from further damage?

Dr. Klenner has used vitamin C in massive doses in 300 consecutive pregnancy cases. (Pregnancy, too, is stress). He believes that failure to give this vitamin to pregnant women amounts almost to malpractice. His patients experience no anemia. Leg cramps occurred in fewer than 3 percent and then only when the patient had run out of vitamin C. Abdominal marks (stretch marks) appear on the abdomens of his patients infrequently and then usually when the women gained too much weight and took too little exercise.

Labor was short and less painful. The perineum was "remarkably elastic even 15 years later." No patients required catheterization. No infections, no cardiac stress, even though 22 of these women had rheumatic heart disease. One patient had been told by another doctor that another pregnancy would be fatal. Under Dr. Klenner's vitamin C treatment, she had two more babies, went back to teaching school and still takes 10 grams of vitamin C daily.

After delivering a famous family of quadruplets, Dr. Klenner started the babies on 50 milligrams of vitamin C the first day and increased it as time went on. The ten children of another couple are all healthy and good looking today, says Dr. Klenner, and are referred to as "the vitamin C babies."

Dr. Klenner treats snake bite and insect bites with injected vitamin C. He believes that all diabetics should be taking massive doses of it. Lack of the vitamin is responsible for the slow healing of a diabetic's wounds, he believes. The vitamin also helps the diabetic to make better use of insulin. And it helps the liver to deal with carbohydrates. Sixty percent of all Klenner's diabetic patients can be controlled with only diet and vitamin C—as much as 10 grams daily. The other 40 percent need less insulin and less oral medication if they are taking massive doses of the vitamin.

Dentists tell Dr. Klenner that 500 milligrams of vitamin C prevent shock and weakness after tooth extractions. He once watched an operation in which the intestines were so weak and "glued together" that any effort to separate them resulted in tearing them. The surgeon mended 20 such tears, then closed the abdomen as a hopeless situation. Two grams of vitamin C were injected every hour for 48 hours, then 4 times a day. In one week the patient was discharged. "She has outlived her surgeon for many years," says Klenner.

He gives massive doses of vitamin C for mononucleosis. As does a famous Tulane urologist, he gives 1½ grams of vitamin C daily to prevent bladder cancer when it is threatening, to prevent a recurrence. Klenner believes that vitamin C is the "anti-cancer vitamin". Ascorbic acid will control myelocytic leukemia, provided 25 to 30 grams are taken orally each day, he says. Why not? Many disease conditions are cured by giving 5 million to 100,000 million units of penicillin as an intravenous drip over 4 to 6 weeks. "How long must we wait," he asks, "for someone to start continuous ascorbic acid drip for two to three months giving 100 to 300 grams each day for various malignant conditions?"

He treats overdoses of drugs with vitamin C. Also tetanus, in combination with a drug. Two cases of trichinosis were treated with vitamin C and a B vitamin. Corneal injury, chicken pox and sunburn are also treated with vitamin C. He treats alcoholics suffering from overdoses of antabuse. He tells of doctors who use vitamin C for treating glaucoma, fever blisters, arthritis, shingles and poisoning from heavy metals like cadmium or lead. He reminds us that plenty of vitamin C prevents the build-up of cholesterol in the blood. "Ten grams of vitamin C or more each day and then eat all the eggs you want," he says.

Will massive doses of vitamin C cause kidney stones? The urine of someone taking massive doses of vitamin C will be so acid that formation of stones will be impossible, he says. Furthermore, vitamin C induces urination, so there is no chance that urine will collect and remain in the bladder—one of the possible causes of bladder and kidney stones.

Dr. Klenner is not talking theoretically here. He gives his patients these dosages, he reports on the results. It is hard to refute his case histories and tell him his own patients so treated are not alive and well, when he sees them frequently and knows their condition.

There seems to be no ulterior motive for him to use vitamin C as he does, if it does not perform as he says. Doctors who never cure any patients usually do not stay successful for very long. Dr. Klenner is not selling vitamin C. He has no commerical reason for promoting its use.

If you want to take vitamin C in large doses, there seems

to be no reason not to. If you have any unpleasant side-effect, reduce the dosage. People differ. Perhaps you need less than others to overcome or prevent whatever condition you are trying to relieve. Perhaps you need more than others. Don't expect miraculous overnight cures. Your body may have been getting along on very little vitamin C for many years. If you smoke or are exposed to cigarette smoke or certain other harmful air pollutants, the vitamin C you take is destroyed very rapidly in rendering these pollutants harmless. Stress, including disease of any kind or fatigue or emotional stress, greatly increases your need for vitamin C.

It is available at your health food store in just about any potency you may desire.

CHAPTER 30

Vitamin C,
Circulatory Disorders
and Diabetes

MEDICAL EVIDENCE IS rapidly accumulating that vitamin C may be a powerful agent in lowering blood cholesterol and preventing the hardening of the arteries that often results following such high levels of the fatty substance.

Medical World News (September 13, 1974) told the story of a British physician's observations and experiments in relation to vitamin C. Dr. Constance Spittle is consultant pathologist at the Pinderlands General Hospital in Wakefield, England. Dr. Spittle believes that hardening of the arteries is a disease of vitamin C deficiency. She also believes that getting large doses of the vitamin may help to prevent deep vein thrombosis—the crisis that so often follows major surgery.

Dr. Spittle started her research on vitamin C during a period when she was experimenting with a diet consisting of nothing but fresh fruits and vegetables. The diet failed utterly to sustain her and she had to give it up, but she discovered, while she was on the diet, that the levels of cholesterol in her blood declined from 240 milligrams percent to 160 milligrams percent at the end of her experiment.

She thought this must be the result of a diet in which there was no cholesterol, for completely vegetarian foods do not contain this fatty substance. But after she returned to her former diet, her cholesterol levels continued to decline. She added large amounts of fresh fruits and vegetables to her diet. The cholesterol levels continued to decline. Then she boiled all the fruits and vegetables thoroughly before eating them. The cholesterol levels began to climb once again. Apparently something essential was destroyed in the boiling process. Could it be vitamin C? It is well known that the vitamin is destroyed when fresh foods are cooked too long.

She persuaded some of her colleagues to try an experiment. She gave them one gram (1,000 milligrams) of vitamin C daily for six weeks and took regular measurements of their cholesterol levels. In some the levels dropped. In others they were increased. She had begun to suspect that vitamin C might be related to preventing the plaques that appear on the inside of blood vessels and produce hardening of the arteries. In some of them the cholesterol levels went up. In others they dropped.

But it seemed that the lower cholesterol levels occurred in young people. They rose in older people, especially those suffering from hardening of the arteries. Dr. Spittle believes there is a good reason for this. Vitamin C, she says, has the job of collecting the cholesterol in arteries and transporting it to the liver where it is transformed into certain digestive juices which help to digest fats.

In young people, says Dr. Spittle, where there is little cholesterol in their arteries, there is a net flow from the blood to the liver. But in older people whose arteries are more "furred," or lined, with cholesterol deposits, the vitamin C pulls out more cholesterol from the arteries than it can readily transport to the liver, so the blood levels go up. In those with fully developed hardening of the arteries, the situation is worst.

But eventually the vitamin C will transport this unwanted cholesterol to the liver and this will produce an improvement in the condition of the patient, says Dr. Spittle. She says that many of the patients who suffered from hardening of the arteries told her they felt better during the experiment. They could walk farther without pain or breathlessness. Dr. Spittle says it is futile just to study the levels of cholesterol in blood.

Instead, she says, doctors should study what effects the vitamin C has on the levels. If it pushes them up, then probably the patient was suffering from hardening of the arteries, but the vitamin sent the offending cholesterol on its way to the liver. This means everything should proceed on its normal course. The vitamin C appears to have the important function of loosening cholesterol from artery walls and sending it along to the liver, as well as taking part in the changes that take place in the liver.

But Dr. Spittle also believes that lack of vitamin C may be responsible for starting the whole process of artery hardening to begin with. Plaques of cholesterol form on damaged places in the inner wall of the artery. If this original damage could be prevented, hardening of the arteries might be prevented.

Dr. Spittle believes that vitamin C can and does prevent such damage. Vitamin C is involved in the manufacture of the "cement" or "glue" that holds cells together. This is especially important in the cells that line the arteries. If one is deficient in vitamin C, damaged parts heal slowly and plaques may appear. When there is plenty of vitamin C around, healing is rapid and cholesterol deposits are prevented.

To test her theories on human arteries would require a lifetime, for the individuals tested would have to grow old during the test. So Dr. Spittle is now working on a theory regarding deep vein thrombosis. This is the blood clot that so often forms after surgery when a blood clot snags on the damaged part of a vein.

Using 60 surgery patients as subjects, Dr. Spittle gave 30 of them one gram (1,000 milligrams) of vitamin C daily while the other 30 received a tablet containing nothing. The number of clots in patients taking the vitamin was only half the expected number and these were so minor they could barely be detected. Many surgeons in Dr. Spittle's hospital are now routinely giving their patients vitamin C after surgery, with good results.

In this same hospital the section for treatment of burns has been giving large amounts of vitamin C for six years, to hasten healing. During that time there was only one fatal lung clot and no deep vein thrombosis—"an achievement far out-stripping that seen in other similar units not using vitamin C."

So it seems that by keeping cholesterol moving in the right direction—toward the liver—and by functioning correctly with it, after it arrives in the liver, vitamin C may perhaps prevent hardening of the arteries, keeping the insides of arteries clean and free from plaques or clots. For people with suspected hardening of the arteries, Dr. Spittle recommends one gram of vitamin C daily. She herself takes half a gram with breakfast and eats a lot of fresh fruits and vegetables, all raw, so that their abundant vitamin C content is preserved.

As if to confirm directly Dr. Spittle's research, comes word from Bratislava, Czechoslovakia that Dr. Emil Ginter has reduced high cholesterol levels in middle-aged men and women by giving them 300 milligrams of vitamin C daily. These people were admittedly short on the vitamin because it was during that season of the year when fresh foods were scarce.

At the Institute of Human Research, Dr. Ginter gave the vitamin for 47 days to people chronically short on vitamin C and chronically found to have high cholesterol levels. These levels dropped an average of 33 milligrams percent in 13 subjects. The reactions were most dramatic in those whose cholesterol levels were highest.

In more recent trials, 1,000 milligrams of vitamin C daily decreased blood levels of triglycerides—another worrisome kind of fatty substance often found in quantity where hardening of the arteries threatens. In patients with the highest levels of this fat, a measurement of 308 milligrams percent dropped to 197 milligrams. In those with slightly lower levels an average of 262 milligrams dropped to 236 milligrams.

In his earlier studies with guinea pigs—almost the only animals aside from human beings which do not manufacture their own vitamin C—Dr. Ginter had produced swelling of the inner walls of the artery by depriving the animals of vitamin C for long periods of time. He did not reduce their vitamin C intake low enough for the animals to get scurvy, but just enough to leave them in a subclinical state of scurvy, which many scientists believe may be the situation many human beings find themselves in these days. These animals, too, had raised levels of cholesterol in their blood and in their livers.

Dr. Ginter believes that vitamin C is necessary for processing cholesterol into digestive juices, which is its normal fate in the liver. If there is not enough vitamin C, this process does not go smoothly. Along with Dr. Spittle, Dr. Ginter believes that disorders of fat metabolism and disorders in the wall of the artery and disorders in the coagulating ability of the blood may all be associated with lack of vitamin C and all may contribute to the final problem which is hardening of the arteries and, possibly, eventual heart attacks or strokes.

A possible relationship between vitamin C and the ill effects of alcohol was found by four Scots physicians and reported in *The Lancet* for September 21, 1974. These doctors, from the Stobhill General Hospital, tell us that alcoholics suffer from many nutritional deficiencies. Subclinical scurvy associated with an inadequate intake of vitamin C is common among alcoholics. This means a condition not serious enough to bring on full-blown symptoms of scurvy, but almost that serious.

Vitamin C works with an enzyme in the liver which is concerned with treating alcohol safely and sending it along to be dissolved into harmless metabolites. To see if this theory is correct, the four physicians gave one gram of vitamin C daily for two weeks to a group of volunteers, then gave them alcoholic drinks. Testing the amount of vitamin C in the blood and the amount of alcohol in the blood, they found that, the more vitamin C present, the less alcohol.

Apparently the vitamin had functioned with the liver enzyme to process the alcohol, removing it from the blood. The liver enzyme, called alcohol dehydrogenase, is the principal body enzyme involved in disposing of alcohol, say these authors, so, therefore, it seems that the effective functioning of this enzyme is dependent on being saturated with vitamin C.

Commenting on these findings, *New Scientist* for September 26, 1974 said, "Drinkers may therefore like to add vitamin C to their list of 'professional' remedies."

"Deep vein thrombosis" is the dreaded aftermath of many a surgical experience even in these days when the most skillful methods are used in surgery and recovery rooms. Deep vein thrombosis means a blood clot in some inner area of the body—often the legs or the lungs, which may bring death.

Dr. Spittle relates in the *Lancet* for July 28, 1973 an experiment she performed, with the consent of all patients involved. There were 63 of them, aged 55 to 84—the ages when circulatory disorders become most threatening. Some were prostate patients, some were cancer patients, some faced hip surgery. Twenty of them had already had some circulatory troubles, 17 had had acute heart attacks, 3 had had strokes.

The patients were divided into two groups, one group was given one gram (1,000 milligrams) of vitamin C daily from the day of admission until two weeks after the operation. The other group was given a tablet that looked like the vitamin C tablet but contained nothing. The legs of all patients were scanned with special equipment to detect blood clots. No one in the hospital staff knew which patients were getting the vitamin C.

At the end of the test, after the operations were over and

enough time had elapsed that doctors could be fairly certain blood clots would not develop, the facts were revealed as to which patients got the "nothing" pill and who got the vitamin C. It was found that there were blood clots in the lungs in three patients who did not get the vitamin C, one in the patients who got vitamin C. Eleven patients who did not get vitamin C had signs of coagulation or blood clotting in the legs. Only one who got vitamin C had such symptoms.

Of the 30 patients on vitamin C, one patient had symptoms of abnormal clotting in the legs, 12 of those not getting vitamin C had such symptoms. Three patients who did not get vitamin C had clots in their lungs. None of the vitamin C-treated patients did. No patient getting vitamin C had both legs affected with clots, while 10 of those not getting the vitamin had such symptoms.

We point out once again that no one doing the tests had any idea of which patients got the vitamin, so there could be no bias in their minds when they made their examinations. There is no doubt that the vitamin C performed near miracles in protecting these surgery patients from possible death.

Traditionally it is believed that blood clots after surgery are caused by three things: the blood stagnating in the veins due to inactivity in bed. Getting patients out of bed as soon as possible minimizes this threat. Alterations in the blood vessel walls also affect the formation of blood clots. Dr. Spittle points out that vitamin C provides the ground substance, the very material, of which the blood vessels are made. And, finally, the formation of blood clots depends on how susceptible to coagulation the patient's blood is.

Says Dr. Spittle, the way in which blood coagulates depends on the condition of the blood vessel walls and what the fatty compounds in the walls have done to change this condition. Vitamin C is responsible for the proper metabolism of fat, she states, and gives three medical references for this statement. So, she says, vitamin C prevents blood clots by preventing the conditions in blood vessels which produce blood clots.

She refers to earlier experiments in which a group of elderly people were given vitamin C and the fats in their blood were tested frequently. It took about three months for massive doses of the vitamin to clear the blood of excess fatty material and reduce the triglycerides (certain harmful fats) to normal levels. So, says Dr. Spittle, giving large doses of vitamin C for three months after an operation would practically guarantee absolute protection against serious or fatal blood clots.

Impressed with this doctor's results, other surgeons in her hospital have started to give 500 milligrams of vitamin C to every patient they treat. They have had only three cases of clots in legs and two slight lung crises in six months. In that unit of the hospital which treats burns, one gram (1,000 milligrams) of vitamin C is given routinely to help in the healing process. Over a period of five and a half years only one death from lung clots has occurred in this ward and no leg clots. Involved were 159 patients over the age of 40 years.

Dr. Spittle is recommending that the dose in this hospital be increased to 1,000 milligrams daily.

We want to point out here that surgical patients are not the only ones who are threatened with strokes and blood clots in legs, lungs and elsewhere. Almost anyone past middle-age has seen friends, relatives, neighbors stricken suddenly with disabling or fatal strokes or heart attacks. If large doses of vitamin C are powerful against such incidents in surgical patients, doesn't it seem they would be even more effective in protecting the circulatory health of people not under this special stress?

We are not talking about a glass of orange juice at breakfast or tomato juice at lunch, although these are good food sources of vitamin C. In a happier time, when our distant ancestors lived surrounded by fresh fruits and berries which they ate in large amounts, these foods would have contained enough vitamin C to meet their needs. Today, in our industrialized world, we live surrounded by a thousand and one poisons for which we call on our limited stores of vitamin C to counteract. In the process, vitamin C is exhausted and we may not have enough left to help us through the next crisis.

Surgery is a terrible stress for the living body. In times of stress, animals which make their own vitamin C manufacture many times more of it than when they are free from stress. Why would we be any different? We, almost alone among animals, cannot manufacture our own vitamin C. We must get it in food. Is it not obvious that, under any kind of stress, we need far more vitamin C than we need during normal times? The vitamin C is used up rapidly combatting the elements of stress, so it must be replaced with large amounts of vitamin C at regular intervals.

Dr. George V. Mann, Associate Professor of Biochemistry and Medicine at Vanderbilt University, believes that, in the future, massive doses of vitamin C may be used along with insulin to prevent or delay the circulatory complications of diabetes. This includes hardening of the arteries and all the disorders that may follow in brains, in heart and blood vessels, in kidneys, in eye tissues, and in many other organs of the body.

Insulin is required for the transport of vitamin C or ascorbic acid, into cells of certain tissues. Diabetics lack insulin. Therefore it seems possible that the vitamin is not transported into these cells, resulting in a kind of "local scurvy."

Vitamin C is needed for the manufacture of collagen, the body "glue" that holds cells together. When it is not present in ample amounts, tissues tend to fall apart, resulting in cataract, hemorrhages, and many artery disorders.

Dr. Mann theorizes that possibly the same mechanism that transports blood sugar through cell walls also carries vitamin C. In the case of diabetics, blood sugar levels are too high so the mechanism may not be able to transport vitamin C at the same time. Old people as well as diabetics tend to have high blood sugar levels. Giving both groups very large doses of vitamin C may force the vitamin into the tissues, even though the body's transportation mechanism is defective.

"Isn't it possible, too, Dr. Mann theorizes, that the circulatory disorders and cataracts of old age are also the result of a diminishing insulin effect? True, these groups do not have the classic symptoms of the vitamin C deficiency disease, scurvy, possibly because they have enough insulin and vitamin C to reach certain cells. But the cells which need insulin and vitamin C the most are left in a deficient state.

In his laboratory, Dr. Mann discovered that in the concentrations of blood sugar which diabetics frequently have—up to 800 milligrams percent—the sugar does indeed stop off the transport of vitamin C into cells. The next step, experimentally, is to put diabetic animals on diets deficient in vitamin C to test the degree of harm to circulatory systems, eyes and so on.

A specialist in diabetes at the Joslin Diabetes Foundation thinks that Dr. Mann's theories are interesting. We should have more research on this subject, he believes. Dr. Harold Rifkin of Montefiore Hospital in New York, agrees that the idea should be studied further. He also warns that diabetics taking large doses of vitamin C may find that their urine tests are off, for somehow the vitamin gives false negative tests for diabetics and false positive tests for non-diabetics. Presumably this occurs because the chemical structure of glucose (blood sugar) ($C_6 H_{12} O_6$) and vitamin C ($C_6 H_8 O_6$) are similar enough that tests do not discriminate between them.

A team of British investigators, working independently, announced in *Medical World News* for April 24, 1974 that there is a complex relationship between insulin, glucose and vitamin C metabolism. Dr. W.J.H. Butterfield of Guy's Hospital and his colleagues found, he said, that non-diabetics who were given an injection of insulin showed a significant increase in vitamin C in the surrounding tissues. So it's possible, he thinks, that lack of sufficient vitamin C in diet may reduce the sensitivity of tissues to insulin, thus reducing the body's production of insulin. This would eventually cause diabetes. Obesity causes diabetes by increasing the amount of insulin needed by tissues to dispose of the accumulated glucose or blood sugar.

Using a complicated testing system which they developed, the doctors injected insulin and found a release of vitamin C in every non-diabetic person tested and an increased output of the vitamin after the injection. The diabetics, on the other hand, showed no effect on their vitamin C levels, but did show the definite and expected result of an increase in blood sugar uptake.

The British physicians intend to continue their investigations, especially the part vitamin C may play in retinopathy (disorders of the eye retina) which are frequent complications of diabetes. Their research was reported in *Perspectives in Biology and Medicine*, Winter, 1974.

Although not directly related to diabetes, another piece of vitamin C research (described in *Atherosclerosis*, Volume 19, 1974, pages 191-199) states that the cholesterol level of the blood, the liver and the heart artery decreased when vitamin C was given to laboratory rats along with methionine, an amino acid, or form of protein. Levels of another kind of fat, triglyceride, also decreased in the heart artery and liver. Vitamin C alone brought about some decrease, though not as much as the two substances together. It is noteworthy that rats make their own vitamin C. They were apparently not making enough in their livers to lower levels of fats. So the additional vitamin and amino acid brought about this healthful change.

These recent, very significant pieces of research have been undertaken because of the scientific community's great interest in Dr. Linus Pauling's and Dr. Irwin Stone's theories about our need for much larger amounts of this substance than we usually get in food. Dr. Stone believes we should not call ascorbic acid a vitamin, for vitamins are something essential to health which occur in food. But in almost all other animals but human beings, ascorbic acid is made in the liver. So, on this basis, it should rightfully be called a hormone, which is a substance manufactured by living creatures rather than plants. At some point in prehistoric times we human beings lost our ability to make our own vitamin C.

Diabetics who take large amounts of vitamin C must be very conscious of the effect this substance may have on their urine tests for sugar. A false test may result in giving a dose of insulin that is too large or too small, with drastic results. For non-diabetics there is no reason not to take large doses of vitamin C which may perhaps protect you against ever succumbing to this serious disease.

Four scientists at the University of Padova in Italy reported in the *International Journal of Vitamin and Nutrition Research* that they had withheld vitamin C from guinea pigs until the animals developed a chronic condition of vitamin C deficiency—a sort of subclinical scurvy. Then they measured the amounts of various essential substances in their brains.

They found, sure enough, that there were very definite and important changes which would be bound to affect many brain and nerve functions in the lives of these animals. If the same is true of human beings—and there seems no reason why it should not be—plain lack of enough vitamin C might certainly be a partial cause of many mental disorders, both serious and minor, both acute and chronic.

The liver of guinea pigs (like the liver of human beings) stores vitamin C. But throughout the Italian experiments it was found that changes in the brain were more important than changes in the liver. From this the scientists conclude that the brain is that part of living creatures which suffers most from lack of vitamin C. They pointed out one fact which surfaces in many studies of mental disorder. The copper content of the brain is increased when vitamin C is lacking. "It is well known," say these scientists, "that neurologic and psychiatric damage usually follows increase in brain copper concentrations."

Guinea pigs were used in the Italian experiment because,

as you will remember, they are one of the very few creatures aside from man which do not manufacture their own vitamin C.

Guinea pigs need so much vitamin C for good health that an equivalent amount for the much heavier adult human being would be 5 to 15 grams a day—that is 5,000 milligrams to 15,000 milligrams. And the officially recommended amount for good health is a measly 45 milligrams! Since 1949 biologists have known that the wild gorilla, eating fresh tropical foods all day, gets as much as four to five grams of vitamin C a day. This suggests, says Dr. Pauling in *Executive Health* (Vol.IX, No. 5) "that one or two grams might be needed by man for the best health."

An important statement on vitamin C in relation to strokes appeared in the January 31, 1976 issue of the British medical journal, *The Lancet*.

Dr. Geoffrey Taylor writes about the beginning of the process that leads to strokes—a rupture of the lining of small blood vessels of the brain which leads to degenerative changes in those blood vessels. "I have seen similar vascular changes under the tongues of elderly people," says Dr. Taylor, "and less striking changes in younger people which I have related to low vitamin C levels. These changes are rare in vegetarians who have a lot of vitamin C in their diets and in their blood. Over 200 years ago James Lind described 'varicose veins under the tongue' as a sign of scurvy (the vitamin C-deficiency disease)."

He goes on to say that in guinea pigs as well (one of the few creatures beside human beings that do not manufacture their own vitamin C) induced scurvy produces changes like this: thinning of the walls of the small blood vessels, disappearance of a certain kind of tissue and dilation of small blood vessels with hemorrhages when they are injured.

American observers, he says, have noted that thyroid and adrenal glands are affected by low levels of vitamin C. The fragility of small blood vessels is increased when vitamin C is lacking and the walls of these tiny vessels become much stronger when enough vitamin C is given. Diabetics, he says, probably need more vitamin C than non-diabetics, since they are highly susceptible to circulatory disease.

Many old folks and others who eat "institutional meals," hospital food or instant meals from dispensers have permanently low levels of vitamin C in their blood, because such meals cannot contain much of the vitamin. We know that vegetables kept warm for even a brief time on a steam table lose most of their vitamin C by the time they come to the table.

Dr. Taylor tells us, further, that vitamin C levels are low in hospital patients, in anybody who has just recovered from a cold, anyone who has had a heart attack, who is in shock or suffering from an infection. Deaths from heart attacks and strokes increase in number during winter when the need for vitamin C is greatest and when there is the least vitamin C in daily food.

He says he often notices small hemorrhage (black and blue marks) in the arms of people whose blood pressure has been taken. These marks occur just below the cuff of the blood pressure gage. This suggests, he says, that low levels of vitamin C, especially in people with high blood pressure, can cause similar small hemorrhages in the brain and in the muscle which surrounds the heart, resulting in stroke or heart attack.

Then, too, low levels of vitamin C may disrupt the levels of fatty substances in the blood bringing increased cholesterol in the blood and surrounding tissues. This may be one of the causes of cholesterol deposits in the process of hardening of the arteries, which is present in most circulatory disorders.

All this suggests, says Dr. Taylor, that doctors begin to reassess the significance of low levels of vitamin C which may be chronic or may just occur from time to time. These low levels may be, he says, factors in the cause and prevention of strokes which are one of the most feared of all complications of circulatory disease.

In the March, 1975 issue of the same publication, *The Lancet*, two American doctors report on treating a Parkinson's Disease patient with a drug which is often used in these cases—levodopa.

Parkinson's Disease is a nerve and muscle disorder which may bring tremor of hands, head or arms, a peculiar gait, excessive saliva, muscular rigidity, slowness of movement, difficulty in speaking, bizarre tics and other distressing symptoms. The patient described had shown dramatic improvement in his condition when the drug levodopa was first given. But the drug produced such nausea that he was unable to continue with the treatment. The doctors reduced the dosage. The patient's nausea continued, only a little less than before, but the initial improvement did not. The doctors decided to give vitamin C—one gram a day gradually increasing to 4 grams a day. This is 1,000 milligrams up to 4,000 milligrams. The levodopa dose was decreased.

Almost at once, the doctors say, the nausea disappeared. Within four weeks of taking these large doses of vitamin C, the patient's symptoms were much improved. He was able once again to move his head normally and to play the organ, something he had not been able to do for several years. Salivation also decreased, and his speech and handwriting improved considerably.

The physicians thought that the increased attention they were giving him might be responsible for the improvement. So, without telling the patient what they were doing, they substituted another pill for the vitamin C pill. All the improvement disappeared within two weeks. Excess salivation returned. Nausea returned. Coordination deteriorated. The doctors started the vitamin C pills again and once again improvement began to show within a short time.

The case of one patient is not an indication that all Parkinson patients will respond this way, say Dr. William Sacks and George M. Simpson of the Rockland State Hospital, Orangeburg, New York, but they think that more doctors should try this treatment and see if they get similar results.

There was no indication that the vitamin C was "curing" the Parkinson's Disease. But the drug which brought improvement for the disorder could be safely given if the vitamin accompanied it. This disabling disease is becoming more common. Doctors do not know why. It afflicts chiefly those of middle age or older. It seems a simple and harmless remedy to give large doses of vitamin C along with the only drug which has proved effective in treatment of this disease.

In the December 1966 issue of the *Journal of the American Geriatrics Society,* Dr. Boris Sokoloff and his colleagues at the Florida Southern College describe experiments which seem to show that vitamin C in quite large amounts and for long periods of time will reduce the levels in the blood of certain fatty substances, in most patients.

They tested 62 patients with normal or only moderate deviations from the norm in the amounts of fatty substances in their blood. They then gave them 1½ grams of vitamin C daily for four to five months. There was little or no change in the condition of the blood of these mostly normal people. But in 14 cases of moderately abnormal fat accumulations in the blood there was a "definite trend toward normal values."

Then they turned to another group of patients whose cholesterol levels were extremely high and some of whom were already suffering from heart disease. They gave these folks 2 to 3 grams of vitamin C every day for 1 to 3 years. In 10 there was no change in the condition. But in the 50 other cases there was definite and often marked improvement.

The authors point out that "in old people the requirement for vitamin C is higher than in younger people, the concentration of vitamin C is low. This seems to be one possible reason for the prevalence of strokes and heart attacks in this elderly group." They quote one authority who says, "a gross and often complete deficiency of ascorbic acid frequently exists in the arteries of apparently well-nourished autopsy subjects. Old age seems to accentuate deficiency."

In an earlier article in the *Journal of the American Geriatrics Society*, October, 1965, an Illinois physician reported giving 3 grams of vitamin C daily, along with very large doses of B vitamins to patients suffering from such poor circulation that their feet were constantly cold and other patients who had patches of gangrene and skin discoloration due to circulatory difficulties. In every case, relief was obtained. The vitamins were given two to three times weekly.

We are told officially that practically no one in these United States is deficient in vitamins. And we are told, so long as you get the minimum amount of vitamin C specified to keep you safe from scurvy, that is absolutely all you need and getting any more is a waste of time and money. How do you suppose such a point of view would strike those people described above whose heart and arteries were greatly improved when they were given massive doses of vitamin C?

The amounts given were very large. Dr. Sokoloff gave his seriously ill patients up to 3,000 milligrams a day for three years. This is far more than our government experts declare anyone needs to stay completely well, no matter what their age. There is no mention of any possible harm from vitamin C, since, of course, the vitamin is completely harmless. Whatever is not used by the body is excreted rapidly so that one should space his vitamin C intake throughout the day, rather than taking it all at one time.

In the 19 pages of Dr. Sokoloff's well-documented article, he presents the view that vitamin C in ample quantity is absolutely essential for the "physiological integrity" of the artery walls. And that this vitamin is closely related to the way the body uses the fat in food. He traces this relationship through many different biological processes involving animals and laboratory experiments.

The more fat you eat, especially animal fat rich in cholesterol, the more vitamin C you may need. This is such a new idea as to be almost revolutionary. Dr. Sokoloff's research does not invalidate all the earlier findings. It just adds one more note of hope for those of us who want to avoid heart and artery troubles.

A startling proposal on the possible relationship of vitamin C deficiency to heart failure was made in the conservative pages of *The Lancet*, July 22, 1967. Its author is a Glasgow physician, consultant to a group of hospitals.

Dr. J. Shafer was called to attend two patients with "florid scurvy"—that is, advanced cases of this disorder which has only one cause—lack of vitamin C. During tests, the patients were given electrocardiographs. Significant heart trouble was diagnosed on the basis of these tests. But after a week during which they were given lots of vitamin C, the two patients had no heart symptoms at all. Their cardiographs reverted to normal.

"In the view of the present prevalence of malnutrition among the elderly," he says. Dr. Shafer became concerned about the possibility of lack of vitamin C being responsible for many cases of illness that are diagnosed as heart conditions. In essence, he asks in this important article, what about subclinical scurvy—that is, lack of vitamin C which has not as yet caused the classic, easily recognized symptoms of scurvy, but which may have affected the heart enough to cause abnormal results in heart tests. Is it possible, he asks, that we are treating these people for heart conditions, when all they need is a good strong dose of vitamin C?

He tells us that scientific information on an association of vitamin C deficiency and heart health is scanty. But, he says, scurvy remains a "not uncommon disorder." He says it occurs mostly in people who live alone, those who have peculiar ideas about what foods to eat and those who have diseases of the digestive tract, which necessitate the elimination of vitamin C-rich foods.

He says he uses the term "doctor-caused" scurvy when the disorder occurs in people who have restricted their diets on the advice of their physician, and where the physician has not provided them with a vitamin C supplement. In other words, let's say a doctor has said you must go on a low residue diet and stop eating all fresh raw fruits and vegetables. This is just about the surest way to develop a sub-clinical, if not a full-blown case of scurvy, the disease of vitamin C deficiency, because this vitamin is all but absent from foods other than those which have been forbidden. A physician who is aware of this will give a patient a vitamin C supplement. But if he isn't and if the patient hasn't enough knowledge of nutrition to know that he must have a good source of vitamin C, how can the vitamin deficiency be prevented?

Dr. Shafer tells us that an investigation of people who have certain disorders of malabsorption, like steatorrhea, has shown that they are all short on vitamin C even though they are getting plenty of it in their diets. They just don't absorb it, because their condition prevents the absorption of many vital elements in food. He quotes another expert as saying that he suggests that "a profitable approach would be to regard all patients affected with gastroduodenal disorders as possibly in a 'sub-clinical scorbutic' condition." He goes on to say that doctors now know that abnormalities of heart action may be present during operations or the taking of anesthetics and one reason for this may be a previous deficiency in vitamin C.

Let's see now. How many people do you suppose there are in our country who are affected with gastro-duodenal disorders? A million? Ten million? Since a great many such victims don't even go to doctors there seems to be no way of estimating the number. Whatever it is, one scientific researcher at least believes that all of them may be short on vitamin C, to such an extent that they may be in a sub-clinical state of scurvy and may be courting heart disorders as a result.

Is it possible, asks Dr. Shafer, in *The Lancet*, that large doses of vitamin C act like a drug in calming the hearts of scurvy victims? He reminds his readers that if vitamin C is given with digitalis, a heart drug, it prevents or minimizes the changes in heart action which the drug brings on and it allows the patient to continue to take digitalis in spite of the appearance of bad side effects from the drug.

A Penn State biologist told a meeting of the Federation of American Scientists for Experimental Biology recently that experiments in his laboratory had shown that a certain form of vitamin C flushes cholesterol from the inner walls of arteries, preventing hardening of the arteries.

Said Dr. Ralph Mumma, "The present results raise the speculation that large doses of some form of ascorbic acid might one day be used to remit—or prevent— atherosclerosis in human beings." Atherosclerosis is the medical term for hardening of the arteries which probably brings on the heart and circulatory complications that are becoming more and more common among people who are middle-aged or older.

In the past years Soviet scientists have claimed that they could prevent unwanted cholesterol accumulations with large doses of vitamin C. Official American medicine was skeptical. Now, however, Dr. Mumma has pointed out that his experiments appear to confirm the Soviet experiments. They were showing that vitamin C made the walls of arteries less permeable, hence prevented the cholesterol from permeating them and collecting there, then hardening into plaques which narrow the walls of arteries so that blood cannot pass through easily.

Surveys have shown that modern Western diets with their large amounts of fat and sugar tend to produce heart attacks and other circulatory ills. Smoking has also been related to these disorders. And stress. A diet rich in fats and sweets would probably be lacking in vitamin C. Fresh fruit does not occupy much space on a menu which features rich, heavily-sweetened desserts. Smoking destroys vitamin C in the blood. Stress uses up vitamin C which is stored in the adrenal glands, those organs which take a beating when we are under stress.

Could not all these related facts have something to do with our modern high incidence of heart attacks? Is it not possible that plenty of vitamin C, in fresh raw fruits and vegetables, along with natural food supplements of high potency, could prevent, or help to prevent the ravages of hardening of the arteries?

New evidence of the relationship between vitamin C and circulatory disorders appeared in the January, 1970 issue of *The American Journal of Clinical Nutrition*. It now seems probable that deficiency in vitamin C may be one of the most important causes of hardening of the coronary artery which is the basic cause of most heart attacks.

Carl F. Shaffer, M.D., reviews medical literature on this subject and tells us that, in animal experiments, the formation of the fatty deposits on the inside of arteries can be reversed by giving the animals vitamin C. Even after only three days of vitamin C therapy, the guinea pigs completely lost their "hard" fatty deposits inside arteries. The deposits continued to decline as long as the vitamin was given.

There is general agreement, says Dr. Shaffer, that vitamin C plays a major role in assuring the health of the lining of arteries. A deficiency in vitamin C produces in guinea pigs a condition that is just like hardening of the arteries in human beings. Correcting the deficiency corrects the condition. Anything that disturbs vitamin C availability, either locally or throughout the animal's body, results in injury to the wall of the artery and the fatty deposits begin at once to form.

"Coronary atherosclerosis (hardening) therefore, appears to be, in part, a possible result of deficient ingestion of ascorbic acid (vitamin C)," says Dr. Shaffer.

He goes on to talk about abnormal electrocardiograms in people suffering from scurvy. Once they have gotten lots of the vitamin for several weeks, the electrocardiogram returns to normal. "The possibility was considered that such abnormalities may develop in those persons with subclinical deficiency, especially in relation to the prevalence of malnutrition among the elderly," he says.

What about cholesterol? Guinea pigs with normal

cholesterol levels and without any deposits of fat on the walls of their arteries develop conditions like human hardening of the arteries when they are made deficient in vitamin C. The cholesterol and other fat in their diets seem to have nothing at all to do with it.

When the inner wall of the artery is injured by lack of vitamin C, one must consider hemorrhage (stroke), thrombosis (blood clots) and deposits of calcium, says Dr. Shaffer. The general medical consensus at present is that these all result mostly from eating too much fat. Research with animals appears to show that it may be caused by too little vitamin C.

He summarizes his observations thus:

1. A main function of vitamin C is to help in the manufacture of the substance which holds our cells together and forms collagen.

2. One part of hardening of the arteries is all the processes that occur around the formation of collagen in the fatty lining of arteries.

3. Hardening of the arteries has been caused in laboratory animals with normal blood levels of cholesterol and no fatty deposits on the insides of their arteries. You do this by withholding vitamin C.

4. Deficiency in vitamin C is much more common among older folks who suffer most from hardening of the arteries, heart attacks, and other circulatory troubles.

5. He believes that the vitamin C deficiency may be only one part of the complex number of things that may be involved in producing hardening of the arteries.

CHAPTER 31

Colds, Vitamin C
and Linus Pauling

IN LATE 1970 Dr. Linus Pauling, twice winner of a Nobel prize and the most distinguished and respected biologist alive today, published a book called *Vitamin C and the Common Cold*. In it he recommended taking very large doses of vitamin C to prevent colds and to shorten the duration of the after effects.

Dr. Pauling's book made nutritional history. He was defended and attacked in many scientific and medical publications, in many newspapers and magazines of general circulation. There were those who tried to intimidate him, those who laughed, those who scorned, those who said he was out of his field of specialty and hence had no competence.

Dr. Pauling's book deserves serious reading by anyone interested in health and nutrition. Its critics managed to ignore the most important part of his theory which is, simply, that human beings may have inherited, down through all the ages, a need for far larger amounts of vitamin C than we are currently getting. Dr. Pauling has calculated the amount of vitamin C that might have been in the daily fare of our early ancestors and finds that it approaches the very large amount of vitamin C he himself takes every day. He recommends that everyone attempt to prevent colds for himself by taking large doses of vitamin C daily. Even if colds are not prevented, they can be considerably shortened and after effects avoided by massive doses of vitamin C, says Dr. Pauling.

In the intervening years, many experiments have been done to negate or confirm Pauling's theory. Some of these have failed. Many have succeeded. And now many thousands of people are regularly taking vitamin C to prevent colds and to treat their side effects, with great success. Dr. Pauling began his research on vitamin C because of the work of a chemist named Irwin Stone who has devoted his life to studying everything available in medical and scientific literature on the subject.

Dr. Stone is the author of a book *The Healing Factor— Vitamin C Against Disease* in which he deals with almost every plague with which modern industrialized man is afflicted. In alphabetical order they are: aging, allergies, asthma and hay fever, arthritis and rheumatism, bacterial infection, cancer, colds, diabetes and its opposite, low blood sugar, eye disorders like glaucoma and cataract, heart and circulatory disorders, kidney and bladder diseases, mental illness, poisoning by chemicals and metals like lead and mercury, pollution and smoking, ulcers, virus infections and wounds.

There is convincing evidence in the book that all of these conditions may improve by the simple addition to one's food supplements of massive doses of vitamin C. The evidence comes from animal and human experimentation. Much of the research was done in early years just after the discovery and synthesis of vitamin C, when the official cynical viewpoint on vitamins had not developed. There was, instead, great enthusiasm for trying all kinds of experiments with this newly acquired substance which is completely harmless and apparently so powerful in its action on the body.

The largest part of Dr. Stone's testimony on vitamin C is involved with its function in relation to collagen, the physiological "cement" that holds us together. Vitamin C is the essential ingredient of collagen. "Collagen is the body's most important structural substance." It is the ground substance, or cement, that supports and holds the tissues and organs together. It is the substance in the bones that provides the toughness and flexibility and prevents brittleness. Without it the body would just disintegrate or dissolve away.

"It comprises about one-third of the body's total weight of protein and is the most extensive tissue system. It is the substance that strengthens the arteries and veins, supports the muscles, toughens the ligaments and bones, supplies the scar tissue for healing wounds and keeps the youthful skin tissues soft, firm, supple and wrinkle-free.

"When ascorbic acid (vitamin C) is lacking, it is the disturbance in collagen formation that causes the fearful effects of scurvy—the brittle bones that fracture on the slightest impact, the weakened arteries that rupture and hemorrhage, the incapacitating muscle weakness, the affected joints that are too painful to move, the teeth that fall out, and the wounds and sores that never heal. Suboptimal amounts of ascorbic acid over prolonged periods during the early and middle years, by its effect of producing poor quality collagen, may be the factor in later life that causes the high incidence of arthritis and joint diseases, broken hips, and heart and vascular diseases that cause sudden death, and the strokes that bring on senility. Collagen is intimately connected with the entire aging process," says Dr. Stone.

Let's talk in detail about just one chapter in the book—cancer, the disease whose very name strikes terror in the heart of anyone alive in modern America. Over half a million people develop cancer every year in this country. More than 280,000 will die of it next year. More than 700,000 people are under treatment for cancer at any given time. At present the official, orthodox treatment involves radiation, surgery or drug therapy.

Dr. Stone reminds us that any of these three methods of treatment present the body with intense biological stress.

This depletes the patient's body of vitamin C. When rats, which manufacture their own vitamin C, are exposed to cancer-producing substances, they immediately begin to manufacture vast amounts of vitamin C as protection. Dr. Stone tells us of experiments in which guinea pigs were exposed to cancer-causing substances. Those which were given ample amounts of vitamin C developed the disease later than animals on vitamin C deficient diets. Guinea pigs, like man, do not make their own vitamin C. They must get it in food.

Dr. Stone quotes National Cancer Institute scientists as saying that vitamin C destroys cancer cells, that it is harmless to animals in extremely large doses—which would correspond to 350 milligrams of the vitamin for a human being. And, finally, they say, "In our view, the future of effective cancer chemotherapy will not rest on the use of host-toxic compounds now so widely employed but upon virtually host nontoxic compounds that are lethal to cancer cells, of which ascorbate (vitamin C)... represents an excellent prototype example."

Then, says Dr. Stone, in the screening program that has gone on at the National Cancer Institute for many years to find new cancer-killing substances, vitamin C has been "bypassed, excluded from consideration, and never tested for its cancer-killing properties. The reason given for not screening ascorbic acid is even more fantastic—ascorbic acid was too non-toxic to fit into their program!"

Then follow four pages of evidence of the effectiveness of vitamin C in cases of cancer, and the power of vitamin C against some cancer-causing agents, the very inadequate amounts of the vitamin that have been used in most unsuccessful trials and finally one astonishing story of a 71-year-old man with leukemia who took up to 42 grams of vitamin C daily "because he felt better when he took these large doses." Whenever, at his doctor's insistence, he stopped taking the vitamin, his symptoms returned. They disappeared when he once again began the vitamin therapy.

Dr. Stone asks, "If megascorbic (large doses of vitamin C) therapy could do so much for an aged leukemic with so many other complications, what could it do for the young, uncomplicated leukemic? The answer to this question could be obtained easily and each day lost may mean more lives wasted. At the present time, millions of dollars are spent in screening all sorts of poisonous chemicals for use in leukemia, while a harmless substance like ascorbic acid, with so much potential, lies around neglected and ignored."

CHAPTER 32

Plenty of Vitamin C
May Prevent
Bladder Cancer

CANCER OF THE urinary bladder appears to be an increasing threat as the toxins in our environment accumulate at a frightening pace and less and less is known about their potential for causing cancer. The body has defense mechanisms for disposing of poisons. It eliminates them as rapidly as possible. One method is to excrete them in urine. So it seems possible that many of the poisons to which we are exposed daily find their way to the kidney, then to the bladder by way of the ureter, which is the connecting tube between these two organs.

It might surprise you to hear that some substances suspected of causing bladder cancer are things some of us use every day, some of us use at every meal. The June 23, 1973 issue of the *Canadian Medical Journal* contained an article on the subject by Balfour M. Mount of the Department of Urology at the Royal Victoria Hospital and the Department of Surgery at McGill University in Montreal.

Dr. Mount tells us the earliest discovery of a relationship between environmental poisons and bladder cancer came in 1895 when a German physician tied the high incidence of bladder cancer among workers in the dye industry to the chemicals they were working with. His discovery resulted in laws to protect workers against such exposure. Since then many chemicals have been incriminated as causes of bladder cancer and a number of others are suspected agents.

Here is a list of industrial chemicals which are known to produce bladder cancer in human beings: 2-naphthylamine, benzidine, 4-aminodiphenyl, Chlornaphazine, 2-bis- (2-chloroethyl) aminonaphthylamine, 1-naphthylamine, Diphenylamine, Auramine, Rosanaline (fuchsin), Dianaisidine, N-1-naphthylthiourea. We are told that there are at present some 1.8 million manmade chemicals at large in the environment and 400 new ones are introduced every year. How many more of these may turn out to be cancer-causing to human beings is anybody's guess at the moment.

Here are other substances now being evaluated for their possible cancer-causing qualities: pain killers that contain phenacetin, artificial sweeteners, Cyclophosphamide, and chemicals which interfere with tryptophan metabolism (this is an amino acid or form of protein.) Also suspected of being cancer-causing are these bracken fern, tobacco, viruses and coffee. Does that surprise you?

Dr. Mount tells us that the incidence of bladder cancer in smokers is approximately twice that of non-smokers. The prospects for recovery are much worse in those who continue to smoke, than it is in non-smokers or those who have stopped smoking. There seems to be no relationship to cigar or pipe smoking. No one knows exactly how tobacco brings about bladder cancer. There may be carcinogenic (cancer-causing) substances in the tobacco smoke itself. This seems to us to be very likely since arsenic is used to spray the tobacco leaf, along with many other pesticides which also may be cancer-causing. Undoubtedly some residue of these poisons remains in the tobacco.

There is also the possibility that the way in which smoking causes bladder cancer is the ability of even one cigarette to lower vitamin C levels in the blood and urine. "Patients in the bladder tumor population should be advised to stop smoking cigarettes," says Dr. Mount. This is, of course, easier said than done. Surely everyone knows by now that smoking is harmful in many ways, but an increasing number of people continue to smoke and an increasing number of people are addicted to smoking to such a degree that they find it impossible to stop and maintain any equilibrium in their personal lives.

Dr. Mount says that sufficiently high levels of vitamin C can be obtained in the urine by taking 500 milligrams of vitamin C three times a day at intervals during the day. He quotes Dr. Jorgen Schlegel of the Tulane University Department of Urology who has been making this advice to his bladder patients for many years. Dr. Schlegel practically guarantees that there will be no recurrence of the cancer if this prescription is faithfully followed for life.

It is most interesting that cancer patients in general, as well as people "at risk" from bladder cancer, and the elderly, as well as smokers all have low blood levels of vitamin C, says Dr. Mount. Does that suggest to you an excellent way that all of these groups might fortify themselves against many disorders and possibly prevent cancer—simply by taking enough vitamin C to flood all their tissues with the vitamin!

One and a half grams, which is 1,500 milligrams, taken in three doses throughout the day is completely harmless, says Dr. Mount, and free from the complications which he feels may result from larger doses than that—complications involving oxalic acid in the urine. We would point out that physicians who regularly use much larger doses of vitamin C daily and prescribe it for their patients do not find that the oxalic acid in their urine presents any problem.

Another vitamin is mentioned by Dr. Mount as possibly preventive of bladder cancer—vitamin B6 or pyridoxine. The vitamin tends to restore the bladder cancer victim's tryptophan metabolism to normal. About half of all patients with bladder cancer excrete elevated amounts of the breakdown products of this amino acid, which is believed to be cancer-causing.

Is it possible that some abnormality in the body's use of tryptophan may be one cause of bladder cancer? We do not know, but Dr. Mount quotes a famous cancer researcher, Dr. W.C. Hueper, as saying that it is an "unproved but interesting speculation." Another researcher believes that it is a good case of circumstantial evidence. Dr. Mount says, "it seems reasonable to proceed with a prophylactic regimen of 200 milligrams of pyridoxine daily which is non-toxic and may rectify the whole metabolic picture where some cancer-causing chemicals are concerned." We would point out that the officially recommended daily level of pyridoxine is only two milligrams daily, so he is recommending one hundred times this amount. However, it seems reasonable to take extraordinary measures in situations which are extraordinary.

What about artificial sweeteners? Cyclamates were recently withdrawn from the market when they caused bladder cancers in rats in quite large doses. There is no evidence that they cause tumors in human beings. Implanting saccharin in the bodies of rats also produces cancer, but there is no evidence that the sweetener, taken by mouth, is cancer-causing in human beings.

Dr. Mount quotes one researcher as saying that it will be difficult indeed to set up an experiment in which one group of human beings taking saccharin is studied in contrast with a control group not taking it, since, he says, at least 75 percent of all Americans have at one time or another taken saccharin. However, the Ninth National Cancer Conference recommended "in the interim, and on the basis of the correlative data presented here, it would appear most prudent at this time to limit utilization of saccharin to diabetics, the severely obese, and others with specific medical problems."

Pain killers which contain phenacetin are everywhere. It is an ingredient of most advertised pain remedies and cold remedies. It is advertised for all kinds of not very serious aches and pains like headaches, neuralgias and pain associated with the menstrual cycle. Evidence from Sweden and Australia indicates that there is an increased incidence of bladder cancer among people who use these pain killers to excess.

No one knows for certain that the villain is actually the phenacetin, but its formula is close to that of another chemical known to be cancer-causing. There is also a risk of kidney damage when this drug is used. Dr. Mount says patients "at risk" from bladder cancer should avoid these and all other pain killers.

And now about coffee. A Harvard University researcher was trying to find out more about the relationship of smoking and occupational exposure to chemicals which cause bladder cancer. He found, to his surprise, that there is a greater incidence of bladder cancer among those men and women who drink coffee. The association of coffee with this kind of cancer was especially strong in the group he studied who did not smoke and who were not exposed in their work to industrial substances known to cause bladder cancer. "This report," says Dr. Mount, "should remind us of the continuing need to be on the alert to the possibility of carcinogens in our environment."

There is not much comfort for those of us who used to smoke and who smoke no longer. It's well known that cancers sometimes take many years to develop, after exposure to the cancer-causing agent. There is not much encouragement in telling ourselves that, well, we don't actually drink much coffee. It seems likely that people who smoke tend to drink more coffee than non-smokers, since both coffee and cigarettes disrupt blood sugar levels in such a devastating way that the poor victim must reinforce his failing sense of well-being by alternating his props—cigarettes and coffee. If indeed the coffee link to bladder cancer is as strong as that of cigarettes, then this kind of person is most likely to succumb to this extremely disabling and serious condition.

What can the health seeker do to protect himself or herself against this threat? First of all, obviously, stop smoking if you smoke. Stop smoking if you have to shut yourself up in a room and go "cold turkey" as other drug addicts must.

It will help greatly if you will, at the same time, break those other harmful habits which contribute to your addiction to smoking. Stop eating sugar or anything that contains it. Eat lots and lots of high protein foods. Eat them at frequent intervals during the day so that you never succumb to that agonizing "all-gone" feeling which is the symptom of low blood sugar.

Stop drinking coffee. If you must taper off, it's probably wise to switch to decaffeinated coffee or tea, although both, of course, contain caffeine—strong tea almost as much as strong coffee. Switch to milk, switch to fruit juice, or to herb teas. But stop drinking coffee. Don't take pain killers. Most especially don't get into the habit of taking them regularly for any slight headache or joint stiffness. Next time you suffer from any such slight indisposition, go outside and take a long, vigorous walk in the fresh air and see if you don't feel better at once.

And, finally, get yourself some vitamin C in high potencies and take it every day. If you have been a confirmed smoker and coffee drinker for many years, this expedient becomes even more important. You can perhaps prevent any bladder trouble before it gets started. Get yourself some pyridoxine and take it in the quantities suggested.

You can perhaps help to prevent any bladder troubles in the future. In any case, both pyridoxine and vitamin C are harmless in these amounts and may, who knows, bring many other health benefits which you aren't even expecting!

CHAPTER 33

Vitamin C for
Your Back Troubles

BACK PAIN SEEMS to afflict just about everybody at one time of life or another. Statistics collected by writers on the subject seem to show that during any given year, 28 million Americans may stagger into their doctors' offices doubled up with pain in (usually) the lower back region. Since President Kennedy's famous rocking chair made its appearance in the White House, lower back pain has become fashionable. In almost any gathering at least some people present can boast of their sacroiliac or "slipped disc" complications.

There seem to be three main reasons for today's epidemic of back troubles. First is the structure of the human back which readily lends itself to poor alignment. We were probably meant to walk on all-fours, as other mammals do. When our early ancestors began to walk upright, the spinal column had to absorb all the extra work and accommodation. Somehow this curiously complicated string of bones and nerves had to become adjusted to carrying weights, walking on hard surfaces, bending suddenly to pick up heavy loads, sitting all day working at a desk or machine, riding all day and/or night in a jogging truck or autombile. We further complicated things by wearing shoes with heels which throw us even further off balance. And we became, over the past 40 years or so, almost sedentary.

And that brings us to the second probable cause of most back troubles—we just don't move around enough.

Dr. James Greenwood, Jr., Professor of Neurosurgery at Baylor College of Medicine and Chief of Neurosurgery at the Methodist Hospital in Houston, Texas, says in *Executive Health*, Volume X, No. 12 that spinal discs, the joints that accompany them and the ligaments that tie the joints together have no significant blood supply of their own. They are, he says, "dependent upon motion for the introduction and distribution of nutrient fluids." In other words, if you don't move around enough, especially if you don't use your back regularly and intensively all day for all the motions that a back is capable of making, you are doing yourself grave harm. Your back, as well as other parts of you, was meant to move vigorously.

As we of the technological age hand more and more of our hard physical work over to machines, as we ride instead of walking, punch buttons instead of doing laundry or washing dishes, turn a faucet rather than pumping a hand pump, parts of our bodies begin to show stress from not being used enough. A protracted illness or convalescence which confines us to bed for a long time further debilitates muscles and ligaments of our backs. If, unused to heavy exercise, we bend all our energies to snow shoveling or spading up the garden, we are likely to develop one of those locked backs, unable to straighten up without unearthly pain.

A third cause of modern back troubles seems to be a plain deficiency in vitamin C. It's not that we're neglecting our ritual glass of orange juice or tomato juice at breakfast, but that, somehow, in all the stresses and environmental pangs of modern life, we seem to need far, far more vitamin C than we get in the average American diet if we want to keep our backs free from pain.

At least that's the way it seems from the experience of some very knowledgeable physicians who use vitamin C in large doses to treat and prevent orthopedic back troubles. M.L. Riccitelli of New Haven, Connecticut tells us in *The Journal of the American Geriatrics Society,* Volume 20, No. 1 that, in 1964, a doctor named J. Greenwood, Jr., reported that he used high dosage therapy of vitamin C in more than 500 patients with low back pain diagnosed as lumbosacral sprain, disc injury with or without root involvement, or chronic degenerative disc lesions.

"A significant number of patients with early disc lesions were able to avoid surgery," he tells us. And many patients who stopped their vitamin C intake after they improved found they had to return to it if they wanted to continue to avoid their painful symptoms.

Dr. Greenwood gave his patients 500 milligrams of vitamin C daily, in two doses, increasing it to 1,000 milligrams if there was any discomfort on exertion.

The same Dr. Greenwood, in *Executive Health*, tells us that adequate protein in the diet is important in maintaining the integrity of all these complicated mechanisms in the spinal column. But it occurred to him some years ago that deficiency in vitamin C might be just as important. Vitamin C is responsible, after all, for the health of all the connective tissues of the body—that is, the tissues that hold us together.

When he himself developed back trouble in 1957, Dr. Greenwood began to take 100 milligrams of vitamin C three times daily, increasing it to 500 milligrams three times daily which relieved his own pain. He found, surprisingly, that he could also prevent muscle soreness by taking vitamin C before he started on some vigorous camping trip or sailing voyage.

He began to use vitamin C in large doses for his patients. His patients had back pain, sciatica, neck pain and arm pain. Many of the back and leg pain patients came from urologists who were treating them for cystitis or prostatitis—inflammation of the urinary bladder or prostate gland. He thinks that the pain in these cases came from direct deficiency in vitamin C, since it is well known that any infections use up vitamin C rapidly. So not enough was available to safeguard the health of the back and leg muscles and ligaments. As his bladder infection patients continued to take large amounts of vitamin C for their back pains, they found that it cleared up the bladder infections as well. And now, he tells us, many urologists are using vitamin C regularly against infections.

Patients who got over their back problems tended to neglect their vitamin C, and many of them came back several years later with the same complaints. Once again, vitamin C came to the rescue. A friend of Dr. Greenwood's, an orthopedic surgeon, suggested that he try larger doses of the vitamin for better results.

Individual dosage is something that must be worked out by the individual, says Dr. Greenwood. It is impossible to lay down any general rules for dosage that will apply to everyone. He tells the story of a patient of 62 who practices ballet one hour four times a week in a class of much younger students. She had an operation on a ruptured disc years earlier when she was taking 500 milligrams of vitamin C daily to prevent colds. Some knee and back troubles that developed in her ballet classes required 2,000 milligrams a day for relief so that she could return to the class.

Dr. Greenwood refers to Dr. Roger Williams' work on biochemical individuality and says that, in every case, one's own physical make-up should govern the amount of vitamin C needed to correct troubles with backs, legs, necks and arms. What is enough for some member of your family may not be nearly enough for you, and vice versa. Even laboratory animals, bred to be as identical in all their needs as possible show great differences—as much as 20 times—in their need for various vitamins and minerals. Human beings who come from a widely varied stock of ancestors must, perforce, have even greater variability in their needs.

Today, Dr. Greenwood says, he usually starts back pain patients on 1,500 milligrams a day of vitamin C—500 milligrams with each meal. Some patients report stomach irritation, in which case he reduces the dosage. If it needs to be increased to alleviate the back disturbances, he does so. He says that large doses of vitamin C should not be taken on an empty stomach, but during or following meals. Some patients take as much as 4,000 milligrams daily without any stomach complaints.

Vitamin C is necessary for prevention of weakness and degeneration of spinal discs, says Dr. Greenwood. It is also needed for healing strains and injuries and to prevent or alleviate severe muscle soreness due to excessive exercise. He does not claim that vitamin C is the only treatment for strengthening the back, but he insists that it is one important item.

The other most important item, he says, is exercise—regular, daily, mild exercise for "circulation of nutrient fluids and metabolism of discs, tendons, ligaments, joints and all tissues of the body . . . Adequate nutrition, including optimum vitamin C, and daily exercise, will eliminate most back pains, strains and disc ruptures," says Dr. Greenwood.

CHAPTER 34

Vitamin C and
Mental Health

A NEW ZEALAND DOCTOR is conducting a study of the effects of one gram of vitamin C daily in the treatment of chronic schizophrenics in a mental hospital. This is our most serious mental disorder in which patients completely lose touch with reality.

Dr. Michael H. Briggs described his experiments in a letter to the editor of the *British Medical Journal*. He says that patients in mental hospitals may suffer from chronic lack of vitamin C because of poor dietary habits. They simply cannot be made to eat enough fresh raw foods which are our most dependable source of this elusive vitamin.

But, says Dr. Briggs, there is another reason why schizophrenics may be short on vitamin C. It has been found, he says, that these mental patients may have an overabundance of copper in the blood. One investigator has shown that the amounts of copper in blood fluctuate rapidly in emotional states. So when mental patients become agitated, as they may several times a day, the copper content of their blood may increase rapidly.

We do not know how or why this should be, but we do know that copper is very destructive of vitamin C. It burns up vitamin C whenever it comes into contact with it. So it would seem that these disturbed people may lose large amounts of vitamin C each time they have an emotional upset.

Dr. Briggs reports that chronic schizophrenics excrete considerably more vitamin C than other types of mental patients. This, too, would indicate that the copper blood levels brought about by their excitement are causing them to lose vitamin C. The New Zealand investigator believes that being constantly short on vitamin C could lead to an imbalance of other substances in the liver which might allow some unwanted substances to accumulate, leading to mental disturbances.

Thus, lack of vitamin C could lead to a disturbed mental condition, which might cause high levels of copper in the blood which would destroy even more vitamin C, thus setting up a cycle that would condemn the patient to chronic mental illness. Certainly no one should suggest that lack of vitamin C is the only cause or even the main cause of the schizoid type of mental illness. But we are glad to know that doctors are experimenting with vitamins in mental illness rather than devoting themselves entirely to drugs and psychotherapy.

Also we think it is encouraging that researchers are beginning to see that there is an important relation between one's physical health and diet and mental health. For those of us who are not mentally ill the lesson is obvious. Emotional excitement may use up vitamin C. Chronic losses of this kind, along with frequent emotional upsets would lead to something more serious.

This is another reason why we should watch our diets carefully to make certain we are getting enough of the vitamins, and supplement our meals with food supplements to insure that we have no deficiency.

A British psychiatrist, too, has been using vitamin C in the treatment of patients at a mental hospital. Dr. G. Milner's interest was aroused when he read of research indicating that anxiety and excitement tend to destroy the body's supply of vitamin C. He, too, found that patients suffering from schizophrenia have lower levels of vitamin C in their blood, even though they are getting the same amount in their food.

He knows, too, that there is a condition called "subscurvy" in which individuals feel tired, depressed, irritable and complain of vague ill health. They do not have a full-blown case of scurvy (the disease of vitamin C deficiency) with hemorrhaging and painful muscles and all the other symptoms, but one would certainly not say they are in good health.

Why not, said Dr. Milner, try to clarify the situation in regard to vitamin C and mental health, to discover whether lack of this vitamin may have something to do with some of the complaints of mentally ill patients—tiredness, depression and so forth. So he set up an experiment in a mental hospital with the cooperation of 40 male patients, some of whom had been in the hospital as long as 45 years.

Studying these men before the experiment began, he found that 12 of them already had symptoms of vitamin C deficiency which no one had thought of any importance. They had indigestion, tiny hemorrhages on the scalp, bleeding gums and rather horny skin. Those patients who were given vitamin C during the test improved while they were taking the vitamin. All symptoms disappeared.

The doctor divided the patients into two groups, each of whom took a measured dose of a liquid every day for three weeks. Twenty of them were taking one gram of vitamin C. The others were getting nothing but flavored water. No one, including the doctors, patients, and nurses knew which patients had been taking the vitamin until the test was over. Throughout this time, all patients were given psychiatric tests which indicate the patient's frame of mind—whether he is still depressed, manic, paranoid and so on. Nurses, doctors and other hospital personnel made notes on their impressions of each patient's condition—whether or not he had improved.

After the test was completed, it was found that the patients taking the vitamin C had improved considerably, both in the tests and in the opinion of those caring for them.

Even more important, said Dr. Milner, is his discovery that these patients were short on vitamin C even though they were eating a well planned diet in which there was apparently enough vitamin C for a well person.

These people had a greater need for vitamin C than the rest of us. Did their state of "subscurvy" contribute to their mental condition? We do not know. But we do know that they improved immeasurably within three weeks when they were given a daily massive dose of vitamin C, so that all their body tissues were saturated with it.

A letter to the *British Medical Journal*, May 12, 1962, reports on the experience of a Canadian doctor who treated a patient suffering from schizophrenia with one gram of vitamin C every hour for 48 hours—a gigantic dose of this vitamin. At the end of that time she was mentally well. She was discharged and remained mentally well for six months when she died from an unrelated disease.

This psychiatrist was Dr. Abram Hoffer whose work we have referred to many times. Dr. Hoffer works closely with other psychiatrists who use the megavitamin, or orthomolecular method of treatment for schizophrenia, with the Huxley Institute for Biosocial Research and various Schizophrenia Associations, all of whom are involved in the effort to treat this baffling and widespread mental disorder with good nourishing diet, plus large amounts of the B vitamins and vitamin C, along with whatever other therapy may be needed.

Orthomolecular psychiatrists report that treatment is successful in most of their cases, that the earlier the treatment is given the more likely it is to succeed. The vitamins are inexpensive. The treatment involves no long drawn out sessions with the psychiatrist. The patient sees him, goes home, takes his vitamins and visits his psychiatrist every month or every few months.

For more information about this kind of treatment and where it is available, write to: The Huxley Institute for Biosocial Research, 1114 First Avenue, New York City 10021.

CHAPTER 35

Is Vitamin C
Really a Hormone?

MANY COMMENTATORS ON the subject of megadoses (very large doses) of vitamin C do not seem to have realized just why these recommendations are being made. Nor do they understand the reason why a number of distinguished scientists believe we should all be getting far far more of this vitamin—a reason that goes back into pre-history and has to do with what scientists call a "mutation."

A mutation is damage to that part of a living cell which carries biological information on to the next generation. Damage may be caused by radiation, by chemicals or poisons of various sorts. Background radiation, which is present in all parts of the planet, is believed to have caused most of the mutations which result in people being damaged in some way that is inheritable. The damage "runs in families."

Hemophilia, the bleeding disease, is a disorder caused by a mutation. In most instances, the harm that mutation does is to disable or destroy an enzyme. Enzymes are those complicated chemical substances which make things happen in our bodies. A mutation which occurred way back in human history and affected every human being alive at that time must have damaged an enzyme. Therefore, it would disable the body's efficiency in this regard.

Irwin Stone, the scientist who has been putting together the puzzle of vitamin C for 40 years, tells us a mutation came about millions of years ago which is responsible for the fact that human beings cannot make their own vitamin C as almost all animals do. In *The Journal of Orthomolecular Medicine,* Volume 1, numbers 2 and 3, he reviews prehistorical times and shows us just how it came about that we all have this serious disadvantage of not being able to make our own vitamin C.

"About 165 million years ago," he says, "when Nature had the evolution of the more active and stressful mammals in view, an important morphological and physiological decision had to be made." It seems that reptiles manufactured vitamin C in their kidneys. These sluggish animals could easily put this strain on their kidneys, since they needed little vitamin C. But when mammals came along, they needed much more vitamin C than the kidneys were capable of making, so the liver undertook this job.

All mammals which manufacture their own vitamin C (and that includes almost all of them, except human beings) made this transition from kidney to liver or they simply did not survive. Presumably the reason is that mammals were subjected to more stress than reptiles, and the more stress any living thing is under the more vitamin C it needs.

Birds, which are midway between reptiles and mammals in the evolution pattern, show a transition between the two body sources of vitamin C. The more ancient orders, like ducks, pigeons and hawks, make their vitamin C in their kidneys as the reptiles do. Of the birds which evolved more recently—song birds, for example—some are still making vitamin C in their kidneys, others have shifted over to the liver. And a few, like humans, cannot synthesize vitamin C at all.

The primates, from whom we are descended, appeared about 65 million years ago. Like other mammals we should be able to manufacture vitamin C in our livers. But we cannot. And if we do not get enough vitamin C in our food, we die of the disease of scurvy. We and a few other living things are the only living creatures which get scurvy.

Until early in this century, scurvy was considered a disease which affected only human beings. But two scientists, doing some research on beriberi, the disease of thiamine deficiency, put some guinea pigs on a diet which was bound to produce beriberi, they thought, but produced scurvy instead. Since then, guinea pigs have been widely used in investigations on scurvy because they, too, get the disease shortly after all vitamin C-rich foods are removed from their diets. Certain monkeys, too, are susceptible to scurvy.

It was not until 1932 that vitamin C was identified as ascorbic acid, lack of which causes scurvy. And it was not until 1959 that a scientist demonstrated in his laboratory that the reason human beings get scurvy is that they lack an enzyme, L-gulonolactone oxidase, in their livers.

The process of changing blood glucose to vitamin C is arranged in the liver by four enzymes. Human beings have the first three, but they lack the fourth. There is no need to remember the long, difficult name of this enzyme. But it is important to remember that this deficiency exists in all human beings and this lack of an enzyme is what Dr. Stone and Dr. Linus Pauling built their case on.

Working with charts of the various pre-historical ages, Dr. Stone came to the conclusion that the very time when this mutation occurred was a period when many other forms of animal life disappeared—or at any rate, disappeared so far as we know. Recently two astronomers showed that an astronomical event during that period showered the earth with large amounts of cosmic rays, gamma rays and x-rays.

If such an astronomical event did occur, says Dr. Stone, "then the random absorption of some of this high energy radiation may have been instrumental in mutating the primary gene for the synthesis of the enzyme protein, L-gulonolactone oxidase, resulting in an inactive enzyme."

Since these mammals, by virtue of the mutation, were

no longer able to make their own vitamin C, why did they not all die of scurvy? They lived, at that time, in the tropics and they ate large amounts of foods rich in vitamin C. Dr. Pauling has calculated that early man may have eaten as much as 4,000 milligrams of vitamin C every day. Wild fruits and berries were all around, free for the picking. Apparently he spent most of his time eating them.

In those times it may have been advantageous for our ancestors to have lost this enzyme, for the other three enzymes could then get involved in other physiological business. So energy was saved. But human beings didn't stay in the tropics. They moved into colder climates where vitamin C-rich food was scarce and, in winter, almost totally lacking.

"Man still carries this defective gene and it has no survival value for modern Man," says Dr. Stone. "In fact, in the course of prehistory and during historical times, it has been a severe handicap and the side effects of this defective gene have resulted in the deaths of more individuals, caused more sickness and suffering and have changed the course of history more than any other single factor."

So, properly speaking, vitamin C is not a vitamin at all. It is a hormone, manufactured by the liver, except that, of course, we humans have lost the ability to make it. If we want to correct this inherited error, we should supply every human being with the same amount of vitamin C he would be making in his liver, if he still had the capacity to make it.

The rat makes its own vitamin C. Judging from the amount the rat makes every day, human beings need 2,000 to 4,000 milligrams of vitamin C daily. But animals under stress need more vitamin C. When rats are under stress (cold, hunger, fright, hard work, illness, etc.), they make much more vitamin C than they normally would.

Assuming that human beings, too, would make more vitamin C for their increased bodily needs under stress, scientists have studied the rat's production of this vitamin and concluded that human beings under stress should be getting as much as 15,000 milligrams of vitamin C a day—which is more than 250 times the modest 45 milligrams officially recommended as the amount of vitamin C that will keep us healthy!

During all the years of man's prehistory and recorded history, there was no way for him to get these large amounts of vitamin C, unless he lived in the tropics and ate vitamin-C-rich food practically all day long. But now we have vitamin C easily and inexpensively available. No one knows or ever can know how much misery could have been prevented during all those years if human beings had been getting all the vitamin C they should have had.

Could it have prevented the terrible plagues that killed millions of people? Could it have kept everyone in such good health that they would not have succumbed to death from the various kinds of unknown poisons which wiped out whole nations? It is believed, for example, that the Roman Empire was finally destroyed by lead poisoning due to the lead utensils which the Romans used for cooking and storage of food.

Says Dr. Stone, "The vital importance of ascorbic acid (vitamin C) in many phases of human physiology has been underrated for the past 60 years because in 1912, 20 years before its discovery and synthesis, it was designated a vitamin for the treatment of frank, clinical scurvy which was considered a simple dietary disturbance.

"Actually ascorbic acid is a liver metabolite produced in nearly all mammals in large daily amounts. Because of this defective gene, Man is suffering from a mammalian genetic liver-enzyme disease, a true 'inborn error of carbohydrate metabolism' named hypoascorbemia (lack of ascorbic acid). . . . This genetic approach provides the rationale for the use of large daily doses of ascorbic acid and opens wide vistas of research for its application to preventive medicine and therapy."

Dr. Stone's book on vitamin C is called *The Healing Factor, Vitamin C Against Disease*. It is published by Grosset and Dunlap, New York City.

IS VITAMIN C A HORMONE?

Dr. Linus Pauling's book, *Vitamin C and the Common Cold,* is published by W. H. Freeman and Company, 660 Market Street, San Francisco 94104. It contains more information on the mutational theory of Dr. Stone's.

CHAPTER 36

Vitamin C and "The Pill"

WE HAVE A large file of material collected from many parts of the world showing evidence of possible harm in susceptible women who are taking contraceptives. Most of this seems to be related to circulatory troubles: strokes and other circulatory problems which occur in women so young that such complications should be expected only far in the future, if at all.

Now we have a study of sixty-three women showing that those who have been on The Pill for a year or more have less concentration of vitamin C in their white blood corpuscles than women not taking any contraceptives. Vera Joyce McLeroy and Harold Eugene Schendel of Florida State University describe the tests they made on a matched group of 126 women whose diets were carefully studied, as well as the supplements they took. Some of the subjects were taking as much as 200 milligrams of vitamin C daily in supplements.

Vitamin C supplements had a considerable effect on the vitamin C present in the blood cells of the women who were not taking oral contraceptives. The more vitamin C they took daily the higher the level tended to be. But in the case of the women on The Pill it didn't seem to matter how much vitamin C they took. Reserves of the vitamin did not increase in their white blood cells.

This kind of measurement is used because the amount of vitamin C in white blood cells is generally considered the best index of the body level of this vitamin. These blood cells are one part of the body's protection against infection. They are sent at once to any part of the body which is fighting off infection and the vitamin C is used up in the course of the battle.

It didn't make any difference what Pill was being used by the women surveyed. Say the authors, "it appears that ascorbic acid (vitamin C) supplementation is unable to maintain adequate or normal concentrations of this vitamin in the tissues of women taking oral contraceptives."

It seems that vitamin C supplies are closely related to the menstrual cycle in women. There are changes in the concentration of the vitamin during stages of the cycle. The greatest concentration of vitamin C appears to be present during ovulation, the time when the woman is most fertile. The amounts of vitamin C in women taking The Pill appeared to be less variable than in those who were not using The Pill.

The authors do not know why or how The Pill influences what happens to vitamin C in the body. They speculate that perhaps the sex hormones in The Pill may change the intestinal tissues in such a way that less vitamin C is absorbed. Or possibly the greater accumulation of sex hormones may stimulate the utilization of the vitamin so that it disappears more rapidly from the body. Or, possibly, the vitamin is shifted to the other tissues when the sex hormones are present. Regardless of the reason, there seems to be no doubt that The Pill does have important implications for the availability of vitamin C where it is most needed in the body. It may not be there, in large enough quantities in a woman who has been on contraceptives for a year or more.

What to do? There seems to be abundant evidence of possible health troubles from oral contraceptives, and the vitamin C facts are only the most recent of many experiments and observations which have disclosed damage to health. If the individual cannot be persuaded to give up The Pill, perhaps the best plan would be to increase the daily intake of vitamin C, and perhaps all other vitamins as well, to prevent any possible lack in any health emergency. Vitamin C and all the B vitamins are harmless in any amounts, apparently. They have been used by physicians and psychiatrists in enormous doses with no unpleasant symptoms. Vitamin A has produced unfortunate symptoms in extremely large doses—more than 100,000 units daily in adults and less than that in children.

CHAPTER 37

Smoking and
Vitamin C

DR. IRWIN STONE, world champion of vitamin C and its beneficial effects on a variety of health problems, has written a brilliant article on smoking in relation to vitamin C. It appears in the *Journal of Orthomolecular Psychiatry,* Volume 5, No. 1, 1976. This is the publication of that group of far-sighted and innovative professional men who are treating schizophrenics and other mentally ill patients with massive doses of vitamins, minerals and special diets.

Dr. Stone begins by saying that, of course, the best way to avoid all health problems brought on by smoking is not to smoke. But for those people who cannot or will not stop smoking, he produces well-documented evidence covering many years of experimentation and observation showing that large amounts of vitamin C are the best protection against harm from smoking. Those of us who do not smoke can also learn a lot from this article about maintaining better health with vitamin C.

Tobacco smoke is full of poisons. Tar and nicotine are only two. Cyanide is another; and carbon monoxide; as well as arsenic and cadmium. Enough vitamin C taken by the smoker will detoxify these and the many other poisons in smoke, thus possibly preventing or postponing the fatal damage that has destroyed so many cigarette smokers.

Countless experiments have shown that vitamin C, in large enough doses, detoxifies many poisons: strychnine, ozone, sulfa drugs, nitrates, phosphorus, coal tar dyes, mercury, chromates and many industrial pollutants.

Says Dr. Stone, "The literature concerning this (detoxification) is so voluminous that adequate treatment would require much more space..." He gives us a lot of references to this material—all of it from respected scientific journals, he tells us that tobacco smoke has been suspected as a cause of bladder cancer since 1931. The 1964 *Report of the Surgeon General* on smoking concluded that there is an association between bladder cancer and smoking.

Many researchers in the past 40 years have worked with this theory. They have found that smoking does indeed put certain cancer-causing substances into the bladder. They also showed that the formation of these substances could be entirely prevented by giving enough vitamin C. One group of scientists found that the cancer-causing substance was present in large amounts in the bladders of cancer patients, in somewhat lesser amounts in the bladders of smokers and much less in the bladders of non-smokers. They also found that giving one and a half grams (1,500 milligrams) of vitamin C every day completely prevented the formation of the cancer-causing substance.

They advise their patients to take large amounts of vitamin C to prevent the recurrence of cancer. Obviously, says Stone, "it would seem implicit from their work that if the smokers had sufficiently high levels of ascorbate (vitamin C) in their urine, the bladder cancer would not have appeared in the first place."

Think of the thousands of victims of bladder cancer who could have been saved by this simple expedient of swallowing a bit of vitamin C every day!

So much for vitamin C's power in preventing cancer. How does it happen that the smoker does not have enough vitamin C in his blood to prevent this disease? Mostly it happens because vitamin C is destroyed in the process of detoxifying poisons. And tobacco smoke is a poison. So the more you smoke, the less vitamin C you have to fortify you against the harmful effects of smoking.

When you smoke, you suffer from smoker's scurvy, meaning a chronic deficiency in this essential substance, which makes you vulnerable to many more diseases like fragile blood vessels (which could lead to stroke), a tendency to hemorrhage, fewer white blood cells to fight off infections, abnormal immunity responses and improper functioning of all those body enzyme systems in which vitamin C plays a part.

For the past 40 years scientists have been showing, in laboratories that tobacco smoke depletes the body of vitamin C. Dr. Stone presents the evidence from 17 such studies. It is impossible to refute. In test tubes, in animals, in human beings, the addition of only small amounts of tobacco smoke destroys vitamin C wholesale. Smokers consistently have lesser amounts of vitamin C in their blood than non-smokers. The longer you have smoked and the more cigarettes you smoke per day, the less vitamin C you have in your blood.

Testing on men and women, one group of scientists found that heavy smoking has the same effect on the amount of vitamin C in the blood as increasing the chronological age by some 40 years! One experimenter theorized that the decrease in vitamin C is one of the causes of early hardening of the arteries in smokers. This is the condition which heralds a lot of circulatory troubles.

In smokers the vitamin C drops in the adrenal glands (which protect you from stress), in the kidneys, the heart, the liver, the spleen and the brain. It follows that the function of all these organs is disrupted and disordered. The vitamin C doesn't just happen to be there. It is there because that organ needs the vitamin C to function. The less vitamin C that organ has to work with, the less efficiently it will work. In smokers who were also alcoholics, investigators found almost no vitamin C at all. The combination of the two poisons destroyed it all.

The reason for all this goes back to the original investigations by Dr. Stone which demonstrated that, millions of years ago, the ancestor of all human beings lost the ability to make vitamin C in the liver. All other animals, except man, guinea pigs and apes, can manufacture this vitamin in the liver and do manufacture it in very large amounts. When the animal is under stress, it manufactures many, many times more vitamin C than when there is little or no stress. Shouldn't the same thing apply to human beings?

A goat, for instance, which weighs about what an adult human weighs, produces as much as 13,300 milligrams of vitamin C every day to meet its health needs. The official recommended daily allowance for an adult human being has been set as 45 milligrams. Why? Why have not our health officials set their recommendations at levels to approximate those of animals which make their own vitamin C?

The reason is that official medicine has been brainwashed into believing that the only recognizable symptom of vitamin C deficiency is scurvy—the terrible disease which wiped out millions of human beings over past centuries. Scurvy is the last step before death from vitamin C deficiency, says Dr. Stone. In no way should we decide that just enough vitamin C to keep us from dying of scurvy is all we need. It seems reasonable, does it not, that we need approximately the same amount of vitamin C other animals need for ordinary good health. As we have seen, one animal, the goat, makes for itself almost 14,000 milligrams more vitamin C than our official estimate specifies. Subclinical scurvy in human beings is the result.

Then, too, goats and horses, dogs and cats, whose livers are all busily manufacturing immense amounts of vitamin C, don't smoke, don't drink or expose themselves to the thousand and one other poisons to which most of us are exposed every day. So for this reason as well, it would seem advisable to get far, far more of this essential substance than animals seem to need for good health.

SMOKING AND VITAMIN C

Dr. Stone believes, as do most of the physicians and psychiatrists who are treating patients with what is called orthomolecular medicine, that we should all be getting far more vitamin C than we get. The more exposure we have to poisons, the more vitamin C we should get.

Smokers who cannot or will not stop smoking should at least protect their health with large amounts of vitamin C. If they work at a job where they are exposed to air pollutants, if they drive to work in horrendous traffic jams, if they breathe the tobacco smoke of others all day long, if they are taking dangerous drugs of any kind, it's fairly certain their vitamin C stores may be depleted by the time they get to work in the morning.

How much vitamin C should one take? Dr. Stone believes that the average human being who is not under stress needs as much as 5 to 20 grams of vitamin C daily (5,000 to 20,000 milligrams). A smoker, he says, should take three to five grams more than that for every pack of cigarettes he or she smokes. That's how terrible the danger from smoking is and that's how easy it is to give yourself at least some small protection against this poison.

CHAPTER 38

A Miscellany
on Vitamin C

No one knows just what causes polyps of the colon or how to treat them. They are a type of tumor which may be harmless, but may progress to become cancerous.

Now we hear of a breakthrough. From the Medical College of Wisconsin comes word that doctors have been using vitamin C in large doses to treat patients with one type of colonic polyp. The patients all had what is called familial polyposis—a rare inherited condition which produces many polyps.

All but one of the eight patients treated had previously undergone surgery to remove the polyps, but had had recurrences. Dr. Jerome J. DeCosse, professor and chairman of surgery at the college, headed the research team. He said that half of the children who inherit this disease will develop many polyps by the time they are teenagers. If the polyps are untreated, victims of this disorder die before the age of 40.

If the number of polyps can be reduced, there is a good chance that cancer of the colon can be prevented. And it appears that vitamin C is the agent which brings this improvement about. Note that we said the vitamin is used in massive doses.

It doesn't seem likely that many physicians know as yet

about Dr. DeCosse's research, nor does it seem important if they do. Vitamin C is harmless in massive doses. Some physicians regularly give it to their patients throughout their lifetimes with nothing but excellent results. There is no reason why someone threatened with trouble from intestinal polyps should not make vitamin C a regular part of every day's vitamin intake. If the doctor is providing some other treatment, ask him if there is any reason why vitamin C should not be taken at the same time.

Chances are he'll say no, "but you're wasting your money." Dr. DeCosse didn't seem to feel that he was wasting his patients' money when he treated their polyps with vitamin C. Undoubtedly, there will be a furor in the medical journals, as there was over vitamin C for treating colds. Doctors who have never tried it and researchers who are not interested in anything new that is not a drug will probably pounce on this information and try to prove that the Wisconsin people just didn't know what they were doing, or the experiment wasn't "controlled," or something of the sort. Arguments will fly back and forth.

Fortunately, we need not wait till the issue is decided. It seems to us that anyone faced with the possibility of cancer of the colon should be willing to try anything harmless that promises relief. If the problem is specifically polyps, then by all means try vitamin C—in massive doses. Dr. DeCosse used three grams (3,000 mg.) daily for up to 13 months.

Meanwhile, never forget that a great deal of research shows a clear relationship between the health of the colon and the amount of fiber in the diet. People who live in countries where the diet is loaded with fiber—lots of fruits and vegetables and only wholegrain cereals and breads—have almost no colonic problems of any kind, but, as soon as they move to our part of the world and begin to eat our bland, over-processed foods, they begin to develop the same elimination problems we have, with all the complications that accompany them.

So put fiber into your diet. The easiest way is to get

bran—plain, unprocessed bran—and eat considerable quantities of it every day—several tablespoons to start with, increasing the amount gradually. You can add it to wholegrain cereals, bake it into bread, put it into salads, casseroles, meat loaves and so on. If the problem is specifically polyps, then by all means get some vitamin C and give it a try.

What's wrong when you have a sore mouth? Is there anything you can do nutritionally to improve the situation?

It is quite possible, first of all, that your sore mouth may be caused chiefly by nutritional deficiencies. You can prevent such disorders easily by making sure that your diet contains the missing nutrients. Mouth tissues are among the first tissues of the body to give warning of nutritional deficiencies.

First of all, there's vitamin B. The entire B complex of vitamins is usually involved. Here are some fairly common causes of sore mouths which can be remedied with plenty of B vitamins. Glossodynia is pain or a burning sensation in the tongue. Chronic inflammation of the lining of the mouth, ulceration of the tissues of cheeks, gums or tongue, a tendency toward a "bald" or glossy looking tongue, gingivitis or bleeding of the gums, leukoplakia (white patches on the lining of the mouth), and many more conditions may respond to vitamin therapy.

A sore, swollen, red tongue can result from lack of one or several of the B vitamins—pyridoxine, thiamine or riboflavin. Long, wide fissures at the corners of the mouth can occur as a result of deficiency in riboflavin, which is vitamin B2. Fissures like this may also occur from badly fitting dentures or allergies to denture material, chewing gum, lipstick or other substances that come in contact with the mouth. Iron deficiency anemia has also caused this condition.

In pellagra, which is the disease of deficiency in another B vitamin, niacin, the tongue is smooth, red and painful and there is a burning sensation in the mouth. If you are short on the B vitamin pyridoxine you are likely to experience some of these same symptoms—inflammation of the mouth tissues, and fissures at the corners of the mouth.

Deficiency in vitamin B12 and/or folic acid, another B vitamin, brings many kinds of mouth disorders, as well as digestive and nervous complications of a very serious nature. Other mouth conditions which indicate deficiencies in B vitamins are a beefy red or magenta colored tongue or a shiny tongue, a tongue with deep indentations in it or notches around the edges where it has pushed against your teeth. Canker sores and sore spots around the edges of the tongue can also appear as a result of not getting enough of the vitamin B complex.

Or possibly vitamin C. The necessity of this nutrient for the health of mouth and gum tissues has been known since early days when scurvy tormented and often killed millions of people. Scurvy is the disease of vitamin C deficiency. One of the earliest symptoms of scurvy is bleeding gums and loose teeth. As the disease progresses, gums become spongy, swollen, dark red in color and the teeth become so loose that they finally fall out.

Not many of us who are otherwise healthy have scurvy these days, but mouth symptoms which are symptomatic of scurvy occur with dismal frequency in many people. Bleeding gums are extremely common. Large doses of vitamin C can stop the bleeding. Loose teeth can be tightened and gums rendered much more healthy simply by adding enough vitamin C to meals and to food supplements.

In *The American Journal of Clinical Nutrition* for July, 1974 two researchers, from Northern Arizona University and Loma Linda University School of Medicine, describe their experiments which seem to show the benefits of doses of vitamin C which are far, far larger than those which prevent scurvy.

Dr. Larry G. Thaete and J. Norman Grim worked with three groups of guinea pigs, which are one species of animal aside from human beings which do not manufacture their own vitamin C. These little animals, like human beings, must get enough of it in their food or they develop scurvy. One set of guinea pigs was put on a diet with no vitamin C. They rapidly proceeded to get scurvy. The second was given just enough vitamin C to prevent scurvy, but no more. The third group was given 100 times more vitamin C than is needed to prevent scurvy.

At the end of the experiment a study was made of the mouth tissues of all three groups. The health of these tissues improved in direct proportion to the amount of vitamin C the animals had received. In those which had developed scurvy, mouth tissues were in very bad shape. In those which got just enough vitamin C to prevent scurvy, gums, tongue and mouth linings were in a little better shape, but not much.

In those animals which had been given 100 times the amount of vitamin C which would prevent scurvy, mouth tissues were flourishing. "It is concluded," say these authors, "that for the maintenance of optimum physical integrity of buccal epithelial cells (mouth-lining cells), ascorbic acid may be necessary in larger doses than the minimum required for the prevention of scurvy. It is proposed that doses up to 100 times the minimum may be beneficial."

Three people we know take vitamin C for fever blisters. One man tells us he can produce fever blisters merely by drinking a lot of coffee and not getting enough sleep. He can prevent and/or control them by getting seven hours sleep a night, limiting himself to three cups of coffee a day and taking vitamin C.

"If I catch it in time," he says, "it can be prevented from developing." He takes 1,000 milligrams of vitamin C every few hours. He also tries to balance his diet with plenty of minerals and other vitamins.

A woman friend takes 150 milligrams of vitamin C every three hours when she feels that a fever blister is threatening. Although she was very susceptible to these pesty things all her life, she has had no more than three during the years she has been using large doses of vitamin C and that was at times when she had run out of vitamin C. It also helps, she says, to stay away from sugar.

A Wisconsin health seeker takes calcium and vitamin C to prevent fever blisters. Taking a lot of vitamin C may cause her mouth to become sore, but when she adds calcium, the soreness and the fever blister disappear. She takes calcium made from oyster shells.

If you have a sore mouth, it's quite possible that something other than vitamin deficiency may be responsible. Bad teeth, poorly fitting dentures, allergies, malocclusion, personal habits like grinding or gritting your teeth—all these and many more causes might be involved. Even so, until you have discovered the actual cause and treated it, there is no reason not to apply all the knowledge we have about vitamin deficiencies and sore mouth. If your sore mouth is caused by nutritional deficiency you can certainly get things back to normal by wise eating and by getting plenty of the B vitamins and vitamin C. If something other than nutritional deficiency has been your trouble, the extra vitamins will be helpful anyway in keeping you in good nutritional health.

Dr. Herbert Sprince of Jefferson Medical College has found that vitamin C protects the body against a substance which develops in the bodies of those who drink alcohol and smoke cigarettes. The substance goes by the name of acetaldehyde. In drinkers this substance has been found in alcoholic heart disease, alcoholic degeneration of the brain, addiction to alcohol and the special susceptibility of certain groups to alcoholism. It may also be involved in lung diseases caused by alcoholism. The same poison, in cigarette smoke, is responsible for causing both heart disease and lung disease.

Dr. Sprince and his colleagues at Jefferson gave large doses of vitamin C, along with vitamin B1, thiamine. These facts give some hope to people hopelessly addicted to either smoking or alcohol. They should not be looked upon as excuses to continue to smoke and drink. But until these folks can summon the required stamina to stop, the vitamins will give some protection, so that physical damage may be less.

In *Executive Health* for December, 1975, Dr. Pauling tells us of a study in San Mateo County, California, which showed that people with a low intake of vitamin C had a death rate from all causes—mainly heart disease and cancer—which was 2½ times that of people who took some vitamin C. The study involved 577 people—all over the age of 50. And the protective power of vitamin C showed itself, even though the amount taken of vitamin C was only about 100 milligrams daily!

Says Pauling, "I am now willing to predict that people who take the optimum amount of vitamin C may well have, at each age, only one-quarter as much illness and chance of dying as those who do not take extra vitamin C. This way of improving one's health will not, I believe, be ignored much longer."

As anyone knows who has cared for a bed-ridden invalid or a paraplegic, pressure sores are likely to be the most serious complication. These are sores that develop on the back or buttocks, in areas which are in constant contact with the bed. In older folks especially such sores are hard to heal. They may last for many months and become badly infected wounds that drain the resistance of the patient.

A group of medical men in Manchester, England has conducted experiments showing that patients treated with vitamin C had a reduction in pressure-sore area of 84 percent, compared to patients who did not get added vitamin C, with a reduction of only 42.7 percent.

The 20 patients suffered from arthritis, broken hips, strokes, broken pelvis, ulcers, prostate trouble, diverticular disease, circulatory complications. All had the same hospital diet. Half the patients were given 500 milligrams of vitamin C twice daily. The other half got a pill which looked just like the vitamin C tablet, but contained nothing. The areas of pressure sores were assessed by photography and other means. The amount of vitamin C in each patient's white blood cells was also assessed. Those who got the extra vitamin C had much higher levels than those who did not.

The authors tell us they know that many studies have shown very low levels of vitamin C in older patients, both in hospitals and at home. Then, too, they remind us that vitamin C is essential for the formation of collagen, the "glue" that holds our cells together. And in the absence of enough vitamin C, certain proteins are not used by the body. Certainly, say these authors, their experiment showed that 1,000 milligrams of vitamin C daily improved the pressure sore areas immeasurably, but, they go on, one must also consider anemia, prolonged protein deficiency and other factors as partial reasons for pressure sores and other disabilities.

We cannot help but wonder why there should be any hemming and hawing about such an important matter as this. These patients are suffering agonies from pressure sores. Why should anyone withhold vitamin C if there is even a slight chance that it might help? It is hardly more expensive than water, especially in comparison to the high priced drugs most hospital patients are given. It is completely harmless. If doctors were to give it in 4,000 or 5,000 milligram doses perhaps they could prevent pressure sores entirely. And who knows what other benefits might show up—like much faster bone healing, fewer circulatory troubles, fewer strokes and so on. The British experiment was reported in *The Lancet* for September 7, 1974.

And in *The Lancet* for October 12, 1974 Dr. Abram Hoffer of Saskatchewan writes on the subject of "wasting" vitamin C. He says that a patient who takes very large doses of vitamin C may excrete much of it in his urine, but this does not prove that the vitamin was "wasted." If you take 100 milligrams, your body may use only 50 milligrams and excrete the other 50. But if you take 1,000 milligrams, the body may excrete 800 milligrams and retain 200. "Certain processes may require these larger doses," says Dr. Hoffer. "It has been suggested that to saturate the leukemic cells in a patient with this condition may require 7,000 milligrams per day. If less is given the avidity of these cells for vitamin C causes the scorbutic (scurvy) symptoms in the rest of the body (black and blue patches, fragile blood vessels and bleeding gums). Pauling has outlined the scientific evidence for his view that increasing doses of an important nutrient can produce increasing vigor and growth in living cells, even though some of the nutrient is wasted." He goes on to point out that perhaps the reason why penicillin must be given in such immense doses to achieve its effects may be that much of it is "wasted."

"The question then is not whether it is wasted but whether it is effective," he goes on. "When there is general consensus that a substance is therapeutic, there is little discussion of waste. But with ascorbic acid (vitamin C) there is no such consensus. Many physicians equate consensus with efficacy. This often delays for many years the proper examination of a new therapeutic idea because consensus may require up to 40 years."

How right he is! All this nit-picking over vitamin C appears to be just nit-picking, nothing more. Many thousands of people are now taking massive doses of this vitamin daily with nothing but beneficial results. Why, in dealing with very sick people, should doctors hesitate for a moment to add this powerful, harmless and inexpensive nutrient to whatever other treatment they give? We cannot help but believe the reason is purely monetary. Nobody can patent vitamin C and make huge profits out of selling it, so drug companies are just not interested in promoting it. And, generally speaking, doctors rely on drug advertising for their information on treating patients.

Pediatrics for July 1974 reports on a serious bone disorder, osteogenesis imperfecta, in which bones fracture following only minor bumps or bruises. Researchers gave these patients 1,000 to 2,000 milligrams of vitamin C daily and found they had less tendency to break bones. Why not go a step farther, gentlemen, and suggest that we all take vitamin C to prevent a tendency toward bone-breaking, especially if the tendency runs in the family? And what's wrong with giving far more than 2,000 milligrams just to see if these fracture-prone patients can manage to get by with no more fractures at all? Maybe larger doses are required.

Two African scientists reported in *Nature* for August 4, 1972 that vitamin C is low in the blood corpuscles of women who take oral contraceptives. The lack of vitamin C appeared to be related to the fact that the vitamin C was taken by mouth, for, when the hormone was injected, the levels of vitamin C were not affected. We have pointed out in other chapters that women who take The Pill should get all the protection they can by increasing their intake of various vitamins, including several B vitamins. Now vitamin C should be added to this list.

Vitamin C prevents liver damage. Large doses of vitamin C given to laboratory mice protected their livers against damage when they were given chemicals which usually produce liver damage. *The Journal of the National Cancer Institute* reported this experiment in their April, 1973 issue. Surely everyone working the field of cancer research knows by now that we are surrounded by chemicals of many kinds which produce liver damage. What in the world is wrong with recommending that all of us increase our intake of vitamin C accordingly, just so that we get whatever protection we can from this inexpensive vitamin?

Dr. T. S. Wilson at Barncoose Hospital in Redruth, England, recently surveyed the vitamin C status of elderly patients being admitted to his hospital. Then he noted what course their health took from then on. He reported in *Gerontologia Clinica,* volume 14, page 17, 1972, that the elderly men and women with higher levels of vitamin C upon admission had longer lives than those with lower levels of vitamin C. The low vitamin C levels did not seem to produce any specific illness or condition of ill health. But, just the same, the folks with lower levels of the vitamin died sooner from all diseases.

A British biochemist, Dr. Sherry Lewin of London Northeast Polytechnic, has proposed a theory on why vitamin C is effective in many of the ways it appears to be effective. He also proposes that it is most effective if it is taken in rather small doses during the day (rather than in one or two larger doses) and if it is accompanied by a glass of grapefruit juice. We suppose orange juice would be just as good, since the important thing about the juice is its citric acid content.

Says *New Scientist* for November 29, 1973, he has convinced himself that the vitamin is effective in the relief and cure of angina, the agonizing pain of which torments some victims of heart attacks. But Dr. Lewin's observations on angina pain were apparently on himself, so he does not consider them to be final scientific proof.

He asked instead how high intakes of vitamin C work in the body. And he asked it in the prestigious pages of *Comparative Biochemistry and Physiology,* Volume 46B, page 427. He suggests that two forms of the vitamin (the oxidized and the unoxidized) may maintain a crucial balance of oxidation and reduction in the cells that produce antibodies to disease.

Then, too, he theorizes, the effect of vitamin C on water in fluids in the body may influence the ability of virus particles to form properly (and colds are caused by viruses, remember). Then he thinks that the vitamin's ability to combine with mineral substances may enable it to excrete harmful minerals from the body and thus control or reverse the production of those fatty calcium deposits on the insides of arteries which produce circulatory disease.

If all these things are so, why, then, have some tests with vitamin C not proved its ability to fight virus diseases, to expel toxins from the body and to relieve hardening of the arteries? In many cases the experimenters have given the vitamin in the form of sodium ascorbate in order to disguise its taste. In this form, Dr. Lewin thinks, it may not be as effective, since it may break down in the stomach.

So, to make it more effective, says Dr. Lewin, perhaps

we should be taking ascorbic acid (not the sodium form) and we should be taking a mildly acid beverage like grapefruit juice along with it. Many of us take our vitamin C with orange juice or grapefruit juice and thus we are getting far better results than some researchers in laboratories who are using the wrong form of the vitamin, and no fruit juice.

There is a possibility, says *Medical World News* for October 12, 1973 that rather large amounts of vitamin C may be added to cured meats. The Food and Drug Administration is working with the U.S. Department of Agriculture on experiments to see if adding vitamin C to meats which contain the nitrates or nitrites will make them less likely to cause cancer when they meet up with certain other food elements in the human digestive tract.

The FDA now allows meat processors to add 500 parts per million of vitamin C to delicatessen meats, bacon, ham and other cured meats. Now they are thinking in terms of making it 1,000 parts per million. They are conducting tests to see if this amount can prevent the cancers which are produced in laboratory animals under certain conditions when they eat these additives. So FDA officials may soon announce that all cured meats can or may contain vitamin C to prevent cancer, at the same time they are telling the general public that there is no need for any of us to get any more vitamin C than we need to prevent scurvy! That should be an interesting corner for the FDA bureaucrats to talk themselves out of.

A new Canadian study reports that soldiers given one gram (1,000 milligrams) of vitamin C daily during a two-week Arctic stay had less than half as many colds as their fellow soldiers who were given pills containing nothing. This is the third study in the past two years that supports Linus Pauling's claims that vitamin C in large doses prevents colds, eases cold symtoms and hastens recovery from colds.

The physician who carried out the test pointed out that all the soldiers were similar in respect to age, diet and activity, all living in the same environment. Half of the company were given two half-gram tablets of vitamin C daily. The other half got pills which looked just the same but contained nothing. One-tenth of the first group got colds, while one-fourth of the second group got colds. In two thirds of the tents where colds occurred, only the men on the "nothing" pills got colds. And cold symptoms lasted for a much shorter periods in those men taking the vitamin C. In an earlier Canadian study of 407 volunteers taking vitamin C, 26 percent remained free from colds, while only 18 percent of another 411 subjects not taking the vitamin remained free of colds.

In the *New England Journal of Medicine* for August 24, 1972 a physician writes to the editor about his experience giving large doses of vitamin C to a man who was having trouble seeing —"diminishing visual acuity" Dr. Edward Poser of Chicago calls it. "Lenticular opacities" were causing this poor vision—that is, opaqueness of the lens of the eye—in other words *cataract*. He prescribed four grams (4,000 milligrams) of vitamin C daily for this patient.

Within four months his vision increased from 20/40 to 20/20. Both lenses were clear. The cataracts had disappeared. The doctor told him he could discontinue the vitamin, since the cataracts were gone. The patient said he preferred to continue to take it. And he did, for 13 years, during which time he experienced no unpleasant side effects of any kind—least of all those which some doctors are warning us of—in the nature of kidney stones and so on. And no cataracts.

Says Dr. Poser, "I have prescribed large amounts of ascorbic acid (vitamin C) to many others over a period of years, without any clinical evidence of trouble."

CHAPTER 39

How Much Vitamin C
Do You Need?

IN THE YEARS since massive doses of vitamin C have been prescribed by many physicians and psychiatrists, those researchers who dislike the idea that just plain vitamins can treat or prevent illness have been telling us that we're all wasting our money. Their belittling, disparaging comments suggest that all vitamin C over a dose of perhaps 30 to 100 milligrams is excreted almost immediately in the urine. So all we "faddists" are doing, say these detractors, is to create very expensive urine for ourselves.

At the same time they tell us that vitamin C may bring us harm. They never explain just how this perfectly natural substance, which plays many important roles in the human body, could harm us if it is indeed all excreted within a few hours. Harmful things are usually substances that are stored in the body, accumulating until the total amount overwhelms us.

Those researchers who regularly use vitamin C in very large amounts continually search for some evidence of harm from the vitamin and have been unable to find any. The detractors, too, have never been able to produce any verified cases where large doses of vitamin C have brought anything but benefit.

Now we have a very significant record of tests done in a

school for mentally disturbed patients who were getting extremely large amounts of vitamin C. Four physicians from the Virginia school write in *The Journal of Orthomolecular Psychiatry,* Volume 5, No. 1, about their very careful tests to determine exactly how much vitamin C is excreted in urine.

Foods Highest in Vitamin C

Food	Milligrams of vitamin C
Acerola cherries	1000 milligrams in 100 grams
Asparagus, fresh green	20 in 8 stalks
Beans, green lima	9 in ½ cup
Beet greens, cooked	25 in ½ cup
Broccoli, leaf	90 in ¾ cup
Brussels sprouts	87 in ¾ cup
Cabbage, Chinese, raw	50 in 1 cup
Cabbage, green, raw	50 in 1 cup
Cabbage, inside leaves, raw	50 in 1 cup
Cantaloupe	50 in ½ sm. cantaloupe
Chard, Swiss, cooked	16 in ½ cup
Collards, cooked	70 in ½ cup
Currants, red	40 in 1 cup
Dandelion greens, cooked	18 in 1 cup
Grapefruit, fresh	45 in ½ cup grapefruit
Grapefruit juice, fresh	108 in 1 cup
Grapefruit juice, canned	72 in 1 cup
Guavas	125 in 1 guava
Honeydew melon	90 in ¼ med. honeydew
Kale, cooked	96 in ¾ cup
Kohlrabi	50 in ½ cup
Leeks	25 in ½ cup
Lemon juice	25 in 1 tablespoon
Lime juice	18 in ¼ cup
Liver, beef	30 in 1 slice
Liver, calves	25 in 1 slice
Liver, chicken	25 in ½ cup
Liver, lamb	20 in 1 slice

Ninety-one patients getting from 4 to 48 grams of vitamin C daily were tested. (This is 4,000 to 48,000 milligrams). Thirty-one of these patients were excreting vitamin C. Sixty of them were not. This means, we must assume, that these 60 people needed this much vitamin C daily, or perhaps needed even more than this, since the

Loganberries	35 in 1 cup
Mustard greens, cooked	40 in ½ cup
Orange	50 in 1 med. orange
Orange juice, fresh	120 in 1 cup
Orange juice, canned	80 in 1 cup
Parsley	70 in ½ cup
Parsnips	20 in ½ cup
Peas, fresh cooked	40 in 1 cup
Peppers, green	125 in 1 med. pepper
Peppers, pimiento	95 in 2 med. peppers
Persimmon, Japanese	40 in 1 large persimmon
Pineapple, fresh	17 in ⅔ cup
Pineapple juice, canned	25 in 1 cup
Potatoes, sweet	25 in 1 med. potato
Potatoes, white, baked	20 in 1 med. potato
Radishes	25 in 15 large radishes
Raspberries, black	36 in 1 cup
Raspberries, red	50 in 1 cup
Rose hips	500 to 6000 in 100 grams
Rutabagas	26 in ¾ cup
Spinach, cooked	30 in ½ cup
Strawberries, fresh	50 in ½ cup
Tangerines	48 in 2 med. tangerines
Tomatoes, canned	20 in ½ cup
Tomatoes, fresh	25 in 1 med. tomato
Tomato juice, canned	48 in 1 cup
Turnips, cooked	22 in ½ cup
Turnips, raw	30 in 1 med. turnip
Turnip tops, cooked	40 in ½ cup
Watercress	54 in 1 average bunch

vitamin was doing its job in their cells and was consumed in the process.

Four months later these same patients were tested again. Of 99 tests, 20 patients were excreting vitamin C. The rest were not. Apparently these 79 patients needed this much or more vitamin C. Later tests turned up the fact that about one-fourth of the patients were excreting vitamin C. Later tests showed that 37%, 25%, 34%, and so on were excreting vitamin C, hence getting more than they apparently needed.

During a later period, 149 new patients were admitted to the school. Urine tests showed not a particle of vitamin C in the urine of any of these new patients. Doesn't this demonstrate clearly that these folks were not getting anywhere near the amount of the vitamin that they needed? Could this not be, as orthomolecular psychiatrists believe, one of the causes of their mental and emotional illness— lack of enough vitamin C to make up for the very great stress of their illness?

While these tests were going on, the investigators also tested school personnel—the nurses, doctors and administrative officials. Of twenty-five samples of urine taken, 19 showed ascorbic acid. Six did not. So at least 6 of these supposedly perfectly well individuals were not getting enough vitamin C to be able to spare any to excrete in their urine.

And what about the potential danger of large doses of vitamin C? In this situation all patients were being observed constantly. Tests were constantly being given and symptoms were constantly being checked. Of the entire population of patients who were getting an average of nine grams (9,000 milligrams) of vitamin C daily, not a single sympton of any kind of ill effect could be found. (The average figure of nine grams means, of course, that many of the patients were getting much higher doses, some were getting lower doses.)

Many of the hospital personnel had undoubtedly observed the beneficial results on health from massive doses of vitamin C. Eighteen staff members have been taking from 6 to 18 grams of vitamin C daily for periods up to eight years. These are trained personnel: nurses, doctors and so on. None of them has noticed any unpleasant side effect, any disease or dysfunction since they began taking the vitamin C, hence attributable to these large doses of the vitamin.

Say the authors, "The psychiatric patient is under high stress and obviously requires very large doses of ascorbic acid (vitamin C). The long-term supplementation of ascorbic acid is apparently a very low risk regimen."

Almost alone among living beings, we humans cannot make our own vitamin C in our livers, as practically all other creatures do. Studying the amount of vitamin C other animals make for their own use, researchers like Dr. Irwin Stone have found that they make enormous amounts of the vitamin for their own use.

When these animals are under stress (fear, hard work, cold, disease, etc.) the amount of vitamin C which they manufacture increases greatly. Why should not the same thing be true of human beings? Why should we continue to try to get along on marginal amounts of this wholly beneficial substance, especially when we are under stress? "Stress" is different things to different people. Things which greatly upset some people have almost no stress effect on others. So each of us must determine for ourselves when we are under stress and how great the stress is.

The tests done at the Virginia school seem to demonstrate clearly that the stress of mental illness may consume vast amounts of vitamin C in some patients, less in others. They also seem to show that people who are supposedly healthy like the school personnel need widely varying amounts of this vitamin, some of them far, far more than others. And most important, they show that, no matter how large the dosage, the vitamin is completely beneficial and harmless.

Vitamin D Is...

Fat-soluble, meaning it is stored in the body, hence not essential in food or supplements every day.

Responsible for formation, growth and maintenance of bones and teeth, in combination with calcium and phosphorus, also maintains correct balances of these two minerals in blood.

Present in appreciable amounts in almost no foods. Fish liver oils contain large amounts. Among foods we eat at meals egg yolk, butter, herring, mackerel, sardines, shrimp, tuna contain very small amounts. Sunlight on bare skin produces vitamin D, so spending some time out of doors every day is helpful, especially for infants and children who need vitamin D for bone and tooth formation.

Safe in recommended amounts. Excessive vitamin D produces toxic symptoms: loss of appetite, nausea, thirst, diarrhea and so on. Following the recommendations on the label of any product is a good idea.

Destroyed in the body by mineral oil, as are all other fat-soluble vitamins.

Required officially: 400 International Units for adults and children alike. This is the reason most milk is fortified with 400 units of vitamin D per quart these days.

Available in capsules of not more than 400 International Units and in one-a-day brands.

CHAPTER 40

Vitamin D, the
Sunshine Vitamin

IN A RECENT issue of the *Journal of the American Medical Association* several articles were reprinted from the *Journal* of 1892. Among these was an article on rickets—the bone-deforming disease that crippled so many children during those times. We now know that rickets is caused by deficiency in vitamin D and/or calcium.

Since vitamin D is manufactured by the skin in the presence of sunlight, rickets attacks its victims usually in winter, when the sun's rays are feeble and children are bundled up in many layers of clothing. Today our children are given milk irradiated to produce vitamin D. In addition, many children are given supplements that contain vitamin D.

But in 1892 doctors had never heard of vitamins. They did not know that food contained anything essential except for carbohydrate, protein and fat. So when doctors diagnosed rickets in 1892 they had to come up with some other reason for this painful, disfiguring disorder. Listen to what they said about rickets in 1892.

"The bane of children artificially fed is malnutrition. Most of the malnutrition of infancy takes the form of rickets. While we are not yet in a position to speak authoritatively on the effect of infantile rickets upon the future adult, we are ready to admit that it probably has some effect most likely in increasing the individual's tendency to diseases, diminishing his resisting power, and possibly playing a powerful role in putting him into the great class of defectives. The importance, therefore, of detecting the first signs of rickets is apparent. It is too late to be of the best service to make the diagnosis of rickets when advanced body changes are present. Anybody can make the diagnosis of rickets when the head is squared, the ribs compressed, the abdomen extended, the wrists and ankles broadened, and the long bones bent. So can anybody passing in the train of a tornado tell what has gone before.

"Continuous bowel trouble often leads to rickets; but the earliest sign of the rickets is sweating, particularly at night and about the back of the head. . . . The presence of rickets means that the child has been deprived of some important food element. Usually this is the fat, but not infrequently the proteid (protein) constituents of the diet are deficient. When sterilized or boiled milk constitutes the basis of the food, the form of malnutrition is more apt to be of the scorbutic (scurvy) than the rachitic type. By carefully reviewing the child's diet the particular deficiency can readily be made out.

"By way of treatment, it is first necessary to get the child's stomach and bowels into a normal condition, so that the food administered can be properly digested and absorbed. Then a diet rich in the element which has previously been deficient is to be prescribed. For the infant, protein food cannot be found outside of milk. But for its fats, not only is milk available, but also cod liver oil. This latter substance is usually taken readily by young children, and is well borne. Bouchut considered it as a specific in rickets and when it is considered that fat deficiency is so commonly a cause of this disorder his belief seems well founded.

"The indication for the administration of cod liver oil to the rachitic infant is to be determined entirely by the character of his preceding diet, and not by its present appearance. If the diet has been deficient in fat, fats must now be given it even if the child itself be excessively fat. The fat of the rachitic baby comes from the excessive amounts of sugar and starch upon which it has been fed, and it seems that the organism, at least the growing organism, requires for its complete nourishment food in the shape of fat . . ."

So 75 years ago doctors knew that rickets was caused by something missing from the diet. They thought that codliver oil was beneficial because of the fat it contained never suspecting that it contained something which in extremely small amounts, is far more essential and more powerful—vitamin D.

They thought that rickets indicated that the infant had not been getting enough fat. Note that, even 75 years ago, doctors were well aware of the fact that too much sugar and starch are bad for children and make them fat. It is not the eating of fat which makes people fat, said this long ago doctor. It is the eating of sugar and starch. (How right he was!)

We can learn something very valuable from this voice from long ago. Today official medicine seems to doubt that any disease, except for the very obvious ones like diabetes, is related to one's diet. True, diet may have something to do with heart and circulatory disorders, they opine. But even disorders like muscular dystrophy, whose very name "dystrophy" means malnutrition, are being studied by physicians and researchers from the point of view of something being wrong with the patient's make-up—not his diet!

How do we know, today, that MD and multiple sclerosis and arthritis and Parkinson's Disease are not caused by lack of some nutrient which is needed in small amounts and which is not being supplied by modern diet—just as rickets is caused by a nutrient needed in very small amounts?

Seventy-five years ago doctors had not as yet discovered vitamin D. There is no way of knowing how many nutrients are as yet undiscovered today.

The lesson to be learned is the same lesson that long-ago doctors knew so well—"the bane of children artificially fed is malnutrition." Don't tinker with food! Don't remove parts of it and destroy other parts of it and change other parts of it, for you have no way of knowing what essential elements are disappearing and what the results will be in terms of health.

Modern food technology and processing consist of nothing more than changing and re-making food, while countless food elements, known and unknown, are destroyed in the process. The key to good health lies in eating only wholly natural, unprocessed food. Here nutritive elements have been carefully preserved rather than being destroyed.

A revolutionary scientific theory revealing the basic, elemental importance of vitamin D was described in the August 4, 1967 issue of *Science,* the publication of the American Association for the Advancement of Science. A biochemistry professor at Brandeis University, Dr. W. Farnsworth Lewis, explains how human beings happened to be able to migrate throughout the world, even into very cold regions like the Scandanavian countries, by developing over millions of years, lighter skins, through which the ultraviolet rays of the sun could penetrate.

This provocative theory depends for its proof on the fact that vitamin D is manufactured in certain layers of the skin when the ultraviolet rays of the sun fall on the skin. Dr. Lewis says there is no essential function of ultraviolet rays, so far as man is concerned, aside from the production of vitamin D.

It is vitamin D, you remember, which prevents rickets allowing the bones of babies to develop straight and strong, helping in the incorporation of the minerals calcium and phosphorus into the bone structure. Children who, for whatever reason, do not get enough vitamin D, develop rickets, which means twisted, deformed bones. On the other hand, if children or adults get too much vitamin D they also suffer, for then they absorb too much calcium and it settles in soft tissues like arteries and kidneys.

According to Dr. Lewis, the human body apparently has no mechanism whatever for protecting itself against too much vitamin D. Human beings originally lived in the tropical zone. So how were they protected against getting too much of the intense ultraviolet rays of the tropical sun? Originally they had dark skins, says Dr. Lewis, for deeply pigmented skins do not allow much of the ultraviolet light to pass into the inner layers of the skin.

So just enough vitamin D to prevent rickets is formed, even under tropical sun, in a dark-skinned person. But what happened when he migrated farther north, where the sun's rays contain much less ultraviolet and where many cloudy days obscure the sun entirely in winter?

Apparently he got rickets, says Dr. Lewis. For perhaps millions of years dark-skinned people trying to live in northern countries became so crippled with rickets that they could not hunt or find other food. So generation after generation, only the lighter-skinned individuals among them survived. Eventually these people became the lighter-skinned people of Northern Europe and Scandinavia. It is noteworthy, he says, that the coloring of skin among native peoples becomes lighter as one goes farther away from the equator. Vitamin D formation in skin is the only possible explanation of this, he thinks.

There is only one exception to this general rule: the Eskimos. Here are people who live in the very far North, where the winters are extremely long and dark, where very little of the sun's ultraviolet rays penetrate for most of the year. For warmth the Eskimos must wear thick heavy clothing which also prevents ultraviolet rays from reaching the skin. But rickets is unknown among the Eskimos. The reason? They eat the livers of fish and animals which are the only dependable food source of vitamin D. Therefore, they can keep their rather dark skins which do not allow the sun's rays to penetrate, but yet they avoid rickets. Such is the magic of fish liver oil.

There are many intriguing avenues of thought leading

out from this basic theory. It becomes apparent why light-skinned people must keep themselves well covered from the tropical sun in which dark-skinned people can walk all day without any difficulty. It also becomes apparent why dark-skinned people coming to live in the north must pay strict attention to getting enough vitamin D in a food supplement. If not, children may develop rickets and adults may develop the adult form of rickets which is called osteomalacia, or softening of the bones.

Today's milk, our best source of calcium, is enriched with vitamin D almost everywhere in the Western world. We do this to protect infants from rickets. Since most babies live largely on milk, the vitamin D enrichment program has prevented rickets on a nation-wide scale even among children growing up in slums in the darkest winter months when air pollution prevents the ultraviolet rays of the weak winter sunlight from reaching their skins.

Physicians know well the whole story of vitamin D and rickets, so children who, for some reason, cannot drink milk, are given vitamin D supplements, and most pediatricians advise some vitamin D in a supplement for all infants under their care. What about older people? There is good evidence that we continue to need vitamin D in later life, even though our bones are already formed. We must still absorb calcium and phosphorus for many different body functions and these minerals can be absorbed only if vitamin D is present.

No one knows for sure all the causes of the bone disorder that bothers many older people—osteoporosis. Many physicians believe that lack of calcium in the diet may play a big part in this condition, which results in pain, discomfort and, often broken bones. Some doctors believe that broken hips which many older people experience are not the result of falls, but that the bone breaks first, causing the fall.

We have evidence that vitamin D is often effective in relieving this condition. Three British scientists, reporting in *The Lancet,* volume 2, page 999, 1966 told of their work with 60 elderly women living alone. All of them were over 70, but mentally alert, active and well. None of them was on any special diet.

The doctors studied their bone density. Obviously thin bones tend to break more easily than very dense ones. Diet histories of some of the women showed that those with the lowest vitamin D intakes had the least dense bones—that is, the ones most likely to fracture. Although these women were apparently getting enough calcium and phosphorus—both important for bone health—they did lack vitamin D, which is the third factor, the third arm of the triangle, in the making and maintaining of healthy bones.

An article in *Nutrition Reviews* for February 1969 expressed surprise, almost shock, at the fact that three Greek physicians have reported rickets in a frightening percentage of infants examined in Greece, a land of abundant sunshine, even in winter.

One hundred thirty-seven infants in Athens and 190 in rural areas were given tests to determine the condition of their blood and bones in relation to rickets. All the children were under one year of age and came from middle to lower income families. They were not just children of poor people.

Testing blood for a substance known to indicate rickets, the doctors discovered that 15 percent of the infants had the disease. More than half of these had it so badly that x-rays of their wrists showed the deforming characteristics of rickets. Almost a third of the babies examined had "clinical signs of rickets" which the editors of *Nutrition Reviews* translate as meaning that they may have healed or inactive rickets. Of the 327 babies, only 116 had taken vitamin D in supplements.

All babies who had been exposed to sunlight—even though such exposure was by custom restricted to the face and lower arms—had a slightly lower prevalence of the disease than those not exposed. Breast-fed babies had only one-third as great an incidence as those given formulas. Just to make certain they had made no mistake in diagnosing the disease, the physician authors gave the children with symptoms of rickets vitamin D supplements for a number of weeks, and all their symptoms disappeared.

Why? How is it possible, in a land where sunlight is so plentiful that tourists come from all over the world just to enjoy the fine weather—that infants should suffer from a disease related to lack of sunlight? The authors do not know. They say that many of the ill children had never been seen by a doctor or a nurse, that some of the mothers who had taken their babies to a clinic failed to follow the doctor's orders, or (they say) were never told by their doctors to give the children vitamin D or expose them to sunlight.

Apparently Greek women feel that their infants should be fully clothed at all times, with only the head and upper arms exposed. This is just not enough exposed skin for the sunlight to work its magic upon, especially if the babies are not taken out every day when the sun is shining strongly. The authors tell us that a similar condition was discovered in a southern part of Israel where the babies' clothing was to blame for the rickets, because it prevented exposure to the sun.

The authors believe that a similar survey "would be of interest in those areas, such as the U.S.A., where clinical rickets is very rare yet the prevalence of the subclinical state is at present unknown." In other words, no one has ever done wide-scale tests of blood substances to discover how many babies in any geographical area in our own country may be suffering from a degree of rickets which does not bend arm and leg bones out of shape, deform jaws and hands, but which is rickets nonetheless.

Winter is the time when rickets prevails, especially in smog-darkened cities where high buildings shade the windows and the weather is too cold for the baby to spend much time in the open air, bundled up—let alone with skin exposed to the sun's rays. In most areas milk is enriched with vitamin D, so that babies will not suffer a deficiency.

But some children cannot drink milk, families among the very poor cannot afford milk. So rickets is not a historical curiosity that we can write off casually as a "conquered disease."

As for the older folks, the experts tell us they do not need as much vitamin D as babies, since their bones have stopped growing. But it seems obvious that bones continue to need nourishment, since they lose minerals constantly which must be replaced. So the older folks, too, need vitamin D—especially those who cannot get away to a sunny climate and spend a lengthy winter vacation in a bathing suit at a southern resort. No one has ever come to harm taking vitamin D in recommended amounts to regulate the body's absorption of calcium and phosphorus.

In 1956 the powers-that-be in Scotland decided that they would reduce the amount of vitamin D in milk and other baby foods eaten by infants.

Scotland is a northern country with long winters. It is a rainy country, so that even in summer, there is not nearly so much sunshine as there is in dry southern countries. So it was felt as early as 1939, that foods which make up the largest part of the diets of infants should be fortified with vitamin D. This was done and rickets almost completely disappeared from the medical scene in Scotland.

But in 1956 the reduction in vitamin D fortification was sanctioned, and almost at once the disease began to appear again, according to three child specialists from Glasgow, writing in *The Lancet* for April 13, 1968. They tell us that medical writers knew of this and wrote warning articles about it as early as 1963.

In 1968—12 years after the amount of vitamin D in infant foods was reduced and five years after the first warnings about it three Glasgow specialists have found "severe infantile rickets" in many Glasgow children and have also found x-ray evidence of bone changes possibly due to too little vitamin D in as many as 9 percent of all children x-rayed!

They say, "In spite of an increased awareness of these

problems by local health authority and hospital staff recent studies of nutrition in childhood have demonstrated clearly that a high proportion of young children in Glasgow are still having an inadequate dietary intake of Vitamin D."

They go on to say, "The incidence of florid (obvious) rickets in Glasgow may be only the tip of the iceberg—the real problem may be the extent of lesser degrees of undiagnosed hypovitaminosis D (vitamin D deficiency) in the infant and toddler population of Glasgow, and perhaps the rest of Scotland, if not the whole of the United Kingdom."

The reason for this is indisputable. Vitamin D is almost nonexistent in food. Children—especially poor children and those whose mothers have little or no nutritional education—eat mostly milk and cereals. Milk has little vitamin D, cereals none. By fortifying these foods with the vitamin, rickets can easily be prevented without the necessity of constantly supervising the diet of children or educating their mothers as to what foods they should eat and how much time they should spend in the sunshine.

But as soon as this steady supply of vitamin D is cut off, the babies and children react almost immediately. Their little bones feel the effects almost at once and crippling and deforming begin. Once bones have carried these deformities into adolescence, there is no hope of remedying the situation. The child is permanently deformed. And, in addition to the unsightly leg bones which characterize rickets, all other bones in the body are similarly weakened, so that the individual who has suffered from rickets is permanently weakened in all parts.

The three Glasgow experts tell us that it is fairly easy to diagnose rickets when it has progressed to the advanced stages. There are gross physical changes as well as those that can be seen on x-rays. But, they say, "the problem of detecting minor degrees of vitamin D-deficiency in children has not been satisfactorily solved."

They have been examining all children x-rayed at their hospital for evidence of possible vitamin D deficiency.

They have found in the bones they studied that possibly 9 percent of all these children already have bone changes indicating vitamin D deficiency although one could not see deformed bones by merely examining the children.

They go on to say that no one knows really what any of these children eat or how their eating habits are determined. What they eat is decided by how much money their families have, how much they know about good nutrition, where they can go for advice on nutritional matters, what their families have traditionally eaten, and whether or not suitable and nutritious food is easily available.

Of course, exactly the same thing is true in our country. A recent survey by the Department of Agriculture revealed that about half of all American families are not eating good diets, nutritionally speaking. About 20 percent of them are eating diets classified as "poor"—that is, not containing the amounts of vitamins and minerals which are officially recommended. Vitamin D was not included in this survey since it is assumed that American children get milk and other foods fortified or enriched by vitamin D. Of course, this may not be true of large numbers of our children. No one knows.

In 1956 British pediatricians reported finding a few—not many—cases of children who appeared to be getting too much vitamin D. So they reduced the amount of vitamin D in milk and cereals. Several years ago, a child specialist in the United States published an article asking whether too much vitamin D in the diet of pregnant women might not be responsible for a condition in babies, present at birth, which seemed to be related to an excess of this vitamin. The matter was referred to several committees one of which was the Committee on Nutrition of the American Academy of Pediatrics.

Their report on the subject states that adding vitamin D to milk has virtually eradicated rickets in this country. The disorder which may (or may not) be related to too much intake of vitamin D is extremely rare and may be proven to have nothing to do with vitamin D at all. So the committee states that reducing the amount of vitamin D in our milk and cereals could be justified only if we could be sure that all the millions of babies who depend on it as their only source of the vitamin would not risk rickets.

The best amount of vitamin D for the average infant seems to be about 400 units a day. And the committee suggests that every effort should be made to see that babies get this amount—the amount found in one quart of milk enriched with the vitamin. They also think that vitamin preparations should be very clear in their labeling to indicate that such-and-such an amount (one capsule or one drop or one teaspoon) will provide this amount so that even the least nutritionally conscious young mother will not make mistakes in giving her baby this vitamin.

The Lancet article about what has happened in Scotland should serve as a warning, a very clear warning to everyone in our country, that decisions to limit the amount of essential vitamins in food or in supplements can have very serious and far-reaching results, which were not anticipated when such steps were recommended. Rickets is an extremely serious disease, which, it now seems, may afflict as many as 9 percent of all Scottish children—just as a result of decreasing the amount of this essential vitamin in infant foods.

Officially, no one knows how much vitamin D is needed by adults. *Recommended Dietary Allowances,* the official booklet, states, "The requirement of vitamin D in adult life is not known. The occurrence of deficiency states (though very rare) indicates that a small need exists, but it is considered that the amounts required are so small that under normal circumstances they are met by the vitamin D content of the usual mixed diet and by exposure to sunlight. For persons working at night and for nuns and others whose clothing or customs shield them from sunlight, the regular consumption of vitamin D fortified milk is recommended."

We think there are several assumptions here that deserve to be questioned. First, how much vitamin D is there in "the usual mixed diet?" Liver, canned salmon, sardines, herring and tuna, and egg yolk are just about the only foods that contain any appreciable amount of this vitamin. Apparently nature meant us to get our vitamin D from the sunlight.

In order to do this we must spend considerable time every day in bright sunlight, with quite extensive areas of skin exposed to the sun. Many adults find this not impossible during spring and summer months. In the South, especially at the shore, outdoor life even in winter assures one of getting some exposure of the skin to the sun's rays.

But what about those of us who live in the North? Air pollution in our cities keeps the sun's rays rather well screened out most of the time and especially in winter. Even on bright, clear sunny days in winter it is, of course, impossible to go outdoors without plenty of clothing, so that nothing but a bit of facial skin is exposed to whatever weak, faint rays of the sun may be around.

Ordinary window glass screens out ultraviolet rays of the sun, so sun-bathing indoors in winter does not add to one's vitamin D store. Many older folks seldom go out in winter, for fear of falling on icy sidewalks. Where, then, are all these folks supposed to get the vitamin D that is essential for good health? The function of vitamin D is to promote the absorption of calcium, a mineral we must have for the health of the bones, muscles, heart and many other parts of us.

Milk, fortified with vitamin D, is available almost everywhere. Of course, folks with dairy farms who get their milk right from their own cows do not get the added vitamin D that is in commercial milk. One quart of such fortified milk contains 400 units of vitamin D, the amount that is supposedly enough for infants and children. Youngsters who drink a quart of milk every day will, supposedly, get enough vitamin D along with ample calcium of the milk, to make strong bones and teeth.

But what about those children who don't drink that much milk every day, or don't drink any milk at all? And what of adults who, for some reason, have decided that milk doesn't agree with them or that it is not something adults need? Where will they get their vitamin D, especially in cold weather?

One of the commonest ailments of everyone over the age of 50 in this country is osteoporosis, a softening of the bones which becomes progressively worse as we age, until the spine becomes deformed and hip and leg bones become so softened that falls are to be expected, with broken bones as a consequence. Could not the basic cause of this disorder be a simple lack of calcium and the vitamin D which is necessary to absorb it? It could, certainly, in people who shun milk and don't get out in the sunshine very often.

A New York ophthalmologist treats some eye conditions of old people with massive doses of vitamin D. Dr. Arthur A. Knapp believes that myopia or short-sightedness is not just an eye condition, but is instead a manifestation of vitamin D deficiency. He gave a group of patients vitamin D and calcium supplements over periods ranging from 5 to 28 months and found a decrease in the nearsightedness in more than a third of them, with a definite halt in the process of another 17 percent. Dr. Knapp discussed his treatment at a 1966 meeting of the American Geriatrics Society.

Dr. Knapp also believes that lack of vitamin D and calcium may be related to the formation of cataract although he says not enough research has been done along these lines to prove the facts. Laboratory animals kept on diets deficient in vitamin D and calcium invariably develop cataracts, he says.

So far as human beings are concerned, there are some mighty relevant facts linking vitamin D and calcium lack to cataracts. A certain drug is used to decrease blood calcium in some diseases. It occasionally produces cataracts. Diabetics may suffer from calcium imbalance. They develop cataracts more often than non-diabetics. A condition called "tetany" in which blood calcium is very low often produces cataracts.

Cataracts cause more than 15 percent of all blindness in

the United States. There is no known method of prevention. Should we not insist upon far more research time and money being used for investigating the possibility that vitamin and mineral deficiencies may be at least partly responsible for this tragic condition which afflicts so many of our older folks?

Common sense tells us that the function of the eye is to admit light. Vitamin A and vitamin D are both intimately tied up with how our bodies use light. Vitamin A must be present in the eye to restore a certain pigment that is destroyed by light. And the only way we can really get enough vitamin D to be healthy is to spend a considerable time every day in the sunlight! So doesn't it seem obvious that the good health of the eyes must be closely related to the continuing good supply of these two vitamins which our diets and our way of life may permit?

Should you take vitamin D as a food supplement? Well, how does your intake of this vitamin measure up to your possible requirements? If you spend the winter in a near-tropical climate with a lot of outdoor activity and if you make certain you are getting plenty of calcium from fortified milk, chances are you need not add to your vitamin D supply. Adults officially need 800 milligrams of calcium daily. One eight-ounce glass of milk gives you 250 milligrams of calcium. It is present in small amounts in foods other than dairy products.

If you spend winters in the North and if you spend most of your time indoors, summer and winter, there seems to be

---

Foods Highest in Vitamin D

Vitamin D occurs in extremely small amounts in butter, egg yolk, saltwater fish such as salmon, herring, sardines, liver. Fish liver oil is the richest source. Most milk these days is irradiated to increase its vitamin D content.

---

lots of evidence that adding vitamin D, along with plenty of calcium, to your diet would be beneficial, not only to bones and teeth, but also to the heart muscle which needs calcium, and to the health of the eyes.

So what should we do? Spend long hours in the summer sun to try to get enough vitamin D to last all winter? Suntan is the body's effort to protect the unwise sunbather from getting too much vitamin D. So after you have developed a dark tan you absorb almost no more vitamin D. This is one reason why most physicians feel that deliberate lengthy suntanning is not wise. You should, of course, spend some time in the sun every day, no matter what your age is. Even very elderly folks enjoy a walk along a shaded street in full summer sunlight. The ultraviolet light penetrates even through leafy trees.

But people who, for one reason or another, must stay indoors most of the time and especially those who wear heavy clothing with long sleeves are quite likely to suffer from too little vitamin D the year around. A supplement is the best answer. Vitamin D is fat soluble, meaning that your body stores it. You need not take a supply of it every day. Once a week or even less often is quite suitable.

How much do you need? This depends on your way of life. If you spend a great deal of time outdoors and especially if you are light-skinned, you will probably get enough vitamin D from the sunlight. If your skin is darker or if you must spend long hours indoors, especially in the middle of the day when the sun's rays are strongest or if you work at night then it certainly would be beneficial to add some of the Eskimos' food supplement—fish liver oil—to your daily supplements.

How much is too much? Officially, the estimate is that amounts on the order of 1,000 to 3,000 units per kilogram of weight per day are toxic. A kilogram is about two pounds. So for a 150 pound person, the toxic amount of vitamin D should be somewhere around 100,000 to 200,000 units daily.

Can you get vitamin D in food? The only foods which

contain any appreciable vitamin D are: salt water fish, especially those which are high in body oils like salmon, sardines and herring, liver and liver sausage, egg yolks and summer milk. Most milk and margarine and some butter in this country are fortified with vitamin D. Fish liver oil capsules are completely tasteless, inexpensive and easy to take.

There is at present a feeling among some members of the scientific community that vitamin D should, by rights, be listed as a hormone rather than a vitamin since it is produced by the body through the action of sunlight on the skin. Where it occurs in food, it is there only because the animal produced it for its own use. Until some official decision is made on this matter, vitamin D is still called a vitamin.

CHAPTER 41

We Haven't Conquered Rickets Yet

ALTHOUGH SCIENTISTS, physicians and nutrition experts have known for many years just about all they need to know about vitamin D and its relation to healthy bones and teeth, we are still turning up widespread incidence of rickets in various corners of the globe. Usually it results from misunderstanding of the needs of infants and children when people move from their ancestral homes to new environments. And in the cases described below, there are quite serious implications for some patrons of health food stores who are making their own unleavened bread. For the story involves unleavened bread, as well as lack of vitamin D. And it is not a happy story.

The article in *The Lancet* for May 28, 1976 described a number of cases of florid (that is, serious or fully developed) rickets in a group of young children in Glasgow, Scotland.

Six investigators from the Royal Hospital for Sick Children and University Departments of Biochemistry and Child Health in Glasgow found that 12½ per cent of all the children they examined suffered from rickets, slight to very serious cases. Rickets is a disease of bone development. It causes knock-knees, twisted spines, deformed legs, arms and wrists. Because it can also deform pelvises, it can create untold hardships for women in childbirth if they suffered from rickets when they were babies.

Say the Scots authors, "It is unacceptable that fetal rickets should occur in Glasgow in the 1970's." Why and how did it happen? Practically all the children discovered to have rickets were African or Asian immigrants living in more or less segregated communities in Scotland, eating mostly their traditional food and, many of them, unable to converse in English. They shopped at their own stores, went to movies and church services conducted in their own languages and had little to do with the Scots teachers or nutrition experts or child clinics conducted in English.

But how does it happen that just not knowing the language can produce a serious, deforming disease whose effects will probably persist for a lifetime? The diet of the Asian and African immigrants consists mostly of *chapattis* (pancakes) made from whole-grain flour. With these they eat clarified butter called *ghee*. People in hot countries who have no refrigeration preserve butter by removing all the cloudy part of the melted butter. What is left is pure fat which keeps well, without rancidity, for some time.

The Glasgow doctors speculate that perhaps this cooking process destroyed what little vitamin D the butter contained. There is no vitamin D in wheat flour. So these immigrant children were getting almost no vitamin D. The official Recommended Dietary Allowance for vitamin D in our country is 400 units daily.

The same is true of native Scots children living in Glasgow whose mothers do not realize the value of supplements. Several Scots children with rickets were reported in this same study. In Glasgow a short cartoon film has now been made in the Hindi, Urdu and Panjabi languages emphasizing the importance of giving children suitable foods and supplements of vitamin D. It is shown at meeting places and to older children at school. Leaflets and posters in Asian and African languages are also posted in these communities. The doctors suggest that supplements of 300 units of vitamin D should be made available to immigrant children and should be given daily between the ages of 3 months and 16 years.

They also suggest that the flour used by the immigrants to make their chapattis should be fortified with vitamin D. One of the reasons for this is that the immigrants' diet, which consists almost entirely of wholewheat flour mixed with water and made into pancakes or chapattis contains phytate which has a tendency to unite with calcium and other minerals and cause them to be excreted unused. This is one reason why it is a bad idea to eat only unyeasted bread. When yeast is used to raise wholegrain bread it changes the form of the phytate so that it does not cause this loss of minerals.

But the African and Asian women have no knowledge of making bread with yeast and they are accustomed to eating unyeasted chapattis so they continue to eat them in Scotland. This, combined with the almost total lack of sunshine (which produces vitamin D) and vitamin D in diets creates the calcium deficiency that results in rickets. Vitamin D is very scarce in foods. We were apparently meant by nature to get most of our vitamin D from the sunshine. But how can this be done in a far northern country by people whose skins are genetically developed to exclude sunlight?

Most of us in this country do not have problems of dealing with immigrants and trying to solve their nutritional problems by understanding all these various aspects of vitamin D nutrition which change drastically when the individuals move to another part of the world. However we do have our own problems with vitamin D no matter where we live in the U.S.A.

Rickets afflicted large numbers of children in early America, because no one then understood the cause of the disease. Egg yolk and the bones of fish like salmon, sardines, tuna, mackerel and so on, as well as fish livers, are the only reliable sources of vitamin D in food. There is a bit of vitamin D in butter, milk, cream, cheese, liver and meat and a very small amount in salad oils.

Most dairy milk these days is fortified with vitamin D. The container states on the label that one quart of milk contains 400 International Units of vitamin D. This was recommended to prevent the epidemics of rickets that prevailed in earlier days. But what about people who don't or can't drink milk? Many people these days have been told by their doctors to shun both milk and eggs because of their supposedly harmful cholesterol content. Where will such people get their vitamin D? It is now well known that adults as well as children need vitamin D to keep their bones healthy.

Where can vegetarians who eat no animal products of any kind get their vitamin D, especially if they spend most of their time indoors or in northern climates? A diet which contains no food of animal origin is quite likely to be short on calcium as well, so this is a double hazard in the badly planned vegetarian diet. Vegetarian children who eat no animal products should get their calcium and vitamin D from supplements.

Its vitamin D and calcium content is one very good reason to use plenty of milk, no matter what your age happens to be. Milk is not just a food for infants, any more than eggs are food just for embryo chicks. See that your family gets plenty of milk and other calcium-rich foods such as all kinds of cheese and yogurt.

And see that your family gets plenty of vitamin D. If you live in the south it's much easier, for you usually have plenty of sunlight all winter. But your skin manufactures vitamin D only when it is bare to the sunshine. So don't bundle your children up unless it's really cold. Let them play outdoors all summer with as little as possible between them and the sky. They need not, and should not, stay in the sun long enough to get sunburned. You get plenty of vitamin D just from being in the open air on a sunny day, even if you spend all your time in dappled shade. Sunburn is unwise.

And take a vitamin supplement if you think you are not getting enough vitamin D.

Vitamin E Is...

Fat-soluble, hence stored in the body.

Responsible for health and maintenance of circulatory system, and muscles in general, health of red blood cells, and healthful sex and reproductive life, detoxifying poisons, preventing oxidation of fats in the body.

Present in seeds, wholegrains, wheat germ, wheat bran, all salad oils, liver, eggs. Wheat germ oil is the best source in food. *Safe* in very large amounts. All reports show no disadvantages in extremely large amounts, even when taken over long periods of time.

Destroyed by mineral oil laxatives, iron medications, impaired fat absorption in certain disorders, heat in cooking and long storage in freezers. Iron medication should be taken at a different time from any vitamin E supplement.

Required officially in daily amounts of 12 International Units for adults, less for children.

Available in low or high potencies in one-a-day supplements or individual supplements.

CHAPTER 42

Your Need for
Vitamin E

BECAUSE OF THEIR unpleasant smell, one would think that rancid fats might not be good food. This is correct. Rancid fats are very unhealthful. One reason is that they destroy vitamin E. If you eat fats that are spoiled or rancid, they will quickly destroy any vitamin E in your digestive tract at the same time. Then, too, foods normally rich in Vitamin E which have gone rancid will contain none of the vitamin.

On the other hand, one of the most important functions of vitamin E is to prevent fats from becoming rancid. Fats are spoiled by combining with oxygen. Vitamin E seems to be an anti-oxidant, that is, it prevents this combination and so prevents the fat from becoming rancid. In the same way, this vitamin protects other vitamins, specifically vitamins A and C, as well as certain other fats called the unsaturated fats. This means that if you have plenty of vitamin E in your diet you can get along successfully without suffering so much from lack of these other vitamins, in case they are short in your meals. This is one example of the way vitamins work with and protect one another.

Throughout scientific literature vitamin E is linked over and over again with the name of that substance without which none of us can live for even a minute—oxygen. Vitamin E and oxygen are important to one another. This alone indicates that this vitamin, which has been identified and studied only since 1936, must be essential for all of us.

Studying laboratory animals which have been made deficient in vitamin E, scientists have found that the muscles of these animals seem to need more oxygen than those of normal animals, so they have concluded that plenty of vitamin E in the diet enables us to get along on less oxygen than we would otherwise need. This discovery is very important, especially in modern times when so many things—environmental conditions and physical disorders—conspire to cheat us of much of the oxygen we need. Smoking, for instance, cuts off some of the supply of oxygen to the cells. The indoor, sedentary life most of us lead deprives us of the oxygen we might get in long country walks with fresh, unpolluted air filling our lungs.

Whether because of its relation to oxygen or because of something else as yet undiscovered, vitamin E seems to be involved in what goes on in an astonishing number of places in the body: reproductive system, muscles, brain, nerves, heart and circulatory organs, joints, skin and digestive tract, to name but a few. *An Annotated Bibliography of Vitamin E*, prepared by the Research Laboratories of the Distillation Products Industries, lists 195 pieces of important research reported just in the years 1958 through 1960, in which vitamin E was given to human beings in varying doses to see what the effect would be on whatever disorder they were suffering from.

Some of the researchers reported little or no success. Others were enthusiastic about the results they got. Here are some of the positive reports.

Premature infants with a disorder called scleroderma (a hardening and swelling of the skin) were given vitamin E. Mortality dropped from 75% to 27%. Children with cystic fibrosis of the pancreas were found to have some symptoms just like those of animals which are deficient in vitamin E. The children also had very low levels of the vitamin in their blood. The scientist who reported this discovery in *Pediatrics* in 1958 recommended that children with this disease be given vitamin E routinely.

A Russian scientific journal reported that the incidence of miscarriage was reduced from 46% to 12% in women whose pregnancy was complicated by the Rh factor, when vitamin E was given along with vitamin C and vitamin K. A German scientist reported in 1959 that a certain kind of inherited muscular dystrophy responded well to doses of the B vitamins, vitamin A, C and E (300 milligrams a day). When started soon enough and continued for long enough, he said, this treatment relieved muscular distress and produced improvement. Note that these two physicians gave other vitamins along with vitamin E and have no way of knowing how much this combination of vitamins had to do with their success.

Dr. Evan Shute of Canada, today's outstanding proponent of the use of vitamin E, reported improved muscle strength in two patients with acute polio and 3 out of 14 patients with chronic polio. A South American physician at the National Institute of Public Health in Buenos Aires told of giving large doses of vitamin E to patients in a mental hospital. There was improvement in their mental state and their muscle coordination. Mentally handicapped children, given large doses of vitamin E showed physical and mental improvement, he tells us. He believes that vitamin E plays some part in regulating the glands and also the nervous system.

Reports on heart and blood vessel disorders are many. A Japanese scientist tells of 80 surgical patients. Half of them received vitamin E before an operation. 54% of these vitamin-E-treated patients were declared safe from any possibility of blood clots or hemorrhages after the operation. Of the other group, who were not given any vitamin E, 50% showed dangerously low levels in the substance that regulates blood clotting, so that their chances of suffering blood clots or strokes were much greater than those of the patients who took vitamin E.

Dr. Shute offers most convincing evidence of his belief that vitamin E is a natural anti-clotting agent, that is, that it prevents blood clots and other conditions which may cause strokes. He also thinks it is a vaso-dilator, that is, it opens blood vessels so that plenty of blood can get through. He uses it for patients who have heart trouble, varicose veins, phlebitis, hardening of the arteries, diabetic gangrene, burns, skin grafts and many other conditions, especially those which are the most widespread causes of death today—disorders of the heart and circulatory system. Dr. Shute is an ardent champion of vitamin E. He claims that doctors who are consistently unsuccessful in using it are simply not giving the right dose or are not continuing treatment long enough.

Dr. Shute edits a fine periodical, *The Summary*, which deals chiefly with the use of vitamin E for preventing and treating major disorders. Every issue contains some 50 to 100 articles or abstracts on vitamin E or related subjects, such as fats in the diet, the use of wheat germ oil, and so forth. Here are some notes from the December, 1966 issue.

Vitamin E is used by Dr. Shute in treating a case of pulmonary embolism and thrombophlebitis. These are blood clots—the first in the lungs, the second in the legs. Dr. Shute says that patients respond well to vitamin E. He adds that thrombophlebitis may recur while the patient is being treated with vitamin E. Don't panic, he says. Just increase the dosage. He lets his patients walk and work without regard to the phlebitis present.

Two Brazilian scientists report on heart studies done on rats that were deficient in vitamin E. Of 26 rats, only six normal ones were found. All the rest showed some heart damage when they were tested with electrocardiograms and other devices. Two German researchers report on the action of a water soluble vitamin E solution on the heart tissues of guinea pigs. They found that the vitamin protects the heart from damage by medication, and helps to prevent heart insufficiency. Dr. Shute adds that this paper indicates that vitamin E should be investigated further in hospital clinics.

Other, more recent researches on vitamin E have been

reported in many scientific journals.

A Louisiana State University professor believes he may have found a key for preventing the aging process—vitamin E. Dr. William A. Pryor, a chemistry professor, says in an article in *Scientific American*, August, 1970, that the effects of diets deficient in vitamin E are very similar to effects of radiation damage and aging. In all three instances there is structural damage to the membranes of cells.

Researchers studying cells have found in them some very unstable compounds they call "free radicals" which play an important part in many processes involving oxygen. These substances are involved in some kinds of cancer; radiation damage to cells occurs partly through the action of these rather mysterious substances. Free radicals are formed in the body during the process of oxidizing food and making it into energy. This process is very carefully regulated in the cell by enzymes which control the burning of fats. When free radicals are present, the process is stopped. The oxygen will not react with the enzymes to consume the fat.

But when enough vitamin E is present, the free radicals are restrained and the process goes on in a normal fashion. So the vitamin E protects from harm. If it is not present, the fatty substances collect into a dark brown debris which is called "age pigment." Now it appears they may have nothing to do with aging. Perhaps they are just symptoms of vitamin E deficiency. Dr. Pryor does not mention it, but doesn't it seem possible, too, that vitamin E may also be able to help protect the cell against the ravages of radiation?

Vitamin E along with vitamin A, has been found to protect laboratory animals from some of the damage done by air pollutants in our large cities—the poisons that collect in the air from car exhausts, chimneys and power stations. Animals which had plenty of vitamin E in their diets showed little damage when they were exposed to nitrogen dioxide and ozone, two ever-present pollutants. Animals deficient in the vitamin suffered extensive damage.

In 1969 researchers found that artificial milk formulas fed to human infants produce very low levels of vitamin E which may be responsible for assorted disorders in these little ones. One scientist believes that "crib deaths"—the mysterious death of suffocation of healthy infants in their cribs—may be a result of vitamin E deficiency.

Dr. F. L. Money of Wellington, New Zealand, has been doing experiments with baby pigs. He has found that pigs, kept in pens and fed artificially, are prone to sudden death, just like the "crib deaths" of human infants. When the piglets are examined their hearts and lungs are affected and they bleed into the spinal cord. It is the same with human babies who die. The human babies who die are usually bottle-fed rather than breast-fed.

Dr. Money found that his animals had very low levels of vitamin E and a trace mineral selenium in their blood. He began to give the vitamin and the mineral to pigs in one group, withholding it from those in another group. The animals which were given the supplements did not die. Those which got nothing continued to suffer many mortalities from what Dr. Money calls "sudden death."

The evidence strongly suggests, says Dr. Money, that crib death, like the sudden pen deaths in pigs may be due to dietary lack of vitamin E and/or selenium. We may be able to prevent it simply by giving these two substances to our babies routinely as they are given vitamin D and vitamin C.

A vitamin E deficiency causes muscular dystrophy in monkeys. Lack of the vitamin causes the accumulation of cholesterol in muscles with the crippling effects of dystrophy. Dr. Manford D. Morris of the University of Arkansas, who is working with dystrophic monkeys, stated in 1968 that vitamin E deficiency cannot be the cause of MD in human beings, because "such deficiency in humans is extremely rare, and probably non-existent in the United States." It seems he has not read the surveys showing that vitamin E deficiency may, instead, be very common among Americans.

Athletes don't wait for the researchers to make up their

minds. *Medical World News* reported in May, 1969 that a pitcher on the Giants team credits vitamin E with keeping his pitching arm in shape. He began to take the vitamin after a sore shoulder affected his pitching in 1967.

Premature babies and infants of very low weight at birth are frequently victims of a kind of anemia which does not respond to the usual supplementation with iron. Some time ago the suggestion was made that perhaps the babies might be deficient in vitamin E.

We know that some modern formulas for babies are very high in the unsaturated fats which would increase the need for vitamin E. We know, too, that the milk given to grossly premature babies is usually very low in this protective substance. Vitamin E does not pass through the placental barrier from the pregnant mother to the infant she carries, so most babies are born vitamin E-deficient!

If the baby has the usual birth weight and is not premature, the mother's milk and formula usually correct this deficiency by the end of the first week of life. In the premature baby, however, the deficiency is more pronounced and persistent, according to two Welsh physicians, writing in *International Journal of Vitamin Research*, volume 40, 1970. Dr. M.A. Chadd and A.J. Fraser review the evidence and then tell us about their own experience with premature infants.

They followed the course of 52 infants, some of whom were given vitamin E supplements, others not. No matter what their weight at birth was, all the infants getting vitamin E showed higher blood levels of vitamin E within a week, demonstrating that there was no problem with absorbing the vitamin. And at the usual time when anemia is expected to appear, the babies who got vitamin E showed higher blood levels of iron than those which did not.

In the case of premature babies, whose birth weight was very low the vitamin E made no difference in the tendency to anemia. The doctors feel that perhaps they were not giving enough of the vitamin. They stress the fact that more work needs to be done, to determine what amounts of the vitamin will be most beneficial depending on the baby's weight. They think that the premature ones may have a worse deficiency than the normal ones, hence may need much more of the vitamin.

In a second article in the same journal they tell us of three babies who were "grossly immature" and suffering from symptoms of vitamin E deficiency. They were swollen and suffered from anemia. They had received routine supplements of vitamins, iron, and folic acid, but the condition persisted. They were given 12 milligrams of vitamin E and responded immediately. The swelling went down, the blood picture improved at once.

Say the authors, "It is suggested that vitamin E deficiency be considered in any very small infant who has an anemia within a few weeks of birth."

These researchers do not discuss the diet of the mothers of these children. But if the vitamin E does not pass readily from mother to unborn child, does it not seem possible that this may be because of lack of vitamin E in the mother? Many researchers have shown that modern diets in which refined foods make up a large part, are lacking in this vitamin. Is it not possible that these infants' mothers were just not getting enough of it to pass some along to the babies?

Considering the close relationship of vitamin E to reproductive functions, isn't it possible, too, that lack of vitamin E in the mother's diet may be one of the main reasons for the babies being born prematurely? Veterinarians have known for years that horses and prize animals of many kinds are liable to abort their young or to deliver them prematurely when they are short on vitamin E. Many stock raisers use the vitamin regularly to prevent this condition. Too bad many of our human children are not given the benefit of this beneficent vitamin as valuable stock animals are.

An important finding in relation to vitamin E was reported in *Science* for March 1, 1968. Two researchers at the University of California studied the process of reproduction in rats which had been deprived of vitamin E, although the rest of their diet was complete in every nutrient. They uncovered a very significant difference in the animals which got enough vitamin E and those which did not.

It is well known that sterility is the first indication of vitamin E deficiency in animals. Up to now, no one could even speculate why lack of vitamin E brought sterility. Scientists know that vitamin E is closely related in function to oxygen, in that it protects certain substances in food from oxidizing or becoming rancid. The two California scientists believe that this ability of vitamin E to protect substances from the action of oxygen may be necessary every time a cell divides. And, of course, cell division is the basis for reproduction and the growth of every new living thing.

Studying laboratory animals made deficient in vitamin E, the scientists found that their cells contained a given number of a certain particle in each cell that is not present in quantity when the cell is dividing normally. Animals which were getting plenty of vitamin E had fewer of these particles. They also found that animals raised breathing the regular air of the laboratory had a normal appearance, whereas the cells of those breathing pure oxygen looked more like the cells of animals which did not get enough vitamin E—another indication that too much oxygen was in some way damaging the process of cell division.

This discovery could be a most important nutritional finding. To those of us who are not scientists, it sounds complex and obscure. But when you consider what the implications for good health are, you realize how important this discovery may be.

As the authors say in their article, they may have shown that vitamin E has the basic function of giving direct protection to the apparatus responsible for the division of cells. Now all cells divide, so this finding is not applicable only to problems of reproduction. The cells of children growing from infancy must divide many times to produce that growth. As we grow older, cells wear out and must be replaced by new cells.

Cancer is believed to be a disorder of cell division, where cells have lost the ability to limit their division and continue to divide wildly and profusely. So you can easily see what great importance may be attached to this finding in regard to vitamin E. If indeed, ample amounts of this vitamin are essential to protect the apparatus whereby cells divide, then it is tied in indirectly with life itself and almost every process in life.

We cannot immediately make such a flat statement because this is not the way scientific inquiry works. Other scientists in this field will have to confirm the work of the California people. Scientists in other fields will then have to relate this work to theirs before we finally have a definite scientific fact, accepted generally by most experts on nutrition.

Until this time comes—and it may be years from now—our public spokesmen on matters having to do with daily diet will probably continue to state, as they do now, that all of us get plenty of vitamin E in our daily meals—no matter what we eat, apparently.

CHAPTER 43

What Does
Vitamin E
Do in the Body?

THOSE OF US who use vitamin E daily for good health are often asked, "What specifically does vitamin E do in the body?" First of all, let's point out that there are many essential food elements whose full activity in the body is not known, nor even guessed at by scientists who have made a life work of this study. This is no reason for not continuing to use them and to get them at every day's meals.

But in the case of vitamin E, we know well some of the activities of this vitamin in our body's mechanism. Dr. Evan Shute of the Shute Foundation in Canada gives answers to such questions in volume 24 of his publication *The Summary*.

1. Vitamin E is an antioxidant. It prevents the formation and deposition of a certain harmful form of fatty substances. It is thus an oxidant as well, he goes on to explain, since it can be used to protect living things from too little oxygen. "We tell patients it is like living in an oxygen tent to take vitamin E," says Dr. Shute.

2. Vitamin E is involved in blood clotting or rather in preventing the formation of unwanted blood clots. The clotting of blood is an essential body process. Without it,

we would bleed to death with any slight cut. But, when the clotting mechanism goes out of control blood clots form where they are not wanted and serious or perhaps fatal circulatory complications result. Vitamin E helps to prevent this kind of clot. It also, "eats away" at clots that have already been formed in arteries, if they are fairly fresh. The only other agents capable of preventing such clots are drugs which are very expensive and dangerous as well, since they must be carefully watched and regulated or they may cause hemorrhaging instead of clotting. That can lead to fatal complications, too.

3. Vitamin E enlarges arteries permitting better circulation. "Can any cardiovascular condition not benefit by this?" asks Dr. Shute. One of the most dangerous complications of heart and artery disorders is the narrowing of arteries which leads to hardening of the arteries so that the blood cannot get through.

4. Vitamin E promotes what Dr. Shute calls "collateral circulation" which means simply that, when an artery or a smaller blood vessel is blocked, the vitamin helps the body to create a new artery around the damaged portion. Some patients have been given grafts by surgeons to bypass such useless arteries, but Dr. Shute points out that a natural substance like vitamin E is much preferable to a surgical graft.

5. Vitamin E promotes the formation of new skin in wounds and burns, doing away with the necessity for skin grafting.

Let's be more specific, says Dr. Shute, and he proceeds to list 25 widely differing conditions in which vitamin E has been shown to be effective. He describes the advantages to using the vitamin and lists the number of medical papers available which have been published on each subject.

(This is a handy reference to have for answering those critics of vitamin E who say, "There is no evidence that vitamin E helps prevent or treat any condition of ill health.")

In the field of peripheral vascular disease:

1. Vitamin E is used for gangrene which may help to avoid amputation, may decrease pain or save the other leg. (Eight supporting papers in medical literature.)

2. Phlebitis. This condition is very common especially in cases of legs left long in casts, or after prolonged periods in bed. Vitamin E eases pain and swelling, prevents clots. The problem seldom recurs and accompanying ulcers are almost unknown when vitamin E is given. He lists 57 papers on this subject in medical literature.

3. Indolent ulcers. These are common, neglected, painful. Vitamin E often cures them after years of failure with all other known therapy. There are 61 papers on this subject in medical literature.

4. Burns. "Pain, infection, shock, scars, long months of painful and expensive skin grafting with hideous cosmetic results" are the usual complications. "No advances in treatment for years." Vitamin E relieves pain, promotes the growth of new skin, leaves flexible scars which seldom need grafting. "Such wound healing has never been seen before in the history of medicine. The effect of alpha tocopherol on burns we regard as one of our most fortunate observations," says Dr. Shute.

5. Strokes. These victims are often left hopelessly crippled and helpless for many years. Giving the right amounts of vitamin E can sometimes help rejuvenate old cases and can help to prevent the occurrence of strokes.

6. Varicose veins and eczema. Both these conditions are troublesome, common and usually neglected. Dr. Shute says candidly that they seldom disappear entirely when vitamin E is taken but they do not become worse, there is less itching and pain, less ulceration, less swelling and phlebitis.

7. Buerger's Disease. Sinister and usually hopeless condition in which circulation in legs becomes so bad that recovery is impossible and amputation is needed. "Vitamin E saves many such legs." There are 13 papers in medical literature attesting to this fact.

8. Intermittent Claudication. Cramps in the legs

making it impossible for the patient to walk—a symptom of hardening of the arteries. Vitamin E is widely used for this condition (32 medical papers) and it is just as useful for night-time cramps in legs, also for "little strokes," nephritis, some eye diseases, itchy keloids, thrombocytopanic purpura or hemorrhages, and other conditions related to the healthy condition of the blood.

9. Collagenosis. "There is no other treatment but alpha tocopherol to be considered." This condition involves the steadily progressive scarring of the legs that follows chronic phlebitis. The leg often ulcerates. Vitamin E halts the progress of the disease. It cannot cure it.

10. Scars and trauma. Even scars that are years old may soften and relax under vitamin E therapy. It is used for Depuytren's contracture, Peyronie's disease, stricture of the esophagus or anus or urethra. Vitamin E on fresh wounds prevents contraction, so that they heal smoothly. (30 supportive papers.)

In gyniatrics:

11. Abortion or miscarriage. Vitamin E helps to prevent threatened abortion, premature rupture of membranes, prematurity and abruptio placentae.

12. Female sterility - no effects apparently.

13. Male sterility. Nineteen supportive medical papers indicate that vitamin E improves the quality of the sperm cells, so fathers sire few or no congenitally damaged babies and their wives have fewer habitual abortions.

14. Non-eclamptic late toxemias. Vitamin E is no help in true eclampsia (convulsions or seizures associated with pregnancy) but in the non-convulsive or late type of this condition it is very helpful if used in time. Nineteen doctors have apparently found it so helpful that they have written medical papers on the subject.

15. Dysmenorrhea (lack of menstruation). Occasionally helpful.

16. Kraurosis and other senile vulvular states. "These troublesome senile conditions associated with itching are very common and are often poorly handled by estrogens

(female sex hormones) the usual medication. But alpha tocopherol is very valuable for shrinking tender vaginas due to aging, senile leucorrhea, vulvar pruritis (itching) leukoplakia of the cervix (this is a pre-cancerous condition) and vulva, and dyspareunia in the elderly (painful or difficult intercourse). Alpha tocopherol is also helpful in diabetic and anal pruritis (itching).

17. Chronic cystic mastitis. Very common and frightening. "It is usually controlled brilliantly by alpha tocopherol, avoiding useless mastectomies and endless biopsies and alarm," says Dr. Shute. There are several supportive papers in the medical literature.

18. Birth trauma. "This condition is less apt to be encountered if alpha tocopherol is given to the mother before and during labor," says Dr. Shute. "There is less intercranial bleeding in the infant and forceps marks heal before the mother leaves the hospital, leaving no trace."

CHAPTER 44

Vitamin E in
Circulatory Diseases

HERE ARE SOME questions and answers about vitamin E taken from a little booklet, *Common Questions on Vitamin E and Their Answers* by the staff of the Shute Foundation for Medical Research.

Question: Is vitamin E used to treat varicose veins?

Answer: We originally refused to treat such patients, thinking it was absurd to believe that vitamin E had anything to offer them. But so many patients with such leg conditions, whom we treated for other cardiovascular (heart) diseases, told us how much their varices improved that we finally decided it was worthy of trial, and now we have become thoroughly convinced of its value.

How could it possibly be helpful?

To answer this, one must briefly describe the probable cause of most varicose veins. This description is oversimplified, perhaps, but then there is considerable disagreement among authorities as to the detailed mechanisms involved. Fundamentally there are two sets of leg veins, the superficial set one sees at a glance, and the deep set running through the depths of the great muscles of the leg.

The latter set is designed to carry about 85 to 90 percent of the return flow (of blood) from the feet, the former only

10 to 15 percent. If the deep set becomes obstructed by old phlebitis, for instance, a new load falls on the superficial set which was never designed to handle such an excess.

In the effort to do so the superficial veins distend, dilate, twist and become "varicose" as we say. Then their valves become useless or nearly so, because the valve cusps are pulled apart as the veins enlarge, "communicating veins" from the deep set pour blood into them steadily, and the full weight of a tall column of venous blood bears on the thinned-out walls of the feet and lower legs. At this point we say that the patient has varicose veins in full bloom.

(The Shute book goes on to describe the various operations given by surgeons for varicose veins—injections, tying off and "stripping"—and mentions that such efforts are usually not adequate, as the varicose veins often recur within several years.)

We never advise surgery for varicose veins therefore—except for women who are ashamed of their unsightly big varices—but advise the use of alpha tocopherol (vitamin E) instead. It acts on such legs by an altogether different principle.

It mobilizes collateral or detour circulation about the obstructed veins in the deep parts of the leg. These therefore, take some of the burden off the existing, superficial, varicosed set of veins. The appearance of the latter may or may not be improved—but there is less swelling, less pain and ache in the lower legs and the natural tendency of the veins to worsen should be halted. Sometimes, too, there is an obvious improvement in the appearance of these legs, but we never promise it. That is an "extra" when it occurs.

Certainly everyone with varicose veins should try vitamin E before he considers operation—and should also remember how poor the results of operation usually are. We see people who have had three and four series of such operations, and end exactly where they began.

Question: Should a man with Buerger's Disease take vitamin E?

Answer: He certainly should, for nothing else has much to offer him.

Buerger's Disease affects men nearly exclusively, and consists of a gradual impairment of circulation in the terminal twigs of the arteries of the extremities particularly the legs. This is ascribed to a clotting process there. It often shows itself first in young men (below fifty years of age) who develop recurrent leg thrombosis, or cramps in the legs upon exertion (claudication.)

Tobacco makes it worse, and most of these men are smokers. Women almost never develop this condition. Some recent writers have regarded it as a form of arteriosclerosis (hardening of the arteries). Certainly if it is, it is an unusual type, with certain peculiarities all its own.

The gradual and very painful process of obliteration of circulation in the tips of the toes and fingers may go on to a gangrene which eventually involves all the extremities and leads to multiple amputations. The disease usually attacks the brain and heart eventually, and many of these patients early mention loss of memory and suffer particularly intractable coronary accidents.

Vitamin E in proper dosage gives good and prompt relief of the leg symptoms, including the cramps which develop on walking, the thrombosis or gangrene, but does little for the loss of memory and such. Certainly every Buerger's patient should use vitamin E because alternative treatments are very discouraging, and here is a simple, cheap and effective alternative. It is also absolutely essential to stop tobacco. No one who continues to smoke is apt to get relief. This means stop—not slow down.

(The booklet from which we are quoting is available from the Shute Institute, London, Ontario, Canada. A fuller book on the subject of circulatory disorders and vitamin E is; *The Heart and Vitamin E*, published by the same Institute and available from them).

A common complaint these days is "restless leg syndrome" and cramping in the legs. An article in *Southern Medical Journal*, Volume 61, 1974, describes how the authors treated nine cases of long standing with vitamin E. In seven of these they attained complete control of the complaint. In one they got 75 percent, and 50 percent control in the ninth.

Of 125 patients whom they have treated over the years, they tell us, women outnumbered men two to one. Those over 50 years of age outnumbered those under 50 by four to one. More than half the patients had suffered from leg cramps longer than five years. Many had had cramps for 20 to 30 years or more. About one-fourth of them suffered from cramps every night or several times a night. In two of every three cases the cramps were severe.

About half the patients responded to 300 units or less of vitamin E daily. When they stopped taking the vitamin, the cramps returned, then disappeared again when the vitamin was resumed. Out of 125 cases only two patients received little benefit. In 103 cases the cramps were completely or almost completely controlled, and in 13 the response was regarded as good. The response to vitamin E was usually prompt—within a week.

Dr. Shute tells us that a number of things can interfere with success in using vitamin E to treat cramps. If the product does not contain the amount of vitamin E that it should or if not enough of the vitamin is given. The use of medicinal iron inactivates vitamin E. (If you are taking an iron medication, take it as far away in time as possible from the time you take your vitamin E.)

In a Hungarian medical journal Dr. F. Gerloczy tells of the beneficial effects of vitamin E on a number of people suffering from various circulatory disorders. He gave the vitamin in enormous doses—up to 24,000 milligrams or units daily. In some diseases "spectacular" results were obtained: in 10 cases of thrombosis of the arteries, 16 cases of thrombophlebitis, and 12 out of 15 cases of thromboangitis obliterans (Buerger's Disease). In other cases of circulatory troubles, the doctor reported great relief in some patients, little improvement in others. One patient who had had a leg ulcer for 20 years was healed completely after only six weeks on vitamin therapy internally, plus vitamin E ointment on the skin.

Three Italian physicians used vitamin E to treat complications of hardening of the arteries in old folks. They were suffering from the mental symptoms that sometimes accompany this disease: confusion, loss of memory, dizziness, and generally decreased mental acuteness. Forty eight patients were given six capsules of vitamin E daily. The capsule contained 150 milligrams (units) of vitamin E. Improvement occurred measured by memory, general intellectual status and other evidence of deficient circulation to the brain. Associative memory showed the greatest improvement. Dizziness responded in some cases. All the patients became livelier and more talkative. The doctors plan longer trials and larger doses.

An editorial by Dr. Walter Alvarez in *Geriatrics*, volume 29, 1974 discusses "little strokes," those transient periods which most of us notice from time to time—a moment of confusion or loss of memory, or dizziness. Dr. Evan Shute commenting on these, states that they are "very common and usually are helped greatly by vitamin E."

Intermittent claudication is a circulatory disorder of the legs and feet which makes it almost impossible to walk any distance because of the extreme pain which occurs. A Swedish physician wrote in a Swedish medical journal in 1973 on his study of 47 patients. All suffered from a closing off of the leg circulation due to hardening of the arteries. The doctor gave them 300 milligrams (units) of vitamin E daily and instructed them to exercise as much as possible and to walk daily. There was significant improvement within 4 to 6 months.

In a similar group of patients who did not take vitamin E, two patients had to have their legs amputated, since the disease had progressed so far. After two years of treatment with vitamin E the flow of blood through the legs was greatly improved. The doctor believes that the pain of intermittent claudication is not caused just by the lack of circulation, but by the muscle degeneration which follows.

In September, 1969, two California researchers reported that they had discovered accidentally that vitamin E relieves leg cramps and a complaint called "restless legs." The doctors, who are dermatologists, were told by their patients who had been taking vitamin E for skin conditions, that their leg cramps disappeared while they were taking the vitamin. The skin diseases, too, were slightly relieved, and these were hitherto incurable conditions.

In the January 10, 1972 issue of *The Journal of the American Medical Association*, they told more about their experiences with vitamin E.

Said Dr. Robert F. Cathcart III, of San Mateo, "The increasing interest in vitamin E in California has led to tremendous public self-experimentation. Health food stores sell massive amounts of concentrated vitamin E."

He refers to an article which appeared in a California medical journal where vitamin E in large doses was used successfully for leg cramps and for a condition called "restless legs." He tells us that such symptoms are common among his patients. He began to prescribe vitamin E in doses of 300 units a day, first to patients with leg cramps, then to those complaining of pain in the neck and lower back.

"I would agree," he says, "... that the medication is almost universally effective on ... nocturnal leg cramps. In my opinion it is far more effective and safer to use than quinine or quinine-aminophylline combinations. Certainly the dosage we have been prescribing and the dosages taken by the health food advocates are in excess of anything conceived of being a minimum daily requirement for the vitamin. The amount used is also far in excess of what could possibly be obtained through any reasonable normal diet."

He goes on to say that some patients who stop taking vitamin E are bothered by leg cramps in excess of those they first complained of. But only for a few days. After that, they disappear. It seems that leg cramps come and go among the folks that have them, so some people prefer to continue with the vitamin E doses while others use them just "over a crisis."

He says that other physicians have warned against using vitamin E with patients who have high blood pressure or diabetes. We would point out that Dr. Evan Shute says that patients with some kinds of high blood pressure may find that their pressure rises when they begin to take massive doses of vitamin E. So he suggests that they begin with quite small doses and increase them gradually. The same is true of some diabetics. Other diabetics find they can avoid many of the circulatory troubles that usually accompany this disease, if they take plenty of vitamin E daily.

Dr. Cathcart tells us that some of his patients find their leg cramps begin again if they decrease the dosage to 100 units daily. Others have found, after several months, that they must increase a dosage of 200 units daily to prevent symptoms. The physician says no one has needed more than 300 units. "I would second Ayres and Mihan's observations that massive doses of tocopherol (vitamin E) are extremely effective in the control of idiopathic leg night cramps."

The other physician, Dr. Samuel Ayers, Jr. of Los Angeles, describes his experience with 26 patients who suffered from leg cramps at night, "restless legs" and rectal cramps. All of them obtained relief, he says, with doses of vitamin E ranging from 300 to 400 units daily, and sometimes as high as 800 units.

He says he has written an article for publication documenting 76 cases "with equally good results." Some of these were "restless legs" cases, others had rectal cramps, and one young athlete training for the Olympics had severe cramps following strenuous exercise, including long distance running, swimming and weight-lifting. "All of these patients received prompt and gratifying relief from the oral administration of vitamin E."

If you have spoken to your doctor about taking vitamin E and he has told you, as many doctors do, "It probably won't hurt you but you're wasting your money," perhaps you should refer him to this article in the respected *Journal of the American Medical Association* and suggest that he discover for himself just how effective this remarkable vitamin can be, especially in proper dosage.

On the basis of this story alone, it's possible he might be persuaded to try vitamin E in dosages this large, and even larger, for much more serious complaints like heart trouble and many kinds of circulatory problems, as well as problems with infertility, menopause, miscarriages, varicose veins, thrombophlebitis and so on.

An editorial in the *British Medical Journal* in 1974 (vol. 2, 625) discussed the power of vitamin E in maintaining the membrane of red blood cells. Low levels of vitamin E put circulating red cells "at risk," says the editorial. Children not getting enough protein or vitamin E may suffer from a kind of anemia caused by these two deficiencies. Protein alone does not cure the condition. Vitamin E must be given. Premature infants may suffer from this anemia which results from lack of vitamin E. Treatment with iron seems to worsen the condition.

This brings us to a consideration of medicinal iron in relation to vitamin E. The kind of iron given by doctors to correct iron deficiency anemia tends to destroy vitamin E. So if you are taking an iron "tonic," take your vitamin E at another time, as far removed as possible from the iron pill. That is, take one at bedtime, the other in the morning. Iron which is present in natural food supplements does not behave this way.

The *Journal* reports that lack of vitamin E may be a major feature of the disease called thalassemia. This is a kind of anemia most common among Greek people which is believed to be hereditary. One would think that an hereditary disease could not be treated with a vitamin. But giving vitamin E to six patients restored the red blood cells in every case.

Seven Canadian scientists reported in the *Canadian Journal of Physiology and Pharmacology* (3:384 1974) that in pregnancies ending in stillbirths, the vitamin E content of blood was lower than in normal pregnancies. Studies in animals indicate that a mother who is deficient in vitamin E is more likely to have congenital malformations in her offspring. The authors suggest that "the possibility of a vitamin basis for congenital deformities may be worth testing."

A letter on estrogen (hormone) therapy for women in menopause which appeared in *Journal of the American Medical Assn.* was commented on by Dr. Evan Shute as follows: "We have never believed in 'estrogens forever.' This is especially true since we have seen what estrogens can do to leg veins and to senile vulvovaginitis. Some of the latter are not helped by the local application of estrogens but made worse by them. These need vitamin E, of course."

Canadian doctors studied the vitamin E status of people with various thyroid disorders and reported their findings in the *Journal of Canadian Medical Women's Association.* They found, they said, that vitamin E levels were low in the blood of people whose thyroid glands were overactive. An overactive thyroid gland can result in gross underweight, nervousness, bulging eyes and fast heart beat.

In a recent issue of the *New England Journal of Medicine*, a British Columbia physician reported on the use of vitamin E for relief of angina pectoris. This is the severe chest pain which accompanies certain heart conditions. Says Dr. W. M. Toone, he treated 22 men from 61 to 73 years old. He gave 11 of them a capsule containing nothing at all and to the other 11 he gave capsules of vitamin E (400 units four times daily).

In addition to the vitamin treatment he had already instituted a therapeutic program for these patients in which they gave up smoking, took long walks every day, lost weight, ate meals with low cholesterol and triglyceride content (these are fatty substances) and avoided stress of all kinds. Now keep in mind that all the patients were on this therapy program—not just the ones getting vitamin E.

The doctor studied the 22 men for two years. During this time three patients in each group reduced considerably the amount of nitroglycerin they had to take to relieve the angina pain. In addition, four patients who were getting the vitamin E reduced their nitroglycerin to one or two tablets a month—that is, almost none. No one in the group getting the "dummy" capsule was able to do this. So it appears, says the doctor, that the vitamin E capsules brought such improvement that the patients taking them could eliminate almost entirely the nitroglycerin pain pill which they had been taking regularly.

At the fifth Annual Conference on Trace Substances in Environmental Health, five researchers reported on their treatment of 25 patients with severe coronary atherosclerotic disease. That is, these people were suffering from hardening of the heart artery which often precedes a heart attack. Several of them had already had such an attack.

They were treated for six years with a special regimen of zinc, copper and manganese, along with moderate doses of vitamin E and vitamin C, plus small doses of two hormones.

One patient died. No other patient had had a recurrence of heart complications. Blood and urine levels of trace minerals were normal. There were no side effects from the trace minerals, except in the diabetics. Here the zinc supplement altered their insulin requirements.

Manganese had a sedative and muscle-relaxing effect. Copper and zinc improved assorted skin, arthritic and eye disorders.

This study seemed to show that lowering blood cholesterol levels, treating high blood pressure, reducing obesity and encouraging physical activity may be advisable in treatment of heart and circulatory patients, but no proof has yet been developed that such measures improve the chances of survival for people who have already had heart attacks.

In a letter to *Canadian Family Physician*, volume 19, page 15, 1973, a Canadian physician, Dr. M. Lattey, reports on his personal experience taking vitamin E for paroxysmal auricular fibrillation. This is extremely rapid, irregular and dangerous heart contractions. The doctor began with 400 units of vitamin E which proved to be not enough. He doubled it, took 800 milligrams of vitamin E daily and his heart returned to normal.

He reported that he now is able to exercise without any difficulty and says he has not enjoyed such good health for seven years. He adds that the medical profession should take another look at the use of vitamin E for heart disease.

In a Polish medical journal, *Fortschiritte du Med.*, volume 90, Supplement 913, 1972, a Polish physician reports on 29 patients with many of the heart and artery symptoms which are becoming commonplace among people who live in Western industrialized societies. These patients ranged in age from 38 to 72 years.

Fifteen were suffering from coronary and circulatory problems, plus angina pectoris, myocardial infarct, claudication, fatty liver and high blood levels of fats.

Ten patients had high levels of cholesterol, fatty livers, diabetes and circulatory troubles. Four patients had fatty livers, high levels of cholesterol, obesity and badly functioning thyroid glands.

All were given 6 capsules of vitamin E, with 150 milligrams in each capsule. As their condition improved, this dosage was reduced by half. In all cases, the level of blood fats went down within a few weeks. In some cases, cholesterol levels were lowered by 100 percent or more. In other cases blood fats were lowered by 36 percent, angina pains decreased and claudication became much improved. This condition occurs in patients when they try to walk, with leg arteries blocked with fatty deposits. Diastolic blood pressure fell an average of 15 mm of mercury. There were no harmful side effects.

Purpura means hemorrhages in the skin, mucus membranes and other parts of the body. An article from the *Journal of Vitaminology* (published in Japan) volume 18, page 125, 1972, tells of seven cases of purpura treated with vitamin E. Four hundred to six hundred milligrams of the vitamin were given daily and there was "marked clinical improvement." Six out of the seven cases improved with vitamin E therapy alone.

It is interesting to note that, at the same time, the vitamin improved other conditions as well, such as local swelling (or edema) and skin eruptions. The authors believe this demonstrates that vitamin E prevents damage to capillary walls (the walls of the smallest blood vessels) when this damage is due to drugs, infections and so on.

An Italian physician reported in *Gynecol. Practique*, volume 22, page 501, 1971, that he treated with vitamin E 68 women complaining of menopausal troubles.

He believes, he says, that vitamin E has many beneficial effects, even on the genital organs. It protects the nervous system and muscles, and deters hardening of the arteries. It "tunes the metabolism" of carbohydrates. In Italy vitamin E is widely used in treating aging, he says, and especially hardening of the arteries. Eighty-one percent of the women he treated with vitamin E were helped through a difficult menopause.

These days we hear many warnings about blood cholesterol levels. Cholesterol is a fatty substance which accumulates in arteries and closes them off, creating hardening of the arteries and eventually circulatory troubles. Cholesterol is manufactured by the human liver, so that, when there is little cholesterol in diets the liver makes more. When we eat more cholesterol, the liver makes less.

Now we find, in an article in *Physiology, Chemistry and Physics*, volume 5, 1973, that the fat soluble vitamins A, D, E and K stop the liver from manufacturing too much cholesterol. In animals with muscular dystrophy there was a very high concentration of cholesterol in the blood and muscle of the rabbits. They were also deficient in Vitamin E.

In rabbits fed plenty of vitamin E the cholesterol levels in both blood and muscle were much lower than in those animals fed a diet in which vitamin E was deficient. One scientist has reported that, in human muscular dystrophy, muscles have a higher than normal accumulation of cholesterol. It seems quite possible that lack of vitamin E, along with other factors, may play an important part in human muscular dystrophy. Studies of cholesterol manufactured in the liver of animals on diets deficient in vitamin E suggests strongly that vitamin E participates in controlling cholesterol.

Say the three authors of this article it appears that vitamin E not only influences the production of cholesterol, but also the way it is used by the cells. This leads to the suggestion that lack of enough vitamin E may be one of the causes of high blood levels of cholesterol.

Nutrition Reports International, volume 10, #6, December, 1974, described experiments with mice which indicated that the older the animals are the more vitamin E is needed to protect their tissues from rancid fats caused by oxygen.

CHAPTER 45

A Survey Reveals
Vast Health Improvement
from Vitamin E

IN 1974 *Prevention* magazine asked their readers to answer a questionnaire on vitamin E and its effects on their health. They received 20,000 replies, a magnificent testimony to the loyalty of health seekers who take vitamin E regularly and are willing to take the time and trouble to tell other folks about their experience.

The survey was conducted and studied by Richard A. Passwater, a biochemist, author of a fine book on vitamin therapy—*Supernutrition: The Megavitamin Revolution.* Dr. Passwater states in *Prevention* that a critical level which appears to influence the possibility of developing heart disease is 300 International Units of vitamin E daily. Occasionally, he says, "people taking 200 I.U. of vitamin E daily developed heart disease (generally in the late 80's) or showed little improvement. When they increased their dosage, they experienced improvement. Only one case of heart trouble was reported to have developed at a higher dosage level." This was in the group of people responding to the survey who were 80 years old or older.

"The suggestion emerges," says Dr. Passwater, "that among persons over 80, taking 1200 I.U. or more of vitamin E daily after a heart attack improves chances of complete recovery and that taking 300 I.U. or more of vitamin E daily for 10 years or more reduces the chances of ever developing heart disease. There is also a hint (in the replies that came in) that eating a balanced diet even in absence of vitamin E supplements has a considerable protective effect against heart disease. This survey supports those observations but does not prove them."

In the following issues of *Prevention* Dr. Passwater reviewed comments from people of the various age groups who replied to the survey. Testimony was almost unbelievable—of heart trouble overcome, circulatory symptoms overcome, much more vigor and freedom from pain, as well as many comments on conditions other than circulatory ones, comments which were volunteered by the respondents although they had not been asked to say anything on these ailments.

The 50 to 59-year-old age group consisted of replies from 6,205 men and women. Of these 818 had heart disease. Correlating the replies, Dr. Passwater found that:

1. taking 400 I.U. or more of vitamin E is strongly associated with reducing the incidence of heart disease to one-tenth or less of the risk for this age group in a general population not taking the vitamin.

2. taking 1200 I.U. or more of vitamin E for four years or more is strongly associated with reducing the risk of heart disease to less than one-third of the risk for this age group in the general population.

3. more than 80 per cent of the people who responded to the survey who already have heart conditions (including tachycardia, angina and fibrillation) reported that their condition improved when they used vitamin E.

Here are some striking comments from people in this age group. A woman had two heart attacks 15 years ago, has taken 400 units of vitamin E ever since. No more attacks. Another woman had fibrillation (rapid disorganized heartbeat) and high blood pressure. She has been taking 800 I.U. for 10 years, has had no more attacks and now has a natural heart rhythm. A husband with a heart attack is now taking 1200 units of E, his wife, also victim of a heart attack, takes 800 units daily. The vitamin has lowered their blood pressure and their cholesterol count and "helped both hearts to heal." A woman whose heartbeat was 200 per minute put herself on 800 units of vitamin E when the doctors could do nothing for her. She has been well since.

Of the group of people 60 to 69 years of age who responded to the survey, Dr. Passwater says, "perhaps the single most important age group to study for heart disease is the 60 to 69 year old group. This age group has a high incidence of heart disease and still includes in its numbers those individuals who are destined not to survive beyond the average life span." They had 6,459 replies to the questionnaire of whom 1,543 said they have heart disease. Their replies showed, in general, what the younger group had shown—that 400 units of vitamin E daily for 10 years or more reduces the incidence of heart disease to one-tenth or less of the risk for people not taking the vitamin. Taking 1200 units or more for four years or more seems to reduce the risk of heart disease to less than one-third of the risk for this age group. More than 80 per cent of those with heart trouble reported that the vitamin improved their condition.

Says Dr. Passwater, "You can't take vitamin E as a preventive measure and do everything else wrong. If you smoke, drink, are inactive, overstrain, don't rest or eat properly, taking a pound of vitamin E daily won't completely protect you from heart disease, especially if you are genetically prone to it. However, you could be better off than if you didn't take any vitamin E at all."

Some comments from the respondents in their sixties are illuminating. A woman reported on curing her angina and a heart murmur with 400 units of vitamin E. When she stopped taking the vitamin for six months both these conditions returned. She began again and her problems vanished. A woman with coronary thrombosis and phlebitis reported that both improved greatly when she took vitamin E. A man with three coronary attacks and hardening of the arteries reported that he gave up his nitroglycerin tablets one year after starting vitamin E—800 units daily. Another man testified that a number of friends *who are also M.D.'s have had coronaries and are all taking from 800 to 1200 units of vitamin E daily*. A man with severe pains from angina increased his intake of vitamin E from 100 to 400 units daily with a slight improvement. When he increased it to 800 units, "the improvement was fantastic," he says.

From the group of *Prevention* readers who are in their 70's 4,060 replies were received. The same trend appears in this group: people who have taken 300 or more units of vitamin E daily for ten years or more are not likely to develop heart disease. And neither are people taking 1200 units or more daily for more than three years.

Many of the people in their seventies wrote of pain treated with vitamin E. A 75-year-old man said, "I would awaken every morning early about four or five a.m. with my eyeballs hurting, severe pains in the temples and back of the neck. I was also nauseated. I felt like I was losing my mind. In just two weeks of 800 units of vitamin E the condition improved and has been relieved ever since."

A 74-year-old man with a coronary 30 years ago has been taking 1200 units of vitamin E daily and has had no recurrence. A 75-year-old woman had angina pectoris and weakness of heart valves. She has been taking vitamin E for 22 years; is at present taking 2400 units daily. Her blood pressure has dropped to a healthy 120/80; her cholesterol level is down to 150.

A 71-year-old woman has been taking vitamin E since 1958 after a Mayo Clinic diagnosis of such severe heart damage that she required surgery. She has been taking high doses of vitamin E since 1958, is now taking 600 units daily. Her doctors say she has no heart damage and very little angina pain. A 71-year-old woman had been taking two heart medications plus three kinds of diuretics and had been told by her doctors that she could not ever live without digitalis. She started to take 1000 units of vitamin E daily. By gradually increasing all her vitamin and mineral intake, she is now able to do without any drugs. She now takes 800 units of vitamin E.

Dr. Passwater says, in part, ".... these comments are not accepted as scientific proof that vitamin E prevents or cures heart disease. Rigid controlled studies involving 'double-blind' tests are required for evidence of validity by most scientists. Yet the information is useful. I do not know of any large-scale well-controlled, double-blind test that proves aspirin cures headaches. But physicians and lay people 'know' it does through experience.

"Similarly many physicians know that vitamin E relieves angina pain and prescribe it; others have tried it and not seen the improvement described here, and still other physicians refuse even to try vitamin E. The main obstacle seems to be that many physicians have not considered the dose-time relationship required. They have tried too-little dosage for a too-little time. Now they should test the 300-plus units for 10-plus years, or 1200-plus units for three-plus years."

What about people in their eighties who answered the questionnaire? Here are some comments from them. In this group the same general conditions prevailed—the level of 300 units of vitamin E daily appeared to influence the risk of heart disease. Dr. Passwater believes the figures he collected show that in those over 80, taking 1200 units of vitamin E daily after a heart attack improves chances of complete recovery and taking 300 units daily for ten years or more reduces the chances of having a heart attack.

One 84-year-old woman has been taking vitamin E for 30 years. She has been experimenting with dosage and with other elements in diet and way of life. She is now taking 500-600 units of vitamin E and is in excellent health. An 86-year old man had two heart attacks years ago, began taking 1800 units of vitamin E daily and has now been free of heart attacks for 25 years. An 81-year-old woman with phlebitis and a leg ulcer has been taking vitamin E for 25 years, mostly in doses of 1000 units daily. All her circulatory problems have cleared up. An 81-year old woman had a coronary thrombosis (heart attack caused by a blood clot) 20 years ago. Fifteen years ago she began to take vitamin E and is now in very good health. An 86-year-old man has no more angina pains since he began to take 600 units of vitamin E daily for six years.

Many other fascinating bits of testimony turned up in the *Prevention* survey. Although no questions were asked about conditions other than circulatory ones, a great deal of evidence came in on improvement in other conditions as well. And, most astonishing of all, 70 physicians answered the questionnaire, 66 of whom had been taking vitamin E from one to 29 years. An 89-year-old physician (and isn't that some kind of a record?) treats himself and his patients with vitamin E. He had very serious heart trouble 26 years ago. He has taken 800 units of vitamin E daily for 26 years. A man described as a "well known" New York physician reported to *Prevention* that his last electrocardiogram and blood pressure are normal after two years of taking 1000 units of vitamin E daily after a coronary thrombosis. Another doctor claims he cured his prostatitis with 800 units of vitamin E daily. That's the first such testimony we have ever seen on that condition.

It is cheering indeed to read such valuable and unsolicited remarks from people who had suffered for years from one or another disease. And not one word of any unpleasant side effects from really immense doses of vitamin E. One can only wonder why official medicine does not realize the significance of all this and take another look at the harm they may be doing with pills and surgery when the answer for most people may lie in a small capsule of a perfectly natural substance taken regularly every day for life.

CHAPTER 46

Vitamin E Is Powerful
Against Ulcers
and Open Sores

ONE OF THE most stunning and dramatic stories to come our way recently is the story of the miracles wrought by Vitamin E in treating stubborn ulcers and gangrene which had resisted all medical efforts to cure.

The treatment took place in a small-town hospital in Pennsylvania. It is reported by the nurse in charge. It appears in *The Summary*, for December, 1974. This is a publication of the Shute Foundation for Medical Research in London, Ontario, Canada. The editor is Dr. Evan Shute, long recognized as the world's top expert in the field of vitamin E and its great usefulness to humanity.

The first case is that of a 59-year-old woman with ulceration of the right foot. A diabetic, she was taking no medication when she came to the hospital. The doctors immediately gave her insulin and 800 units of natural vitamin E daily. Then they packed the ulcerated area with cotton saturated in vitamin E. Two months later all wounds were healed.

The second case is that of a 72-year-old woman with partial bowel obstruction and a huge bed sore (decubitus ulcer the doctors call it) which covered most of the upper part of her buttocks. A color photograph reveals a hideous festering sore with blackened areas. The ulcer was treated with daily applications of vitamin E and the patient was given 800 units of vitamin E by mouth every day. Treatment was begun on February 15, 1974 and was completed on August 12, 1974. Says Dorothy Fisher, who wrote this article, "In less than six months there was total healing and the area involved has remained well healed. The area now looks very healthy."

The third case is a 25-year-old man, a paraplegic, crippled in a car accident. Bedfast, he had developed bed sores on the buttocks, in the right leg and left foot. He had been treated without success in five different hospitals and rehabilitation institutions. He was given 400 units of vitamin E daily, plus 250 milligrams of vitamin C and his bed sores were treated topically with vitamin E ointment. One month later his vitamin E and vitamin C dosages were doubled. A month later the vitamin E was increased to 600 units twice daily, later to 800 units twice daily.

He was sent home completely healed and is still taking 400 units of vitamin E daily, along with applications of the ointment to any area threatened with pressure sores.

The fourth case treated by this devoted nurse was a woman of 63 who was operated on for cancer of the rectum. The surgeon performed a colostomy. The opening or stoma which he created for evacuation of the bowel became infected and ulcerated. It and the area around it were treated daily with vitamin E ointment. The patient was given 400 units of vitamin E daily. Within six days all this area of badly ulcerated skin was completely healed.

Color photographs of these cases are printed with this article. It seems almost impossible to believe that any physician, aware of the benefits of vitamin E treatment, would not use it. It also seems incredible that official medicine has never published in any of its journals any material on using vitamin E in this way.

In the same issue of *The Summary*, a Long Island (New York) doctor reports on 20 schizophrenia patients suffering from severe circulatory disorders in their legs. Three had gangrene; one had a perforating ulcer which had never completely healed in two years. She wore orthopedic shoes in an effort to escape the pain from this ulcer. Nine other patients had infected dermatitis on the insides of their legs.

All were diabetic, maintained on strict diets and an oral diabetic pill. "The patients often committed breaches of diet," says Dr. Deliz. They were given 20 to 40 capsules daily of vitamin E (400 units per capsule). The gangrenous areas are healing, he says. "These dramatic results were described by visiting internists as incredible. The patients have been maintained on a daily average of 20 capsules of 400 units each, and four months after healing of the lesions they are well and without leg pain."

An Italian doctor reported in 1973 on experiments with rats in whom he induced bed sores. They had suffered from these for five months, when he gave them 65 milligrams daily of vitamin E. (This is a very large amount for an animal as small as a rat.) Within two weeks of therapy the bed sores were arrested.

In an editorial in *Geriatrics*, volume 29, page 159, 1974, Dr. W.C. Alvarez described what doctors call "little stroke," those common little lapses in memory and speech, with perhaps a moment of dizziness, which afflict many of us as we grow older. Said Dr. Alvarez, these are usually helped greatly by taking vitamin E.

In a fascinating letter to the editor of *Archives of Dermatology*, Volume 108, page 855, 1973, two physicians report using vitamin E for patients suffering from neuralgia which afflicted them after a session of shingles (herpes). The doctors treated 13 patients with oral and topical vitamin E. That is, they gave them vitamin E by mouth and used the ointment on the affected skin. Eleven of these patients had suffered more than six months, 7 for more than one year, one for 13 years and one for 19 years. These two last patients had almost complete relief from pain with the vitamin E treatment. Two were moderately improved and two were slightly improved. The doctors gave dosages of 400 to 1,600 units of vitamin E per day.

One of these patients had angina (the agonizing chest pain that afflicts heart patients). Taking 1,200 units of vitamin E daily she controlled the neuralgia. She also cured the leg cramps she had been suffering from and found that she no longer needed nitroglycerin, the drug she had been taking to control the angina.

Would you believe a 53-year-old diabetic man with a perforating ulcer of the foot (of such seriousness that he could not move the fourth and fifth toes) whose ulcer was healed in two months with no treatment other than vitamin E?

Would you believe a 58-year-old diabetic woman with an ulcer on the sole of her foot and with advanced osteoporosis of the bones of her feet, whose ulcer and a later ulcer in the same foot were healed in a few months with no treatment other than vitamin E?

Would you believe a five-year-old boy, badly burned, with itchy keloid scars whose discomfort was ended within a day after vitamin E ointment was applied locally?

Would you believe a 46-year-old woman, with second and third degree burns on hand and forearm who recovered within a week on vitamin E by mouth and applied locally?

These are only a few of the stunning case histories told in a recent issue of *The Summary*, which is published from time to time by the Shute Foundation for Medical Research. Dr. Evan Shute, who edits *The Summary*, is the foremost champion of vitamin E. He has worked with it for many many years and uses it routinely for treating a multitude of disorders and wounds.

His success with complications of diabetes seems almost miraculous. The 53-year-old man described above had been taking insulin for 15 years. He would not adhere to his diet and was taking large doses of insulin regularly. On 375 units of vitamin E he healed completely in 71 days and could reduce his intake of insulin to about one-third of what it had been. He returned to work.

The diabetic woman, who was obviously suffering from many kinds of malnutrition, including calcium, was given 600 units of vitamin E daily.

Within two months she was allowed to walk on her ulcerated foot. She was healed clinically and by X-ray observation within several months. Her second diabetic ulcer was also healed quickly with vitamin E.

The burned child suffered from keloid scars resulting from skin grafts, so that he could not do his school work. The vitamin E ointment was applied to the scars and, although he was given no vitamin E by mouth, just the ointment cleared all his problems within a day. It seems quite possible that all keloids could be treated successfully with vitamin E, does it not?

The woman who burned her hand was a long-time devotee of vitamin E. She began to take large doses of it immediately after she was burned. Then she wrapped her arm in a bandage and set off for the Shute Clinic. They treated her with saline bubble baths and more vitamin E ointment applied several times a day. She was almost completely recovered within eight days, suffered no pain and had no contracture of the burned area, and no scars.

Dr. Shute says that one of the most mysterious aspects of vitamin E treatment of burns is the relief of pain. "Why there should be such a prompt response is hard to understand," he says. "One would suspect it was a matter of nerve endings in the dermis—but why is this property unique and what is its mechanism? Is it identical all over the body at once? How long does this analgesia persist?"

"When skin grafts fail they are merely repeated, for that is the end of the line," he says. "We rarely send a patient for grafting and never repeat it. Since vitamin E is slightly anti-infective wounds are usually clean, an important factor in the 'take' of grafts."

He tells us further that most burn patients are rushed to a hospital and immediately put into the usual orthodox treatment so it is difficult to teach medical students about the helpfulness of vitamin E, even if anyone at the hospital had any desire to learn. Scars left by the usual treatment, including grafts, can permanently cripple people and end their careers, if the small joints involved are essential parts of their work—as with a surgeon, a musician, or someone doing very fine, intricate work.

For burns of the conjunctiva of the eye, Dr. Shute recommends just cutting open a capsule of 400 to 800 units of vitamin E and pouring the vitamin into the eye. We would add that many readers have reported similar success treating many kinds of wounds, cuts, abrasions, as well as burns. Most of them took large doses of the vitamin by mouth as well as applying it directly to the injured area.

"If vitamin E is useful for burns it should help frostbite or immersion foot and be of great value to aviators and mountain climbers," says Dr. Shute. "I got in touch with Sir Edmund Hilary prior to his last climb in the Himalayas and suggested that alpha tocopherol (vitamin E) be included in their resources on that ascent. He courteously acknowledged my suggestion—but I heard nothing from his doctor. The sequel was tragic, as we all know."

Dr. Shute tells us further that irradiation scars in deep tissues have become very troublesome in some patients treated with X-ray. "Surely," he says, "a scar-lytic (scar-dissolving) substance like alpha tocopherol should be tried for these pitiful people. There seems to be no alternative as yet.

"Burns and cuts often end as keloids and these can be painful or intolerably itchy.... The prompt symptomatic relief by applying vitamin E ointment is hard to explain, but many patients attest to its value. Some of these keloids can be excised or loosened. If this is done the patient should be given alpha tocopherol orally and locally when convalescing, in the well-founded hope of producing a secondary scar that is easier to live with. We often suggest this where major joints such as those in the neck are involved, before there is considerable and irremedial distortion.

"Vitamin E should be in every kitchen for convenient use. Every parent should have it handy for the children. As in coronary attacks, the best results can be achieved only if treatment is prompt."

In treating skin ulcers, Dr. Shute says that at least 60 reports in medical literature mention the help vitamin E has brought, mostly in cases of chronic ulcers. "When everything else has failed," he says, "we suggest alpha tocopherol both orally and locally. The latter is what means most, we suspect. It must be remembered that many people are sensitive to local tocopherol. The latter may induce . . . a rash over part or all of the body. This means one should dilute the ointment or stop its use altogether, continuing with its oral exhibition only."

We have heard from all sides testimony to the helpfulness of vitamin E applied locally in many kinds of trouble. There is no reason it cannot be applied experimentally to almost anything that wrong on the skin. It is easy to apply by puncturing the capsule with a pin or cutting off the end and squeezing out the contents.

CHAPTER 47

Does Vitamin E
Delay Aging?

THE STARTLING EVIDENCE came from human cells kept alive in a laboratory culture. Under normal laboratory conditions such cells might live for 50 generations of cell division. But when a small amount of vitamin E was added, the human cells in the test tube continued to reproduce beyond more than 120 divisions. Then the scientists conducting the research discontinued the experiment.

Drs. Lester Packer and James R. Smith of the University of California stated that the cells appeared to show no signs of old age. They were still completely normal and going on about the healthy business of dividing, just as they had when the experiment began. Scientists generally accept the theory that cells have a built-in lifespan depending on the inheritance of the individual. You inherit a set of cells which will see you through to a healthy old age, other things being equal. Or, because of a long line of short-lived, unhealthy ancestors, you may have inherited a tendency to succumb to many diseases and die at an early age.

But now it seems that the magic of vitamin E may have proved this theory to be false. Perhaps just getting enough and more than enough vitamin E may enable the individual with a poor heritage to live much longer than expected.

DOES VITAMIN E DELAY AGING?

The California scientists deny that their research demonstrates anything like this, of course. According to *The New York Times* for September 2, 1974, they stated that the most immediate benefits of this world-shaking discovery will be to benefit scientists. Now they can keep human cells alive long enough in a laboratory to investigate human genetics and develop ways to tinker with the genetics of human cells. Then, too, researchers can use such long-living cells to evaluate the effects of environmental stress, like pollutants, on cell life.

So, said they, this doesn't mean at all that taking vitamin E will prolong life or will turn the clock back for a 40-year old and make him or her feel like 18. And why not? Well, said another California researcher who has done much work with vitamin E, everybody gets so much vitamin E in their food that the body has large stored reserves to draw upon, hence getting any more would be useless.

This is the kind of argument some scientists use when they are confronted with laboratory experiments which prove beyond a shadow of a doubt that some extraordinary vital substance exists in a given vitamin which performs almost magically on individual cells. Now consider for a moment that the human cell under the microscope which went right on behaving like a young, vital cell way past the time when it should have stopped dividing, apparently contained enough vitamin E to be a healthy cell. There was no indication that these cells were deficient in vitamin E. But when more vitamin E was added, the effects were entirely different from what happened to other cells being studied, which had not been given extra vitamin E. Is it not possible that whole human beings might expect this same effect, since the vitamin affects individual cells that way and since human bodies are nothing but collections of human cells?

Drs. Packer and Smith went on to make two of the most highly contradictory remarks we have ever heard from scientists. "Vitamin E won't extend life in humans," they said, "except in the possible case where humans are subjected to severe environmental pollution." (Aren't we all?) And then they went on to say, according to the *Times*, "Even if vitamin E can't turn a 40-year old into a 14-year old, it might prevent an early death, or brain disease, heart attacks or senility. Of course, we don't know these things at all, yet."

And the two scientists, who have presumably been told for years that we all get plenty of vitamin E in our food, are now taking 200 milligrams of vitamin E daily in capsules!

In the tenth volume of *Executive Health*, Dr. Linus Pauling speaks his mind on vitamin E. As one would expect, it is very much worth listening to.

He begins by outlining the course of vitamin E in present-day medicine. More than 40 years ago three Canadian physicians began to use it in their treatment of disease. These were Drs. Evan and Wilfrid Shute and their father, Dr. R. James Shute. They reported excellent results. But official medicine on this continent refused to accept these results and steadfastly averred that vitamin E has no place in human health in amounts larger than the officially recommended amount of 12 milligrams per day. Says Dr. Pauling, "It is my opinion that the authorities are wrong about vitamin E as they were about vitamin C."

In 1956, Dr. Pauling tells us, a researcher experimented with a diet which contained only three milligrams of vitamin E.

Nine volunteers ate a diet containing only this small amount of vitamin E while a comparable group of volunteers had diets containing 18 milligrams of vitamin E.

Within six months the people getting the small amount of vitamin E began to develop fragile red blood cells resulting in anemia and the concentration of the vitamin in their blood began slowly to decline. The volunteers on larger amounts of vitamin E had no such problems.

Dr. Pauling explains that the main function of vitamin E is its ability to prevent the rancidity or oxidation of fats in the tissues of the body. "Vitamin E is the principal fat-soluble antioxidant," says he, "and vitamin C (ascorbic acid) is the principal water-soluble antioxidant. They probably cooperate in providing protection for our bodies and slowing the aging process."

Dr. Roger J. Williams, distinguished nutrition researcher of the University of Texas, is quoted as saying in his book *Nutrition Against Disease:* "Vitamin E is thought to be the leading agent for the prevention of peroxidation and the free radical production which is associated both with it and with radiation. Vitamin E—along with... other antioxidants—do their jobs in a complicated manner. They protect the body against the damaging products formed when oxygen reacts directly with the highly unsaturated fatty substances which are essential parts of our metabolic machinery.

"We do not know all the details of how these antioxidants do their work in practical situations, and the information probably would not be of interest to laymen anyway. As a practical matter, providing plenty of vitamin E and ascorbic acid (vitamin C)—both harmless antioxidants—is indicated as a possible means of preventing premature aging, especially if one's diet is rich in polyunsaturated acids."

Dr. Williams goes on to describe the brown pigments (like freckles) which are often found on the skin of older people. Such deposits are not just on skin. They are also found in the brain, the heart, the adrenal gland and many other parts of the body. They seem to represent lack of vitamin E, since they are symptoms of rancidity which has not been prevented and which vitamin E and vitamin C can and do prevent.

The stubborn refusal of the medical hierarchy to accept thousands of pieces of evidence of the healthfulness of vitamin E could be settled easily, says Dr. Pauling, by setting up a series of tests in which one large group of heart and circulatory patients are given vitamin E dosages recommended by specialists like the Shutes and other physicians who use the vitamin, while another matched group of volunteers with circulatory problems get the usual medical treatment with no vitamin E. The Shutes themselves can not conduct such trials, he says, since their duty is to treat all their patients with the very best treatment they know, which is of course, vitamin E.

Dr. Pauling quotes Dr. Alton Ochsner, the distinguished surgeon, as saying that for many years he has used vitamin E (100 I.U. three times a day) for surgical patients to prevent blood clots in veins. The vitamin is a "potent inhibitor" of the blood clots which are such a fearful aftermath of surgery in many instances. Drugs which prevent blood clots are likely to bring about hemorrhages unless they are regulated with extreme care. Vitamin E presents no such problems.

A "free radical" is defined as a highly reactive compound in which the central element is linked to an abnormal number of atoms or groups of atoms, along with the presence of at least one unpaired electron. This doesn't mean much to the layman, but free radicals are apparently very destructive of health. One scientist, J.M. Washburn, speculates in *The Gerontologist*, volume 13, page 436, 1973, that free radical reactions in the arteries which carry blood may be the cause of hardening of the arteries. A layer of fat collects on the inner lining of the artery, more fat collects on top of that and the damage that ensues appears to be caused by "free radicals."

Studying animals, this researcher discovered that the liver of an animal on a diet deficient in vitamin E contains a large amount of free radicals—50 times more than would be produced by a damaging amount of radiation. Thus, vitamin E may be very important, says he. Along with other antioxidants it may increase the life span of animals. And, we would add, presumably also human beings.

In line with these findings, it is not surprising to find, in *Chemical and Engineering News* for September 30, 1974, that one scientist treated human cells enriched with vitamin E in a test tube and found that he could prolong their lives for as much as 120 generations of cell division, compared to a span of 50 generations, for untreated cells. The vitamin was apparently acting as an antioxidant in this experiment.

While we cannot, from this, decide finally that getting plenty of vitamin E will enable us all to live longer lives in good health, it does seem wise, does it not, to make certain we get lots of the vitamin at meals and in food supplements, since it seems to have a protective action in so many areas of health, and since it seems to be totally harmless in any amounts?

And finally, here's an account of an experiment reported in the May 1973 *Proceedings of the National Academy of Sciences*. Damage to chromosomes, the genetic material in cells, has been linked to cancer and the aging process. If we could prevent the damage to chromosomes perhaps we could prevent cancer and retard aging.

Vitamin E, vitamin C and two other anti-oxidants have now been shown to reduce damage to chromosomes in blood cells exposed to chemicals known to be cancer-causing. Vitamin E gave 63.8 percent protection against chromosome breakage and vitamin C gave 31.7 percent protection.

The Cleveland Clinic Foundation scientists who conducted the experiment believe, they say, that "The protection against chromosomal breakage provided by antioxidants may have important relationships to aging and carcinogenesis (cancer)."

This means that taking plenty of vitamin C and vitamin E may retard aging and help to prevent cancer. Some scientists believe that the incidence of stomach cancer has declined in this country since most people have been eating cereals which are preserved with chemical antioxidants. So all the news is not bad!

CHAPTER 48

More Evidence
of the Value
# of Vitamin E

STILL MORE EVIDENCE of the helpfulness of vitamin E in preventing aging and in protecting us from environmental pollutants was presented at the 1976 meeting of the American Chemical Society. A Tacoma, Washington scientist described experiments in which he prevented "blow outs" in human red blood cells.

An editor of *Medical Tribune* asked Dr. Jeffrey Bland if this means that people may take vitamin E and live longer, healthier lives. He answered, in their August 18, 1976 issue, by saying that he cannot promise such things definitely. But, he said, you should be able to avoid accelerated aging if you take "the right amount" of vitamin E. And studies are now in progress to determine what that "right amount" may be.

This is how he made his discovery. Exposing a red blood cell to any substance that oxidizes the cholesterol in the cell membrane weakens the membrane and there is a 'blow-out', or a "budded cell". Vitamin E apparently slows this process. The process is enhanced by exposing the cell to oxygen, to the chemical pollutants in smog, to cigarette smoke, x-rays or the sun. These oxidizers change the cholesterol into cholesterol hydroperoxide which does the damage to the cell membrane.

Dr. Bland and his associates gave 24 human volunteers 600 units of vitamin E and then took samples of their blood. A similar number of volunteers gave blood without taking the vitamin E. The cells of both groups were then exposed to light and oxygen for 16 hours. As expected, the cells from those volunteers who had no vitamin E showed a totally budded condition. That is, the cell membranes had been totally destroyed.

But the blood cells from those volunteers who took the vitamin E showed only a small number of budded cells. This seems to indicate that the cell walls were almost completely protected from this kind of destruction by only 600 milligrams of vitamin E. To someone exposed to cigarette smoke, air pollution or any of the other thousands of pollutants which oxidize cell membranes, it appears that just taking vitamin E alone might give an enormous amount of protection.

In a second experiment Dr. Bland mixed some normal red blood samples with some vitamin E and exposed the mixture to light and oxygen. Once again, he tells us, "The cells resisted membrane destruction at the same rate . . . as the cells taken from those donors on the augmented vitamin E diet."

Said Dr. Bland, "The vitamin is a biological antioxidant that sits in the fatty bilayer of the cell membrane" as protection against the effects of "cellular aging." He then recommended that people exposed to smog and/or cigarette smoke take vitamin E as protection against these poisons. Since it is almost impossible to escape these two prevalent toxins in modern life, it seems that he has just recommended, as we do, that everyone should take vitamin E in quite large amounts. We are surely not living in a pristine environment. Every breath of air we take contains pollutants. Most of us, whether we smoke or not, are exposed almost constantly to cigarette smoke, since someone is smoking almost everywhere we go.

Dr. Bland seems to feel there is an upper limit to the amount of vitamin E that is needed to protect us. Not that any vitamin E over this amount would be harmful, just that it wouldn't give us the protection the "right amount" gives. Considering the vast amount of evidence that has appeared in medical and scientific journals, much of which we have collected here, it seems to us that "the right amount" which can possibly be determined in a laboratory has little relevance to the vast majority of us human beings who deal with varying degrees and amounts of pollution and who smoke or do not smoke, and who are otherwise exposed or not exposed to the welter of chemicals that surround us.

In addition to this, there is the question of biological individuality. Each of us is born with a different need for vitamins and minerals and other nutrients. Some of us may need twenty or more times more of these than others. If someone whose needs have always been greater because of inherited tendencies happens to be the person whose exposure to pollutants is very great, surely such a person would need more of the vitamin than someone whose needs from birth are smaller and who somehow manages to escape many pollutants possibly by moving to a remote area, avoiding tobacco smoke and so on.

Should you take 600 milligrams of vitamin E daily in the hope that it may help you to avoid damage from pollution and also early aging? We see no reason why you shouldn't. Should you hope, if you do, that you will live forever and will forever appear to be no older than 25? It doesn't seem likely that such a future can be achieved from taking any vitamin or from following any regimen of diet and supplements. We all age eventually.

But surely it is worthwhile to achieve whatever we can in the way of good health and postponement of disabled old age as long as we can. As it seems quite likely, from Dr. Bland's experiments, and those of many other scientists that as much as 600 milligrams of the vitamin might provide that postponement. Along with a highly nutritious diet, plenty of rest and exercise.

CHAPTER 49

"Eating Crow"
Over Vitamin E

FROM TIME TO TIME some dedicated follower of the "establishment" position on vitamins has a sudden revelation and changes his mind. Such an about-face occurred in a distinguished nutrition expert at a recent symposium on vitamin E.

"I have to eat crow," said M.K. Horwitt, professor of biochemistry at St. Louis University School of Medicine. He was wrong about vitamin E all these years, he went on, for he has been saying what lots of establishment researchers have been saying—that we all get plenty of vitamin E in our meals and there's no reason to add more in the form of a supplement.

But Dr. Horwitt's more recent investigations have turned up such startling facts that he is now recommending up to 800 units of vitamin E as insurance against the blood clots which complicate the lives of heart and circulatory patients. Because of its effect on clotting, some doctors have been recommending large doses of aspirin to their patients, since aspirin is known to affect blood clotting. But vitamin E appears to be a better solution, said Dr. Horwitt.

Vitamin E breaks down in the body into a substance called d-alphatocopherol-quinone which cancels out the work of vitamin K. Vitamin K is busy persuading the blood to coagulate, since this is its role in the body. But, in the case of heart attack victims (or, presumably people who may face such an emergency) the vitamin K is doing too good a job. The blood coagulates too readily.

In Sweden, said Dr. Horwitt, at a symposium of the Vitamin Information Bureau, they tested nine patients who had had heart attacks. Doctors gave them 300 units of vitamin E daily. Within six weeks their "clotting time" tests showed improvement. That is, the chances a blood clot would cause a stroke or heart attack were much less. Support for these Swedish researchers has recently appeared from a coagulation research group in this country, he went on.

Another drug often given to heart patients to prevent blood clots from forming is warfarin. This is effective because it destroys some vitamin K, thus preventing blood clots. But it must be given with great care and frequent blood tests must be taken, for a bit of an overdose can be so effective that hemorrhages take place, since the blood has been "thinned" too much. Strokes can result.

When doctors give warfarin and vitamin E at the same time, the vitamin E makes the drug more powerful so that even less time is needed to get the blood in such a condition that it will not clot. Laboratory scientists have found that rats, too, react this same way. Animals given warfarin show slower blood clotting if they are given, at the same time, either vitamin A, vitamin D or vitamin E.

So Dr. Horwitt recommends that, if doctors give vitamin E while they are giving warfarin or other anti-coagulants, they should decrease the dosage of the drug. It seems obvious, doesn't it, throughout all this discussion, although Dr. Horwitt does not mention it—that the body is trying to tell us that by correctly balancing all essential nutrients, like vitamin A, vitamin D and vitamin E, we need never have to take any drugs! The vitamins themselves will perform their duties of preventing clots from forming (vitamin A, D and E) or protecting the clotting ability of the blood so that we do not bleed to death. And this is the function of vitamin K.

What throws the whole mechanism out of kilter is the catastrophic imbalance created in modern diets when all the vitamin E is removed from the cereal foods that make up perhaps one-fourth of the average diet. And it is never returned. Nor do most of us ever get enough vitamin A to take care of all the functions of that essential nutrient. Human beings originated in the tropics where they got lots of sunshine on their bare skin the year round. The sunshine is converted into vitamin D in the body.

How many of us live in northern climates where sunshine is sparse and feeble for half the year? All of us live with air pollution which shuts off the sun's rays, making vitamin D less available the year round. Taking supplements of these vitamins is, therefore, only replacing the nutrients which our modern way of life has destroyed.

Dr. Horwitt continued his world-shaking address by urging doctors to consider vitamin E rather than other anticoagulants. He also revealed that recent research has found that, in minor deficiencies of vitamin E, certain red blood cells are destroyed 8 to 10 times faster than they should be. These cells are easily examined and tested, he said. But what about other body cells which doctors can't get at to test? Isn't it likely that the same premature destruction is also affecting them?

Vitamin E is known to act as a protector of fats in the body—that is, its antioxidant qualities prevent fats from becoming rancid, hence dangerous. Without enough vitamin E, said Dr. Horwitt, all body cells may not be getting enough antioxidant to protect the fats in these cells. He believes, he says, that the official dietary recommendations for Vitamin E should be reconsidered.

He also noted that vitamin E in pre-processed fatty foods is lost when it is stored in a freezer for any length of time. This suggests that "convenience" foods—TV dinners, cakes, cookies and any kind of fatty food stored for long periods of time—no matter how low the temperature—will lose some vitamin E in storage. So such foods cannot be depended on to provide the essential vitamin E.

Dr. Horwitt is a distinguished specialist in this field of nutrition. This change of heart—this complete switch from opposing vitamin E to wholehearted recommendations of it, taken in supplements every day—is a milestone in the history of this vitamin. Dr. Evan Shute of the Shute Clinic in Canada has been saying for years, of course, that vitamin E is the world's best anti-coagulant. The scientific and medical community has tried to pretend they didn't hear what he was saying. But now Dr. Horwitt has "eaten crow" before an important scientific gathering. Things may change very rapidly.

Another distinguished researcher at the same meeting, Dr. Daniel B. Menzel of Duke University, presented once again the compelling evidence of vitamin E's protective action against certain elements in air pollution. Certain kinds of fats in the lungs are destroyed by ozone and nitrogen oxide, both common ever-present air pollutants in urban localities. Testing lung cells exposed to these pollutants, Dr. Menzel found that 200 milligrams of vitamin E protected these cells against damage.

Then he tested the animals themselves. "Animals deficient in vitamin E died on an average 11.1 days after exposure to one part per million of ozone, while vitamin E supplemented animals died at 17 days," he said. Deficient animals exposed to 33 parts per million nitrogen oxide died after 8.2 days. Animals getting plenty of vitamin E averaged 18.5 days of life—more than twice as long.

He attributed these facts to the vitamin's ability to interfere with the oxidation, or destruction, of natural unsaturated fats in the lungs. Exposure to ozone causes lung cells to become viscous, he said, causing emphysema in the lungs—or cancer in other parts of the body. Getting enough vitamin E can prevent this damage.

Testing 11 human beings, Dr. Menzel found that diets containing 9 milligrams of vitamin E brought destruction to certain red blood cells. After only one week of getting 100 milligrams of vitamin E, this damage disappeared. The cells' resistance to damage was greatly increased, he said, when they were given 200 milligrams of vitamin E daily, and they continued to improve.

"The present dietary intake of vitamin E is inadequate to provide maximal protection against ozonides (ozone)," he said. He also said that vitamin E supplementation might be beneficial in cases of pulmonary hypertension (high blood pressure), vascular (circulatory) disease, pulmonary embolism (a clot in the lung) and disseminating vascular coagulation—that is, many blood clots in various parts of the body.

As our world becomes more and more polluted by mysterious chemical compounds of which we have little knowledge, it seems ever more important to protect ourselves in any way possible from these pollutants which we cannot avoid—millions of them—and the number is increasing every year. All the vitamins are important for this protection. And a good diet is important. Those foods which we recommend avoiding are the same foods which contain the most potentially dangerous additives—the packaged goodies, the candy, soft drinks, TV dinners, mixes—and the "convenience" foods which must be well-protected by chemical additives to remain "fresh" on the shelves.

The individual cells of our bodies, already assailed by the thousands of pollutants in the air, water, drugs, cosmetics, household preparations and chemicals we use at work suffer even more damage from these food chemicals. If there were one or two—but there are many thousands!

Doesn't it seem to you that we should make use of every single protective measure available to us? Vitamin E is one of these.

CHAPTER 50

A Miscellany
on Vitamin E

A DISEASE WITH the jaw-breaking name of dermolytic bullous dermatosis is also one of the most disabling and heart-breaking. It is a skin disorder in which the patient is covered with blisters. To apply and change dressings sometimes requires half a day or more. Skin is so sensitive that some patients cannot endure the touch of anything on the surface of the skin. The blisters break and "weep" continually.

Two New Mexico physicians report on using vitamin E in the treatment of this disease. Writing in *Archives of Dermatology* for August, 1973 they tell us of two sisters who suffered from this excruciating disease. One of the sisters was given a drug which is used to treat this disease, the other was given vitamin E. The vitamin E treatment caused a marked reduction in the formation of blisters while the drug had no such effect.

Then the treatment was reversed and the sister who had gotten the vitamin E was given the drug while the other sister got the vitamin E. Once again the vitamin gave immediate improvement while the drug achieved nothing. The mechanism of the action of vitamin E in this disease is unknown, say the authors, Dr. E.B. Smith and W.M. Michener.

A MISCELLANY ON VITAMIN E

The Summary, December, 1974, published by the Shute Foundation for Nutritional Research in London, Ontario, Canada describes a number of cases of epidermis bullosa. Three cases in three generations of one family were treated with 300 milligrams of vitamin E daily with excellent results.

Two children—a 7-year-old girl and an 8-year-old boy—with epidermis bullosa acquista were treated with vitamin E and improved to such an extent that the little girl could run and skip rope while the boy could play football. The doctors began with doses of 200 units a day and recommended that, for severe eruptions, dosage as high as 800 to 1,600 units should be used. It is noteworthy that the disease improved only as long as the vitamin was given.

Vitamin E is very much involved with the way our bodies use oxygen. Scientists speak of vitamin E as an antioxidant. Now of course we must have oxygen, for it takes part in many essential functions inside cells. But too much oxygen can be harmful. There's a very thin line between what is life-saving and what is harmful.

In the case of premature infants, they must have oxygen therapy or they will die. Giving them oxygen therapy may bring on a serious eye condition called retrolental fibroplasia which may cause blindness. Fifteen years ago this disaster was striking premature infants in epidemic proportions, says *Medical World News* for September 13, 1974. Today doctors have many new methods for preventing the eye disorder, but these improvements have not eliminated the problem. Conditions such as severe myopia (short-sightedness), strabismus (crossed eyes), amblyopia (dimness of vision) and other conditions may develop even if the child does not become permanently blind.

Three Philadelphia physicians, working on the problem, asked themselves whether vitamin E might not help out, since it is known as an antioxidant. That is, it protects foods from oxidation or becoming rancid. It also protects body cells from possible harmful effects of too much oxygen. Is it not possible, said Drs. Lois Johnson, David Schaffer and Thomas R. Boggs, that vitamin E might protect premature infants from the harmful effects of oxygen, given to prevent the eye disease (RLF) which causes blindness. They noted, too, that many premature babies are deficient in vitamin E.

Working with 81 children all of whom were premature and had very small birth weights, they gave 41 of these babies vitamin E injections from the first hours of life until the eye tissues most sensitive to RLF had completely matured or until any active disease had disappeared. They maintained blood levels of the vitamin in this group of babies. The other 40 infants received no vitamin E.

In 22 percent of the treated infants some degree of retrolental fibroplasia occurred, but the non-treated children had a much higher incidence of 37.5 percent. The children treated with vitamin E also had much better scores on severity of disease and the actual number of eyes affected. Among children who developed RLF, 15½ weeks passed before the disease disappeared, if they had received no vitamin E. But children who got the vitamin were disease-free in six weeks.

Following up the children for one year, the physicians found that the condition of the vitamin E-treated babies was better. A veteran specialist in the disease said that vitamin E therapy is still too experimental to be an everyday part of treatment, but the Philadelphia physicians have "charted a sound course." So still another experiment shows the close relation between vitamin E and oxygen.

We uncovered a letter from a Colorado scientist which was published in *The Lancet* for March 1, 1975. Dr. Eldon W. Keinholz of Colorado State University relates his troubles with pain in his knees after strenuous leg work. "The condition became worse," he says, "until in 1973 I was almost unable to complete a hike in nearby mountains because of pain. The problem was identified by an orthopedic surgeon as ligament irritation on lateral and frontal parts of the knee joint. I was recommended to accept the situation since there was no accepted therapy.

"I learned that selenium ingestion has been suggested as a method of relieving some types of arthritis. In January, 1974 I began to ingest gelatin capsules, each containing one milligram of sodium selenite plus 68 milligrams of d-alpha tocopherol succinate (vitamin E). One capsule was taken regularly with meals every third day. A week before a hike in September, 1974 I ran approximately ½ mile each day (as I had done before hikes in previous years) and I increased my selenium and vitamin E intake into one capsule per day. Insofar as I was able to plan the experiment, everything was the same as in previous years with the exception of my selenium and vitamin E intake. I hiked 11 miles in one day, ascending and descending 2,875 feet with absolutely no knee discomfort. This contrasted with past hikes, especially one . . . in which the distance was identical but I only ascended and descended 1,685 feet and knee pain was nearly unbearable during the last 20 percent of the hike . . .

"I hope that the success of this small personal experiment will encourage further research into vitamin E and/or selenium therapy of arthritis problems in human knee joints. However the hazards of selenium supplementation must be borne in mind—one milligram of selenium supplement per day probably approaches the adult human toxicity levels. The vitamin E levels did not exceed those in widespread use."

Selenium occurs generally in those foods which also contain the most vitamin E: wholegrains and other seed foods mostly. When these foods are refined and processed, both the selenium and vitamin E are removed, along with many other vitamins, minerals and trace minerals. So eating only refined cereals and breads almost guarantees a deficiency in both the vitamin and the trace mineral selenium. Interestingly enough, animal experiments have shown that the more vitamin E you get, the less selenium you need. As the vitamin E content of your diet goes up, your need for this trace mineral decreases. You can get along on much less selenium if you are getting plenty of vitamin E.

Recently selenium supplements combined with vitamin E are available at health food stores. One product also contains chromium, another trace mineral which we need in extremely small amounts to help our bodies handle carbohydrates. The amounts of both trace minerals are included in only microgram amounts—extremely small— so there seems to be no hazard associated with them. And both the chromium and the selenium come from brewers yeast which contains another substance which activates the chromium.

Should people with high blood pressure take vitamin E? Dr. Evan Shute tells us that "Some hypertensive patients display a small initial rise of blood pressure when *first suddenly* given *large* doses of vitamin E. As this agent continues to be taken, any elevation of blood pressure may drop—although perhaps not to normal levels. More than anything else a hypertensive fears a stroke, a blood clot or ruptured vessel in the damaged arteries of his brain. There is no safe prophylactic (preventive) agent he can take to ward off this danger but vitamin E. It is his best and safest insurance policy. He needs that policy desperately and should keep his premiums paid every day as long as he lives."

If you begin to take vitamin E for heart and circulatory health, must you continue it indefinitely? Dr. Shute replies to this question as follows: "If one starts to eat bread, he always needs bread. If one starts to eat meat and potatoes the body continues to need them. Vitamin E is just another food. If one begins to take it, he wonders how he ever got along without it. If he stops it, the effect soon wears off, as is true of bread and meat. The influence of any food is usually transient. If the patient stops it, he very soon, in a matter of a few days, returns to much the same conditions as at first, before he took it at all.

"The patient is under no compulsion to take vitamin E at any time, just as one really is not compelled to eat anything.

But people who stop eating regret it, and that is true of vitamin E also. Vitamin E is treatment—not cure—like insulin (for diabetics). The day the diabetic stops his insulin he becomes the same old diabetic he was before he took insulin. This is as true of cardiovascular patients taking vitamin E. In a few days or weeks after it has been stopped, the patient once again is vulnerable and exposed to the steady ravages of his disease ... Vitamin E is not habit forming."

One problem encountered in taking vitamin E is that the vitamin is destroyed in part when it is exposed to medicinal iron in the digestive tract. The literature from the Shute Institute tells us that "One can take organic iron, such as is found in raisins, spinach or in many other foods, or an organic iron salt, at the same time he takes vitamin E and no harm is done to the tocopherol (vitamin E). It is inorganic iron, such as most iron tonics contain, that seems to destroy vitamin E by oxidation.

"If a doctor gives iron because of a profound anemia, for example, he can still give it when vitamin E is being administered by separating the doses of each in the stomach. This is, one can give all his vitamin E at or before breakfast and all his inorganic iron at bedtime—or vice versa. Thus an interval of at least eight hours separates them and the inorganic iron does not oxidize the tocopherols in the stomach.

"Iron can be given by intramuscular injection at any time, of course. It is only iron in the bowel that interacts with vitamin E. If one is taking a vitamin-mineral mixture at the same time as vitamin E, he should be sure to find out if the iron in it is the permissible organic or the improper inorganic type."

When the doctor gives you iron medication, it would be wise then to take it at the other end of the day from when you take your vitamin E. If you are taking a vitamin supplement which also includes iron, the manufacturer undoubtedly knows of the potential destruction of vitamin E if certain compounds of iron are present at the same time, so he has probably put into the supplement only those forms of iron which are organic—that is, they occur in food such as raisins, spinach, wheat germ and so on.

Ever since nutrition scientists discovered that the fatty material cholesterol can collect in blood vessels and gall bladders and cause trouble, they have been warning us away from foods that contain any cholesterol. The only way to avoid circulatory trouble, they say, is to eat only those foods in which there is little or no cholesterol. And some of them continue to say this, even though many highly nutritious foods like eggs and liver are thus eliminated from our diets. Now we have word from *The Journal of Nutrition*, June 1972, that vitamin E changes all that.

Working with laboratory rats, Dr. L.H. Chen and two associates found that animals who were getting little vitamin E had much higher blood levels of cholesterol than those which had plenty of the vitamin. And when vitamin E was added to the former diets, the cholesterol levels promptly dropped. Another aspect of the diet was studied. Animals which were getting low protein diets had higher cholesterol levels than those on high protein diets.

Say the authors, "the interrelationship of dietary protein and vitamin E level in altering serum cholesterol was apparent." Good news! Removing from the diet such excellent foods as liver, meat, eggs and whole milk is almost bound to produce a diet low in protein and low in many other essential elements as well. With plenty of vitamin E supplementation and plenty of protein such deprivations may be entirely unnecessary for disposing of cholesterol healthfully.

In an article in *Postgraduate Medicine*, July, 1968 Dr. Alton Ochsner describes his use of vitamin E post-operatively. This is the famous New Orleans surgeon who was among the first physicians to realize the harm being done by smoking. He had operated on the lung cancers of too many smokers!

Dr. Ochsner states that he has used alpha tocopherol

(vitamin E) routinely for the past 15 years in the treatment of patients who have been subjected to major trauma. None of his patients has had pulmonary embolism. This is the clot in the lung that may prove fatal. It is the most feared aftermath of surgery. Dr. Ochsner has been able to prevent the occurrence of this fatal complication in all his patients since he began to use vitamin E routinely on all surgery patients. Unlike the anti-coagulant drugs which are given to prevent clots, vitamin E poses no threat of hemorrhage. There is no need to keep testing the blood to be certain it is not becoming too "thin." Vitamin E is completely safe.

Dr. Shute comments that in his practice he no longer has any problems with peripheral thrombosis and embolism since he uses vitamin E both before and after operations.

Several other notes on vitamin E came to our attention recently from scientific literature. *Science News*, for December 23, 1972, reporting on "How You Age" stated, in part. "On the hypothesis that aging might be linked with too much oxygen at the tissue or cellular level, Denham Harman of the University of Nebraska School of Medicine has given antioxidants, such as vitamin E, to experimental animals. The antioxidants extended the normal life span of rodents 30 percent."

Harman said, "We don't know whether vitamin E has a good effect or not in humans. We hope to eventually come to some concrete suggestions. We are not at that stage yet."

He, too, it seems, does not read medical literature very carefully or he would have stumbled over countless reports of vitamin E being used successfully for a wide variety of human ailments.

In *Medical World News* for December 8, 1972 a fascinating article described the puzzling relationship between vitamin E and the trace mineral *selenium*. Scientists understand very little about it up to now. But it seems that selenium was the mysterious "factor 3" which sometimes seemed to accompany "pure" vitamin E when it was used in early experiments.

Since then many disorders have been found to respond

to treatment with either selenium or vitamin E or both. When selenium is absent or deficient in soils, dreadful diseases afflict the animals eating food grown on these soils. Yet selenium is highly toxic in amounts just a bit above the necessary levels. Vitamin E, of course, is not.

Dr. Donald F.L. Money of New Zealand's Animal Health Laboratory believes that lack of selenium and/or vitamin E may be responsible for that tragic occurrence called "Sudden Infant Death Syndrome," when a perfectly healthy baby is put to bed and found dead in the morning with symptoms of suffocation. The incidence in bottle-fed babies is about 3 in every thousand births.

There are almost no fatalities among breast-fed babies. Human milk contains up to six times more selenium than cow's milk and about twice as much vitamin E. Possibly these two deficiencies combined produce the fatalities.

It seems you can give rats "stress ulcers" by confining them in a small area in which they can see and smell food and water, but cannot reach it. This is called a "stress apparatus" by scientists. It seems a very cruel kind of experiment to conduct on animals, especially when there is an abundance of opportunity to study just such conditions among human beings.

Be that as it may, the rats in this experiment, conducted at Stanford University, were confined in this stressful way with food and water available for one hour only, every 47 hours. This went on for 12 days. Half of the rats were given 50 milligrams of vitamin E twice a day, while the other half received a similar solution but containing no vitamins. This is an extremely large amount of vitamin E for a creature as small as a rat.

At the end of the experiment the scientists found that rating for "stress" ulcers in the stomachs of the vitamin E-fed rats was 1.92 on a scale from 1 to 4, while the rats which had received no vitamin were rated at 3.42. So the rats deprived of the vitamin had 1½ times more trouble with ulcers than the ones getting the vitamin.

We don't know if this experiment applies also to

"stressed" human beings. The scientists say, "Vitamin E seems to have significant preventive properties in relation to the ulceration process." And they think much more research should be done along these lines. So do we. How do you feel about it, over there in your own "stress apparatus" which, these days, seems to consist of mounting frustrations with almost every aspect of our technological society? Doesn't it seem that vitamin E might help?

According to Dr. Evan Shute, vitamin E is helpful in preventing arteriosclerosis, or hardening of the arteries. This condition is most likely to develop in diabetics, in patients with too little activity of the thyroid gland and in some families predisposed to high levels of cholesterol in blood.

Other animals than human beings suffer from hardening of the arteries. Recently scientists discovered that a disease not unlike that of human beings occurs in hens. In these birds a combination of vitamin A and E has been quite effective in preventing hardening of the arteries and relieving its symptoms.

And for people who have already developed symptoms of hardening of the arteries such as leg cramps (claudication) or cold feet or gangrene or angina pectoris, vitamin E has much to offer. We cannot say for certain that arteriosclerotic disorders in the brain can be helped by vitamin E since such symptoms are not generally recognized until too late. Brain tissues cannot be regenerated. However, says Dr. Shute, "We all have more brain, more heart, more liver, more kidney, and more lung than we need for survival. Hence one can cut out a lung or a kidney and the patient goes on as before. In the same way we have great reserves of unused blood vessels to be called on in emergency or as we grow older. These are mobilized by alpha tocopherol (vitamin E) as by nothing else we know, and so can preserve tissues otherwise deprived of adequate arterial circulation.

"Vitamin E is uniquely able to do this, it has special powers of enabling the body tissue to make better use of whatever oxygen they receive. This is really equivalent to providing them with more oxygen. In short, alpha tocopherol helps tissues to breathe, and this can be vital in relieving pain or improving functional activity. In fact, it may make the difference between life and death of a tissue or even of a person."

CHAPTER 51

How Much
Vitamin E
Do You Need?

OFFICIALLY, WE ARE told that a minimum of 10 to 30 milligrams of vitamin E daily should be sufficient for most adults. And we are told that "The estimated average daily adult consumption of vitamin E has been calculated to be about 14 milligrams."

Some time ago a survey was conducted by four researchers who chose food from a supermarket which, they thought, might be typical of the food we Americans eat every day for breakfast, lunch and dinner. They made a special effort, however, to include as many foods as possible that are rich in vitamin E—salad oils, for example, and margarine, butter and mayonnaise.

They planned menus for eight days, and, by careful investigation in a laboratory, found out just how much vitamin E each day's menus contained. They were very well-planned, highly nutritious menus—far bigger meals than most of us eat, probably.

A typical breakfast, for instance was tomato juice, cooked cereal, two slices of ham, one egg, two slices of whole grain bread with margarine, coffee with cream and sugar. How many people you know eat that big a breakfast? Lunches and dinners were equally well planned, with an eye to including as many foods as possible in which vitamin E is abundant.

They found that the daily average intake of vitamin E was only 7.4 milligrams, or just about half the amount that has been officially announced as the average daily intake of the average American. The authors of the survey say in their article in the *American Journal of Clinical Nutrition*, July, 1965, that it indicates the possibility of relatively low vitamin E intake in a portion of the population. We'd say it certainly indicates that even if you eat well planned meals with nothing much but their vitamin E content in mind you will still be getting only half the amount officially recommended for you.

How does this happen? Have human beings always been short on vitamin E? No, of course not. The richest source of vitamin E is the germ of cereals—that little nubbin which is removed when we process grains to make white flour or commercial cereals. At present it is estimated that about half of our meals consist of foods made of sugar and these highly processed grains, from which all the vitamin E has been removed. It's no wonder that large numbers of us are probably not getting even the 7.4 milligrams of vitamin E which turned up in the survey described above.

Another reason for a possible shortage in vitamin E is that many of the foods we eat today have been frozen. If we eat commercially processed foods which have been fried in deep fat, these foods contain almost no vitamin E at all, for it is destroyed in the fat when they are frozen.

In a letter to *Chemical and Engineering News* for October 9 1972, a reader protests a previous article in which it was stated that the only demonstrated function of vitamin E in man is as an antioxidant. Richard A. Passwater lists a number of other functions performed by this vitamin in the human body. Then he objects to another statement made in the earlier article—that vitamin E deficiency is practically unknown in man.

"It may be unknown," he says, "but borderline

deficiencies may exist in more than half our population, if the arbitary 20-30 milligrams per day RDA established by the Food and Nutrition Board of the National Research Council is used as a guideline. Surveys... indicate typical diets may contain less than 7 milligrams a day of vitamin E. These surveys do not consider the vitamin losses due to preparation or storage, nor analytical problems. Blood level measurements are inconclusive... An antioxidant deficiency state existed in 90 percent of those studied.

"As vitamin E deficiency in animals leads to tissue degradation and gross changes in biochemistry, we should err on the high intake side, rather than the low.

"Today's typical vitamin E consumption is only a fraction of that of 50 years ago, even when adjusted for lipid intake. Degermination, bleaching, processing and longer storage periods have depleted foods. The long-term effects of this, along with decreased (physical) activity and other factors may explain our worsening morbidity/mortality rates of cardiovascular disease and other diseases.

"In conclusion it is difficult to assess, but borderline vitamin E deficiencies are widespread, based on both the RDA and the diene test (for antioxidants). It is difficult to assume that the long-term consequences are not a major problem."

The Journal of the American Geriatrics Society for August, 1974 published an article by E. Cheraskin, MD, DMD, W.M. Ringsdorf, Jr., DMD, and B.S. Hicks on "Eating Habits of the Dentist and His Wife: Daily Consumption of Vitamin E." They tell us that they collected information from a group of 369 dentists and 288 wives on what they ate every day for one week. They kept very careful records, with special attention to the frequency with which they ate certain foods—in this case, foods in which there is lots of vitamin E.

The information was analyzed by a computer. The results were discussed with the people involved. They were told of the relationship between good nutrition and good health, especially, in this case, getting enough vitamin E.

They were told how they could increase their intake of vitamin E and why they should.

About one year later, the survey was made again. Every participant kept account of every food eaten during one week. Similar surveys were taken every year for four years for the same group of people, so that the researchers now have a good idea of just what foods are eaten daily by each member of this group and how much vitamin E is contained in each day's diet.

At the same time, the same group of volunteers were being given certain tests to determine just what their condition was in regard to heart and circulatory health. Some of them showed improved health in this area. Others showed no improvement or little improvement. These facts were then correlated with the amounts of vitamin E which each individual got in his daily diet. It's hard to imagine a more comprehensive and convincing way to arrive at the facts.

One object was to see if those who had not been getting enough vitamin E would increase their intake after a period of nutritional education. Another object was to see if an increase in the amount of vitamin E in the daily diet would improve heart and circulatory health and if a decrease in the amount of vitamin E in the daily diet would cause lack of improvement or even a turn for the worse in heart and circulatory health.

The results are enlightening. First of all the Alabama scientists found that there was a wide range of vitamin E intake among the volunteer dentists and their wives. Among the dentists, some got as little as 6 units of vitamin E daily, some as much as 212 units. Forty-six percent of all the dentists got, at meals, less than 30 units daily, which was the recommended daily allowance until recently. Their wives also got widely varying amounts of vitamin E. Some got as little as 4 units, others as much as 213. Forty-five percent of the wives were getting less than the 25 units daily which were until recently recommended by federal experts.

How did they do after the nutritional education course?

The average amount of daily intake of vitamin E at the beginning of the test was 21 units in a selected group of 84 paired subjects. At the second visit, after the nutritional instruction, these same people were getting an average of 51 units. And at the third visit they were getting 127 units of vitamin E. So there is no doubt that a simple course of instruction in nutrition can improve the intake of nutrients among those who wish to show improvement. In other words, it's perfectly possible to learn how to get more of a given vitamin at meals, if you want to.

And what happened to the health of the people who arranged their eating patterns so that they got more vitamin E? You have perhaps guessed what happened. As the intake of vitamin E went up, so did the heart and circulatory health improve. When the intake went up only slightly there was little or no noticeable improvement. But when daily intake went up considerably, there was considerable improvement in circulatory conditions.

This was determined, incidentally, by use of the Cornell Medical Index Questionnaire on which various facts in regard to heart and circulation are recorded.

The Alabama researchers report that the dose of vitamin E seems to be very important in regard to benefits received. Dosages twice as high as those officially recommended appeared to be the most beneficial. As we have pointed out in other chapters of this book, The National Academy of Sciences—National Research Council, which sets these standards, lowered their estimate of daily needs for vitamin E in their latest booklet, *Recommended Dietary Allowances*. They lowered it from 30 to 25 units for men and women respectively to 15 to 12 units. Their reason was, generally speaking, that there does not appear to be any national deficiency in vitamin E and it appears that all of us get at least this much in our food.

On the contrary, the Alabama test showed that almost half of us may not be getting this basic requirement. It also shows that the more vitamin E you get, apparently, the more improvement there will be in your circulatory health.

And remember that the subjects of this test were dentists and their wives—people who would, one imagines, have a fairly good basic education in nutrition, unlike most of the rest of us.

In a previous article these Alabama doctors showed much the same thing in regard to refined carbohydrates, using the same group of professional men as volunteers. The less of the refined carbohydrates eaten, the better the health of the subjects. The more refined carbohydrates eaten, the worse the general condition of health, as determined by the Cornell test.

Now we find the same general condition in regard to vitamin E. The better the diet eaten—that is, the more vitamin E it contains—the better the cardiovascular health. And as the diet grows worse, just in regard to vitamin E, the circulatory health declines.

How can you improve your intake of vitamin E? The best sources of this fat-soluble vitamin are seeds, cereals and their oils. But they must, of course be wholegrain, for refining and bleaching of cereals destroys vitamin E wholesale. And nothing is done to replace what has been lost from white flour and commercially refined cereals.

Here are some of the best food sources of vitamin E. Think of them in relation to the amount of each that you might eat in the course of a day. You eat liver and oatmeal in average servings. You eat a serving of peas or baked beans, brown rice, turnip or other greens at a meal. All these contain ample vitamin E. Although soybean oil along with other salad oils, is very rich in vitamin E, you cannot get down "a serving" of soybean oil at one meal, and you shouldn't. Salad oils are highly concentrated foods. But you can and should use them in smaller quantities wherever appropriate—in salads, for instance, and recipes where you might otherwise use butter or hydrogenated shortening.

As might be expected, wholegrains contain more vitamin E than white flour or processed cereals, since most of the vitamin E in grains is concentrated in the germ and bran which are removed during processing. Adding insult to injury, bleaching of flour to make it chalky white destroys the last of whatever vitamin E was in the white flour or processed cereal to begin with. The two parts of the grain which are removed, the germ and the bran, are rich sources of vitamin E.

A serving of wheat germ (3½ ounces) contains 27 units of vitamin E. All whole, unrefined seeds contain it, as well as green leafy vegetables and eggs. There are, of course, many food supplements containing vitamin E. It is possible to take it in very large amounts if you feel that you need it. And there is much research in medical journals showing the health advantages to large doses of vitamin E.

In *The American Journal of Clinical Nutrition* for September, 1972 Karen C. Davis of the Agricultural Experiment Station, University of Idaho, tells us about the amount of vitamin E in baby's diets in this country.

As might be expected she found that the situation in regard to vitamin E in commercial baby food is chaotic, completely chaotic. Since American parents spent $344,700,000 for baby foods every year, it is apparent that most babies are fed out of drug store bottles and supermarket cartons. Breast feeding being generally considered too inconvenient most babies live on formulas which are bought at the store. It's also too inconvenient to prepare baby's formula at home apparently.

Because of the nationwide scare over cholesterol, commercial baby's formulas these days are loaded with unsaturated fats, rather than good, old saturated fats that come in human milk and cow's milk. But unsaturated fats must be accompanied by very sizable amounts of vitamin E or they create a deficiency in this vitamin. And most of the commercial formulas Dr. Davis studied contained little or no vitamin E.

So, in consultation with a local pediatrician, she designed complete all-day feeding schedules for babies of different ages using 23 different commercial formulas, plus fruit, cereal and vegetables. And she carefully calculated the amount of vitamin E the infants might get from such diets. She found that the minimum amount of vitamin E was 1.38 milligrams, the maximum was 14.92 milligrams, depending on which formulas were used!

She came to the conclusion that the range of vitamin E varies so greatly that "it becomes a matter of real concern to choose formulas and foods that are adequate with respect to both vitamin E and the ratio of vitamin E to the unsaturated fats. ... Baby foods generally do not supply much vitamin," she says, mostly because the cereals are all refined cereals, and fruits and vegetables are not very good sources of the vitamin. So, she says, we should fortify the commercial formulas with vitamin E. Some of them are already fortified but probably have too little of the vitamin.

Interestingly enough, whenever cereal appears on her list of foods, the infant always gets one teaspoon of sugar, plain white sugar, along with the cereal—just to make sure,

Vitamin E Content of Some Common Foods

Food	Vitamin E in one serving
	mg.
Beef	0.63
Liver	1.62
Haddock	1.20
Baked potato	0.05
Baked beans	1.16
Fresh peas	1.73
Whole wheat bread, 4 slices	2.2
Oatmeal	3.23
Corn oil margarine, 1 tablespoon	2.60
Mayonnaise, 1 tablespoon	3.16
Wheat germ, ½ cup	11.0

we guess, that the child will be addicted to sugar by the time he can toddle. Or maybe pediatricians and nutritionists simply do not know that children have no need of added sugar, don't especially like it but very soon become addicted to the taste. Adults apparently go right on assuming that babies are born with the same perverted sense of taste their parents have developed, over the years, in regard to sugar and salt.

What to do? We suggest if there's a new baby at your home, that breast-feeding is infinitely superior to any formula and that all babies should be breast-fed as long as possible. We also suggest that homemade formulas are infinitely superior to commercial ones, that they should be made of cow's milk or goat milk diluted to make them as nearly identical to human breast milk as possible and that early foods should include cooked cereals with as much vitamin E as possible, as well as egg yolk and pureed meat along with fruits and vegetables.

For more information on breast feeding, write to: La Leche League, 9616 Minneapolis Ave., Franklin Park, Ill 60131.

And finally, *Nutrition Reviews* for March, 1972 reported on the great difficulty found in trying to calculate the amount of vitamin E actually in food. The article tells of testing the diets of 40 ambulant patients in a hospital. Twenty-nine of the forty diets contained less than five milligrams of vitamin E per day. (Remember, this is a hospital where, supposedly, highly trained nutrition experts plan the meals!)

Part of the reason for all the confusion, said the article, is simply that the same food may contain widely varying amounts of vitamin E depending on where and when it is bought.

The other day in an animal feed store, we saw gallon cans of wheat germ oil, enriched with considerable amounts of vitamin E, vitamin A and vitamin D. These preparations are available for use in the diets of cows, horses and other valuable stock animals. The stock raiser cannot take any chances on poor health in his animals. It's too costly.

So even though they are eating the best possible diet, even though they suffer from almost none of the daily stresses to health which we human beings suffer from, stock animals are regularly plied with massive doses of the fat soluble vitamins. Nobody—least of all the FDA—says a reproachful word.

But the minute anybody suggests in print that perhaps human beings, too, might benefit from the addition of vitamin supplements to their diets, a hue and a cry goes up from every regulatory bureau in Washington.

"What are you saying!" they shout. "Don't you know that every American eating 'the average American diet' is already getting enough vitamins and minerals? Why waste your money buying vitamins?"

Gentlemen, the hard-headed raisers of prize horses and cows don't consider vitamin supplements a waste of money. Why do you?

For a list of some common foods which contain vitamin E, refer to the chart on page 396.

CHAPTER 52

How Can You Tell Synthetic Vitamin E From Natural Vitamin E?

THERE IS A way to tell natural from synthetic vitamin E. It is outlined here by a spokesman from Eastman Chemical Company which manufactures much of the natural vitamin E we see in food supplements. Although some of this discussion is a bit difficult for a non-chemist to follow, the basic way to determine at a glance the difference between natural and synthetic vitamin E is clearly indicated.

Vitamin E was discovered in 1922 in the course of biochemical research with laboratory animals. Over the years, thousands of scientific papers have been published on the subject. Much research on it is still going on in well-respected laboratories around the world.

Despite this half century of research, much less is known about the extent of the biological role of vitamin E than of a number of other vitamins.

In research, the effects of a lack of a vitamin can be studied by controlling the diet fed to animals. However, vitamin E is unusual in the large variation of effects among animal species from insufficient vitamin E.

For example, in male rats the lack of vitamin E results in

sterility; in calves, heart failure; in lambs paralysis of the hind quarters; in chicks, leakage from the capillaries and brain deterioration, and in milk cows, bad flavored milk.

Even deciding on the recommended daily allowance of vitamin E is complicated. It depends very much on what else the animal is getting. For example, in cat food switching from one kind of fish product to another resulted in greatly increased need for vitamin E. When these increased needs were not met, pets died...

To serve the human need to make one's own choices, the marketplace offers such things as dietary supplements in such forms as capsules, tablets and liquids. Some of these are represented as "natural" in origin in contrast with "synthetic."

As one of the companies that supplies manufacturers of these products with the naturally derived form of vitamin E, we want to explain what we mean by "naturally derived" and how to make sure you get it.

The particular kind of molecule that gives vitamin E effects is a structure of carbon, hydrogen and oxygen atoms. Molecules composed of these atoms are called "organic" because of a belief among early chemists that a certain category of substances could come only from living organisms. Today, scientists know how to make millions of kinds of "organic" molecules that never occur in nature, in addition to other thousands that do occur in nature. A "synthetic" molecule may be absolutely identical in every known property with one made by the body of a plant or a creature other than a human chemist.

It may be. It may also be slightly different. The difference, if any, may not matter for some purposes. For others it may matter.

Look at a glove for the right hand and its mate for the left hand. Same design, same material, but different. Molecules made by nature can differ from otherwise identical ones made by the chemist in just this property of "handedness." Only certain molecular structures have handedness, just as some familiar objects like dishes, for example, have no inbuilt handedness, while gloves and screw threads do have it. Vitamin E molecules have it, too.

When factories make molecules, the processes have to be efficient. Efficient methods of quantity production leave it to chance whether the parts of each individual molecule will be assembled left-handed or right-handed where either twist is possible. Nature, using subtle methods, tends to put them together with all the same twist.

In the case of vitamin E, a difference in twist makes a difference in biological potency. This is officially recognized in National Formulary's definition of the International Unit of vitamin E, the unit required by regulatory authorities for stating vitamin E potency on labels. It recognizes that handedness affects potency, just as one of a person's hands is stronger than the other.

One milligram of the synthetic vitamin E, dl-Alpha tocopheryl acetate, is equal to one International Unit of vitamin E. The two letters "d" and "l" in combination is a chemist's way of indicating that the molecules are built on both the left-handed and right-handed pattern.

The same National Formulary goes on to specify that one milligram of d-Alpha tocopheryl acetate equals 1.36 International Units (36% more).

It takes careful reading to note the difference in those chemical names:

dl-Alpha tocopheryl acetate
d-Alpha tocopheryl acetate

That small "l" results in a lower potency. When it is NOT there you are being informed that the molecules have indeed all been assembled nature's way.

This doesn't mean that it is necessarily a better nutrient. It just means that less of it is required to do whatever essential biochemical job is to be done in your body by the vitamin E. It doesn't say that the chemist hasn't tinkered with the molecule nature made. The absence of that little "l" doesn't even prove that nature actually built those particular molecules, although actually building them in a laboratory from their constituent atoms would have been exorbitantly expensive. If the consumer wants "d" rather than "dl" it is far more practical to let nature do the molecule building out in the field where she makes vegetable oil.

If, for reasons of your own, you prefer the naturally derived form of vitamin E, just look at the label carefully. Find that little "d" that goes with tocopheryl (sometimes it's tocopherol). Be sure that it applies to all the vitamin E in the product. If there is a little "l" after the little "d," there is vitamin E in it that did not start out from natural vegetable oils, whatever else may be stated about natural oils contained.

Not that synthetic vitamin E would harm you.

It's just that you have a right to know.

Vitamin K Is...

Fat-soluble, hence stored in the body.

Responsible for maintenance of the blood's clotting system.

Without vitamin K we would bleed to death with the slightest scratch. So a deficiency in vitamin K results in a tendency to bleed or hemorrhage.

Present in cabbage, cauliflower, soybeans, spinach, liver, kidney, wholegrains, wheat germ, wheat bran, egg yolk, potatoes, tomatoes.

Usually safe in large amounts. Given by doctors to prevent bleeding, it may eventually cause clotting, though it is safer than drugs given for this purpose.

Destroyed by mineral oil laxatives, impaired absorption of fat in the intestine, antibiotics given by mouth, certain liver disorders.

Required officially as an essential nutrient. But no official recommendation given, for this vitamin is manufactured by bacteria in the human intestine. Vitamin K may be given to newborns, since their intestinal bacteria are not yet established.

Not available in supplements since it is assumed that the body makes its own.

CHAPTER 53

Vitamin K Stands
for Well-Ordered
"Koagulation"

TWO WORRISOME CIRCUMSTANCES of modern life are the
reasons why we are especially concerned about vitamin K.
First, the fact that coronary thrombosis is a leading cause
of death, and "strokes" take an additional toll of life, as well
as crippling and disabling many thousands each year. The
second reason for our concern is that the FDA has recently
granted permission for the irradiation of various foods and
we are promised that eventually almost everything we eat
will be irradiated.

Why do these two circumstances worry us so and what
do they have to do with vitamin K? Vitamin K is so-called
because it is involved chiefly with the process of blood
coagulation. The letter K stands for Koagulation—the
spelling of this word in Danish. The vitamin was discovered
by a Danish scientist. Vitamin K is necessary for
manufacturing, in the liver, the substance which causes
blood to coagulate normally. Without vitamin K we would
bleed to death.

In fact, many newly-born children do not survive
precisely because their small bodies are lacking in this

important substance during the early days of life. Many obstetricians now give vitamin K to pregnant women to prevent any hemorrhaging accident in their newly-born children. The reasons why any prospective mother might be deficient in vitamin K are abundant. If her liver does not function well this may interfere with the manufacture of the coagulation substance by vitamin K in this organ.

If she suffers from some disease affecting the digestive tract, she may not absorb the vitamin from her food. Sprue, diarrhea, dysentery, colitis, and other disorders of this kind prevent the absorption of many vitamins. If she has been taking mineral oil, the fat-soluble vitamin K in her digestive tract would be destroyed, along with the other fat-soluble vitamins A, D and E. Bile is essential for the absorption of vitamin K, so if some disorder prevents the presence of bile in the intestine, vitamin K will not be absorbed.

Strokes are, of course, hemorrhages of blood vessels. We do not know what causes them. But it seems quite possible that one cause may be lack of vitamin K. That is, lack of the substance in the blood which helps it to clot in the way it is supposed to when some small blood vessel is broken. Coronary thrombosis may be caused by a blood clot in the main artery of the heart. After such an attack, the patient is usually given some anticoagulant drug—that is, a drug which interferes with the process of coagulation so that further clots will not form. These drugs must be administered with great care, for serious accidents can occur when the blood loses some of its ability to clot.

Vitamin K can be given to help regulate this delicate balance, since it will provide materials to help the natural and healthful clotting process.

So we see that this vitamin is absolutely essential to health. The older we are the more important becomes an ample supply of vitamin K because it is in these later years that problems with the circulatory system become most troublesome. Also, as we become older, we tend to have more problems with the proper absorption of food elements. Up until quite recently we were told that vitamin

K is manufactured by helpful bacteria in the intestine, so it isn't necessary to have a certain supply in the diet.

Such conclusions were arrived at by studying laboratory animals. We do not know, however, how much of this information can be applied directly to all human beings. There is, we must not forget, the problem of decreased numbers of helpful bacteria in the human intestine as a result of the antibiotic drugs which are given so widely these days. Antibiotics and sulfa drugs destroy bacteria, both harmful and helpful. So anyone who has been taking these drugs is quite likely to be unable to synthesize any vitamin in his digestive tract. The helpful bacteria must first be re-established there, preferably by daily intake of considerable quantities of yogurt or other products which contain the same helpful bacteria yogurt contains.

The October 11, 1965 issue of *The Journal of the American Medical Association* printed an aricle by an Arizona physician which seems to show that we cannot depend on intestinal bacteria for manufacturing our own vitamin K, but must get it in our food. Dr. John A. Udall gave human volunteers diets completely lacking in vitamin K and found that the normal clotting ability of the blood decreased almost at once.

By giving vitamin K he could raise the level of this substance. As soon as he took vitamin K out of the diet, it decreased once more. He concluded, "Foods, rather than intestinal bacterial synthesis, probably provide most vitamin K for humans." Doesn't it seem as though some official body should take cognizance of this fact and set some official standard for the amount of vitamin K we should be getting in our diets?

Instead, *Recommended Dietary Allowances*, 1968, states: "Because of the lack of reliable information concerning human intakes of vitamin K and because of other factors shown to be operative in experimental animals, but not yet evaluated in man, an absolute daily allowance for this vitamin has not been established."

In the 1964 edition, the National Academy of Sciences

said: "A daily allowance for vitamin K cannot be established because of the wide but inconsistent distribution of the vitamin in the diet and the variability of intestinal flora (bacteria) and absorption activity from person to person." In other words, if you are eating a nourishing diet and if your ability to absorb vitamins has not been impaired by taking drugs and/or mineral oil, then you may be getting enough of this fat-soluble vitamin.

Now for our second worry in regard to this vitamin. The Army and the Atomic Energy Commission have been experimenting with irradiated foods—that is, perishable foods sterilized by subjecting them to massive doses of radiation. It seems that such foods will keep, without refrigeration, for several months. This is economical. Many of the earlier experiments showed damage to animals who ate these foods. A professor at the St. Louis University School of Medicine reported in *Federation Proceedings*, December, 1961, that laboratory animals which were fed a diet, 35 percent of which consisted of irradiated foods, died of hemorrhage. Animals given a supplement of vitamin K did not succumb to hemorrhaging.

It is known that radiating food destroys its vitamin K. Now we know that, unless enough vitamin K is obtained in foods and supplements other than the irradiated ones, hemorrhaging and possible death will result. The St. Louis physician adds that there are many mysteries surrounding vitamin K which he hopes will be speedily resolved.

One of the mysteries, we would add, is the fact that anybody authorized the radiation of foods, declaring that no harm could come to anyone from eating them. So far as vitamin K is concerned, it seems that this may be true, provided you are getting plenty of vitamin K in other foods to make up for the vitamin K destroyed in the radiation process. How do you know that you are? Since there is no official estimate of the amount of viatmin K needed by the average person, how could anyone safely work out this problem for himself?

There seems to be little activity on irradiated foods in this country at present. Public resistance to the idea of eating foods which had been so treated was apparently responsible for closing factories and cutting off research funds by the government. The Netherlands, Israel and the Soviet Union are proceeding with plans to irradiate foods in the future, we are told in a *New York Times* article, September 9, 1971.

Vitamin K is abundant in "the average diet," we are told by experts. Is it? Check over the list of foods below and see for yourself. As you read the list, think of all the surveys that have been done showing that a great many older folks are trying to nourish themselves on tea and toast with a little processed cereal and cookies.

How much vitamin K would such a diet provide for these older people, those who are most susceptible to circulatory disorders? How many times have you read of the appalling diets of many of our young people, who eat no breakfast, have sketchy hamburger, soft drink and potato chip lunches and badly planned dinners? How much vitamin K would such a diet contain?

It is true, apparently, that only a very small amount of vitamin K is necessary to maintain the normal clotting ability of the blood. But you must get this vitamin K in your diet—nothing else can take its place. And your digestive tract must be in such good shape that you will absorb it all.

Keep well in mind in planning everyday meals just which foods contain most vitamin K. Green leafy vegetables are excellent sources. Since they contain many other essential vitamins and minerals as well, make them part of every day's menus. For someone who can't eat them either cooked or raw, because of plain dislike or because of some condition of ill health, use a juicer. But get plenty of these green leafy vegetables. Wheat bran and wheat germ are other fine sources.

Foods that contain most vitamin K are: pork liver, soybean oil, spinach, kale, carrot tops, cabbage, alfalfa and other green leafy vegetables, cauliflower, tomatoes, egg-yolk, corn, mushrooms, oats, peas, potatoes, soybeans, strawberries, wheat bran and wheat germ.

Suggested Further Reading

Adams, Ruth and Frank Murray, *Body, Mind and the B Vitamins,* Larchmont Books, New York, 1972.

Adams, Ruth and Frank Murray, *Vitamin C, the Powerhouse Vitamin,* Larchmont Books, New York, 1972.

Adams, Ruth and Frank Murray, *Vitamin E, Wonder Worker of the 70's?,* Larchmont Books, New York, 1971.

Adams, Ruth and Frank Murray, *Minerals: Kill or Cure?,* Larchmont Books, New York, 1974.

Bailey, Herbert, *Vitamin E, Your Key to a Healthy Heart,* ARCO Books, New York, 1964.

Bailey, Herbert, *The Vitamin Pioneers,* Rodale Press, Emmaus, Pa., 1968.

Bibliography of Vitamin E, 1965-1967, Distillation Products Industries, Rochester, New York, 1968.

Bicknell, Franklin and Frederick Prescott, *Vitamins in Medicine,* Lee Foundation for Nutritional Research, Milwaukee, Wisconsin, 1942.

Burkitt, D. P. and H. C. Trowell, Ed., *Refined Carbohydrate Foods and Disease,* Academic Press, New York, 1975.

Cheraskin, Dr. E., and Dr. W. M. Ringsdorf, Jr., *New Hope for Incurable Diseases,* Exposition Press, Jericho, New York, 1971.

Cheraskin, Dr. E. and Dr. W. M. Ringsdorf, Jr. with Arline Brecher, *Psychodietetics,* Stein and Day, New York, 1974.

Cleave, T. L., *The Saccharine Disease,* Keats Publishing

Co., New Canaan, Conn., 1975.

Davis, Adelle, *Let's Get Well,* Harcourt, Brace and World, New York, 1965.

Ellis, John M., M.D. and James Presley, *Vitamin B6, The Doctor's Report,* Harper and Row, New York, 1973.

Food, the Handbook of Agriculture, U.S. Department of Agriculture, Washington, D. C., 1959.

Hawkins, David and Linus Pauling, *Orthomolecular Psychiatry,* W. H. Freeman, San Francisco, 1973.

Heinz Handbook of Nutrition, McGraw-Hill Company, New York, 1959.

Hoffer, Abram and Humphrey Osmond, *How to Live With Schizophrenia,* University Books, New Hyde Park, New York, 1966.

Kaufman, William, *The Common Form of Niacinamide Deficiency Disease: Aniacinamidosis,* Yale University Press, Bridgeport, Conn., 1943.

Newbold, H. L. *Meganutrients for Your Nerves,* Peter H. Wyden, Publisher, New York, 1975.

Passwater, Richard, *Supernutrition: Megavitamin Revolution,* The Dial Press, New York, 1975.

Pauling, Linus, *Vitamin C and the Common Cold,* Bantam Books, New York, 1971.

Pfeiffer, Carl C., Ph.D., M.D., *Mental and Elemental Nutrients,* Keats Publishing Co., New Canaan, Conn., 1975.

Recommended Dietary Allowances, Eighth Edition, 1974, National Academy of Sciences, Washington, D. C.

Régnier, Edmé, *There is a Cure for the Common Cold,* Parker Publishing Co., West Nyack, New York, 1971.

Rosenberg, Dr. Harold and A. N. Feldzamen, Ph.D., *The Doctor's Book of Vitamin Therapy,* G. P. Putnam's, New York, 1974.

Shute, Evan and Wilfrid, *Alpha Tocopherol in Cardiovascular Disease,* Ryerson Press, Toronto, Canada, 1954.

Shute Institute for Clinical and Laboratory Medicine, *The Summary,* a Periodical of Abstracts of Relevant

Medical Literature, The Shute Foundation for Medical Research, London, Canada.

Shute Institute, Medical Staff, *Common Questions of Vitamin E and Their Answers,* Shute Foundation for Medical Research, London, Canada, 1961.

Shute Institute, Medical Staff, *The Heart and Vitamin E,* The Shute Foundation for Medical Research, London, Canada, 1961.

Shute, Wilfrid E., M.D. *The Complete Updated Vitamin E Book,* Keats Publishing Co., New Canaan, Conn., 1975.

Shute, Wilfrid E. and Harald J. Taub, *Vitamin E for Ailing and Healthy Hearts,* Pyramid House, New York, 1970.

Stone, Irwin, *The Healing Factor; "Vitamin C" Against Disease,* Grosset and Dunlap, New York, 1972.

Williams, Roger J., *Biochemical Individuality,* John Wiley and Sons, New York, 1956.

Williams, Roger J., *Nutrition Against Disease,* Pitman Publishing Corporation, New York, 1971.

Williams, Roger J., *Nutrition in a Nutshell,* Doubleday and Company, 1962.

Yudkin, John, *Sweet and Dangerous,* Peter H. Wyden, New York, 1972.

Index

A

Abdomen, complaints in, 27, 108, 118, 158, 193

Absorption, malabsorption, of food, 22, 29, 30, 37, 71, 99, 125, 154, 161, 175, 176, 180, 182, 244, 406

Acetaldehyde, 129, 287

Acidosis, 50, 166

Acne, 85, 123, 158

Adrenal glands, adrenalin, 93, 108, 131, 133, 157, 191, 193, 238, 279

Adreno-chrome, 131

Aging, 79, 110, 249, 327, 349, 364ff., 370ff., 385

Air pollution, 21, 71, 222, 225, 281, 308, 327, 370, 376

Alcohol, alcoholism, 35, 50, 60, 111, 117, 119, 121, 125, 128, 137, 155, 161, 173, 180, 208, 224, 230, 279, 287

Alcoholics Anonymous, 137

Alcoholism, the Nutritional Approach, 199

Allergies, 12, 40, 60, 147, 190, 191, 196, 219, 249, 284, 287

Alpha tocopherol (see Vitamin E)

Alvarez, Dr. Walter, 342, 359

Amblyopia, 35

American Academy of Pediatrics, 311

American Association for the Advancement of Science, 77, 304

American Cancer Society, 74

American Chemical Society, 370

The American Journal of Clinical Nutrition, 66, 125, 246, 285, 390, 395

American Journal of Diseases of Children, 154

American Medical Association, 121, 204

American Society of Plastic and Reconstructive Surgeons, 82

Amino acids, 34, 62, 129, 130, 136, 140, 155, 156, 165, 206, 236, 254

An Annotated Bibliography of Vitamin E, 324

Anemia (see also Iron Deficiency Anemia, Pernicious Anemia, etc.) 29, 30, 63, 108, 109, 111, 123, 125, 155, 157, 158, 168, 176, 180, 182, 183, 191, 216, 222, 284, 289, 329, 345, 366, 383

Anemia, iron deficiency, 21, 30

Anemia, megaloblastic, 184

Anemia, pernicious, 29, 45, 108, 125, 172, 175

Anemia, sickle-cell, 182

Angina pectoris (see also Heart Disease), 292, 346, 348, 360

Ankles (see also Feet), 119

Ansbacher units, 44

Antabuse, 224

Antibiotics, 35, 36, 88, 99, 112, 119, 125, 166, 210

Antibodies, 191, 196, 292

Anti-convulsants, 182

Antihistamines, 36

Antioxidants, 36, 323, 333, 366

Anus, 28, 123, 337

Anxiety, worry, 21, 27

416

N

National Academy of Sciences, 16, 25, 69, 407
National Cancer Institute, 73, 75, 77, 124, 251
National Formulary, 401
National Institute of Arthritis and Metabolic Diseases, 94
National Institutes of Health, 61
National Research Council, National Academy of Sciences, 16, 391, 393
National Resources Defense Council Newsletter, 215
Nausea, 108, 136, 158
Nebraska, University of, School of Medicine, 385
Nephritis, 208, 336
Nerves, nervousness, nerve disorders, etc., 21, 27, 28, 93, 107, 108, 115, 118, 123, 128, 135, 151, 176, 183, 191, 193, 204, 285, 325, 346
Neuralgia, 176, 257, 359
Neuritis, 13, 28, 29, 107, 115, 157, 176
New England Journal of Medicine, 155, 186, 212, 294, 346
New Jersey Neuropsychiatric Institute, 130
New Scientist, 175, 187, 218, 231, 292
New York Academy of Science, 218
New York Medical College, Metropolitan Hospital Center, 125
New York State Journal of Medicine, 89
The New York Times, 66, 73, 90, 365, 409
New Zealand Animal Health Laboratory, 386
Niacin (see Vitamin B3)

Niacinamide (see Vitamin B3), 136, 145, 159
Nicotinamide (see Vitamin B3)
Nicotine, 32, 35, 277
Nicotinic acid (see Vitamin B3), 141
Night blindness, 27, 91, 94, 102, 107
Nitrates, nitrites, 99, 278, 293
Nitrogen dioxide, 71, 327
Nitrogen oxide, 376
Nitroglycerin, 347, 354, 360
Nobel Prize, 248
Noise, 21
Northern Arizona University, 285
Nuclear power plants, 80
Nucleic acids, 197
Nutrition Against Disease, 197, 367
Nutrition and Alcoholism, 199
Nutrition Foundation, 162
Nutrition in a Nutshell, 199
Nutrition Reports International, 350
Nutrition Reviews, 155, 159, 160, 162, 170, 307, 397

O

Oak Ridge National Laboratory, 77
Obesity, overweight, 11, 60, 136, 208, 236, 256, 346, 348
Ochsner, Dr. Alton, 368, 384
Odors, body, 190
Old people, 21, 27, 29, 30, 49, 51, 57, 80, 110, 111, 113, 118, 119, 125, 128, 187, 197, 227, 233, 234, 238, 241, 243, 246, 288, 291, 306, 314, 342, 353, 409
Oliver, Dr. M.F., 141
Orange juice, 21
Orthomolecular psychiatry,

The best books on health and nutrition are from

LARCHMONT BOOKS

Vitamin C, The Powerhouse Vitamin, Conquers More tha
Just Colds, by Adams and Murray, Foreword by Dr. Frederick R
Klenner, 192 pages, $1.50.
Vitamin E, Wonder Worker of the 70's?, by Adams and Murray
Foreword by Dr. Evan V. Shute, 192 pages, $1.25.

Titles from
THE PREVENTIVE HEALTH LIBRARY

Improving Your Health with Vitamin A, by Adams and Murray,
128 pages, $1.25.
Improving Your Health with Vitamin C, by Adams and Murray,
160 pages, $1.50.
Improving Your Health with Vitamin E, by Adams and Murray,
176 pages, $1.50.
Improving Your Health with Calcium & Phosphorus, by
Adams and Murray, 128 pages, $1.25.
Improving Your Health with Niacin (Vitamin B₃), by Adams
and Murray, 128 pages, $1.25.
Improving Your Health with Zinc, by Adams and Murray, 128
pages, $1.25.

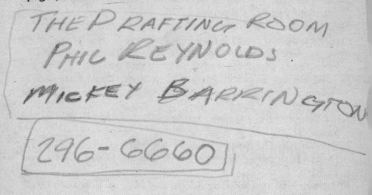

THE DRAFTING ROOM
PHIL REYNOLDS
MICKEY BARRINGTON

296-6660